To my closest Colleague: With

Dan Porte!

ALDOSE REDUCTASE INHIBITION

ALDOSE REDUCTASE INHIBITION

An Approach to the Prevention of Diabetic Complications

Authored by Dushan Dvornik, D.Sc.
Edited by Daniel Porte, M.D.

with
Foreword by Jin H. Kinoshita, Ph.D.
Afterword by J.D. Ward, M.D., F.R.C.P., B.Sc.

Biomedical Information Corporation
a division of McGraw-Hill

First Edition, 1987

Library of Congress Catalog Card Number: 87-71278
Dvornik, Dushan
Porte, Daniel (editor)
Aldose Reductase Inhibition
An Approach to the Prevention of Diabetic Complications

ISBN 0-935404-67-8

Printed in the United States of America.

Foreword

Although the discovery of insulin has had a dramatic effect on prolonging the lives of diabetics, it is obvious that other metabolic factors are at play, because serious secondary complications have become more and more common. Long standing diabetes sufferers are faced with the possible consequences of three major complications: nephropathy, neuropathy, and retinopathy. Insulin treatment by itself cannot prevent these late diabetic complications that can lead to death, amputations, and blindness.

Recently, interest has focused on a metabolic change occurring in diabetes that involves the activation of an enzyme that can adversely affect cell function. Aldose reductase (AR) catalyzes the conversion of glucose to the polyol sorbitol, and the reaction is especially effective when glucose is elevated. This enzyme together with sorbitol dehydrogenase, which converts sorbitol to fructose, constitute the polyol pathway, the two-step reaction that was thought to be confined to the accessory reproductive organs. However, it has now been shown to function in a variety of tissues, especially those targeted by diabetes.

In 1959, Van Heyningen found the presence of sorbitol in the diabetic lens. This discovery led to the polyol-osmotic theory of the formation of diabetic cataracts. It was only natural for scientists to look into the possible involvement of AR in the development of other diabetic complications. There is now growing evidence that AR also may play a role in diabetic neuropathy, nephropathy, retinopathy, and corneal keratopathy as well as cataracts.

Dr. Dushan Dvornik and Dr. Daniel Porte, co-authors of this authoritative textbook, have played key roles in the development of the AR concept. If AR is involved in the tissue abnormalities in diabetes, one obvious approach to prevent the changes must be to find an inhibitor of this enzyme. Dr. Dvornik of Ayerst Laboratories was among the first to recognize the possibility that this approach may lead to a new treatment for diabetics. In 1967, Dr. Dvornik and his associates at Ayerst developed tetramethyleneglutaric acid, an inhibitor of AR effective in preventing lens changes in an organ culture system simulating diabetic conditions in vitro. In 1969, Dr. Dvornik and his colleagues developed another AR inhibitor, alrestatin, which effectively delays the onset of sugar cataracts in rats. This was the first inkling that an AR inhibitor could alter the course of a diabetic complication, and it stimulated other pharmaceutical companies to search for AR inhibitors. Pfizer developed sorbinil, a very effective inhibitor in 1977. AR has a unique property in that a number of chemical compounds of diverse structures could serve as inhibitors. Since then the search has been on for more and more potent AR inhibitors. Ayerst came up with an improved inhibitor, tolrestat, of which you will read a great deal about in this text. These more potent aldose reductase inhibitors have been found not only to delay but actually to prevent cataracts from occurring in diabetic rats. There are additional companies that have developed effective inhibitors that are currently being tested in clinical trials.

Dr. Porte was also involved in an important milestone in the development of an aldose reductase concept in diabetic complications. This occurred in the early 1980s when Dr. Porte at the University of Washington (Seattle) with diabetologists from the University of Chicago and Harvard Medical School published the results of a randomized clinical study that had a great impact on the AR field. Their findings indicated that sorbinil treatment leads to improved nerve conduction velocities of both motor and sensory nerves in diabetics. This was the first clear-cut clinical demonstration that an AR inhibitor can be effective in diabetic patients. The results of this study have raised the priority of AR inhibitor projects at several companies, and as a consequence a cluster of new inhibitors have become available. In addition, the Japanese Diabetes Association held an impressive international symposium on the AR concept in diabetes in October, 1986. It became evident at this meeting that there has been a growing body of evidence building, pointing out that treatment with aldose reductase inhibitors may indeed prove to be a new treatment modality for diabetics.

This informative book written by two distinguished scientists, is being published at a propitious time, when the results of a number of clinical trials with several ARIs are imminent. It will be useful not only to clinicians who are treating diabetics but also to scientists who are active in this area of research.

Jin H. Kinoshita
National Eye Institute
June 1987

Table of Contents

Preface

The concept of aldose reductase inhibition was originally formulated to test Kinoshita's hypothesis that sugar cataract formation is initiated by the osmotic stress caused by intracellular accumulation of polyol produced from excess sugar by the action of aldose reductase. The hypothesis was indeed verified by preventing sugar cataract formation through aldose reductase inhibition in vitro with AY-20,037 (tetramethyleneglutaric acid) and in vivo with AY-22,284, later known as alrestatin. The hypothesis was then extended to other tissues and, as in the lens, alrestatin was found to decrease polyol accumulation in the nerves of diabetic and galactosemic rats. This finding led to the testing of alrestatin in human subjects with diabetic neuropathy and, later, to the conclusion of Fagius and Jameson that "aldose reductase inhibitor treatment may be of value in diabetic polyneuropathy" thus "providing support for the sorbitol pathway hypothesis of diabetic polyneuropathy." The concept was subsequently broadened to include other tissues capable of metabolizing excess glucose via the polyol pathway and, consequently, prone to develop diabetic complications.

The pharmacological approach based on the use of aldose reductase (AR) inhibitors to prevent, arrest, and, possibly, reverse the sequelae of chronic diabetes is particularly attractive because aldose reductase seems to assume a role only in the nonphysiological condition created by diabetes-induced hyperglycemia. In addition, AR inhibitors are meant to decrease the AR-catalyzed conversion of excess glucose to a tolerable intracellular sorbitol level and not to cause complete AR inhibition. In fact, results obtained in animal models of diabetes suggest that AR-containing cells may tolerate some polyol accumulation without loss of functional integrity.

In addition to their potential usefulness as drugs to prevent the progression of diabetic complications, AR inhibitors are also providing a tool to elucidate the degree of AR-induced biochemical, functional, and structural changes and their interaction, which, in a given tissue, define the extent of reversible damage, hence, determining the potential for improvement by controlling AR activity with an inhibitor.

The purpose of this book was to compile the available experimental data deemed useful to position aldose reductase and its inhibition as an approach to the understanding of the initiation of diabetic complications and their prevention. The book was prepared at the request of Dr. John Mullane, in charge of scientific affairs at Ayerst Laboratories, and an ardent supporter of the AR inhibition concept.

I have never written a book and I did not appreciate how much help is needed from others. Now that I know, I wish to thank all those who have helped me, particularly to Dr. Marlene Molinoff for preparing Chapter 1 and for her tactful aid with the style of the other chapters; to Dr. Leslie Humber for preparing Chapter 5;

to Ms. Barbara Boyajian and her staff for the almost endless number of literature searches and references; to Dr. Michael McCaleb for his comments, and to Mrs. Winnie Brown for her devoted, competent, and patient participation in the protracted gestation and the accelerated delivery of a final typed version of the manuscript. I am particularly grateful to Dr. Daniel Porte for bringing his wisdom and vast knowledge of diabetes to the editing of the manuscript at a time when he had so many other commitments.

This book is devoted to all those who share the faith in the potential benefit that subjects with diabetes could derive from treatment with AR inhibitors. Above all, to Dr. Jin Kinoshita, who has formulated the concept of AR inhibition and who has been contributing so very much to its application and refinement; to Dr. Kenneth Gabbay, the first clinical investigator to self-administer and then to test an AR inhibitor, alrestatin, in diabetic patients with neuropathy; to all my colleagues and their associates at Ayerst who were involved in our investigations of AR and its inhibition, especially Drs. Michael Kraml, Nicole Simard-Duquesne, Ermenio Greselin, Jean Dubuc, Ramona Gonzalez, Jane Millen, and Janet Sredy, to Dr. Kazimir Sestanj, who designed and synthesized both alrestatin and tolrestat, and to Drs. David Hicks, Mitchell Cayen, and Eckhardt Ferdinandi, who investigated the metabolic disposition of alrestatin and tolrestat.

Dushan Dvornik

Introduction

A wide range of complications leading to loss of nerve function and sensation, blindness, kidney failure, limb amputation, and death have long been associated with diabetes mellitus of long duration. Until it became possible to treat the hyperglycemia of diabetes with insulin and oral hypoglycemic agents, few diabetics survived long enough to suffer these late complications of the underlying metabolic disorder. As advances in treatment reduced death rates from diabetic coma these complications have now become more frequent and today they provide the major contribution to diabetic morbidity and mortality.

There is little question that chronic hyperglycemia plays the major etiologic role in the pathogenesis of these lesions of nerve, lens, and microvascular tissue. But these conditions, once established, have not, as clinicians know only too well, been susceptible to treatment by subsequent control of blood sugar. This has led to attempts to find a new pharmacologic approach to diabetic complications, one focusing on the role of the enzyme aldose reductase in their pathogenesis.

Aldose reductase, first described in 1956 by Hers, mediates the metabolism of excess glucose to various sugar alcohols, or polyols, via what has come to be known as the polyol pathway. This enzyme has since been identified in a great many mammalian tissues, including all those that are the targets of diabetes-associated complications.

The link between aldose reductase and diabetic lesions was established by Kinoshita and his colleagues at the National Institute of Health in 1962. They demonstrated its mediating role in the production of the diabetic lens, in which the accumulation of the polyol sorbitol as a result of excess glucose in the circulation, and consequent osmotic changes, contribute to cataractogenesis. Further research has addressed the role of aldose reductase in other tissues.

This monograph presents the clinician with a comprehensive review of the experimental and clinical research literature on the polyol pathway and its part in the development of the complications of diabetes as well as the proposed biochemical mechanisms by which these may take place.

The final chapter holds special interest for those charged with the responsibility of treating these conditions in its review of experimental work with aldose-reductase-inhibiting (ARI) agents. It concludes with a presentation of the clinical data, drawn from experience with more than 1,400 patients, which assesses the effectiveness of four ARI pharmacologic compounds in the treatment of diabetic neuropathy—alrestatin, sorbinil, epalrestat and tolrestat.

ALDOSE REDUCTASE INHIBITION

Chapter 1

Complications of Chronic Diabetes in Man and Their Relation to Hyperglycemia

by Marlene S. Molinoff, Ph.D.

SYNOPSIS

This review of the literature of the complications of diabetes of long duration covers the prevalence, incidence, natural history and response to treatment of diabetic neuropathy, nephropathy, eye complications, increased risk of atherosclerosis and limited joint mobility syndrome.

These disabling and often life-threatening conditions affect patients with both insulin-dependent diabetes mellitus (IDDM) and non-insulin-dependent diabetes mellitus (NIDDM), and generally become clinically evident 10 to 20 years after the onset of the disease. As advances in treatment have reduced death rates from diabetic coma from almost 66% before the introduction of insulin to 1% by 1968, the increase in survival has contributed to the rise in the frequency of these manifestations of diabetes of long duration.

Because of their greater frequency and clinical impact, the diabetic neuropathies produce a substantial proportion of the morbidity suffered by individuals with diabetes. The most serious of these involve sensory disturbances, motor weaknesses and autonomic dysfunctions, often producing neuropathic foot ulcers which can lead, eventually, to amputation, and a number of cardiovascular, gastrointestinal and urogenital disorders.

In diabetic polyneuropathy, axonal degeneration, segmental demyelination and other histopathologic changes in peripheral nerves produce a wide variety of clinical manifestations and electrophysiologic dysfunctions. These are related to the duration of diabetes and the degree of hyperglycemia. Lacking a pharmacologic compound capable of interfering with these pathophysiologies, treatment is nonspecific and symptomatic, and includes efforts to achieve control of glycemia. This is also the case with the autonomic neuropathies. In diabetic mononeuropathy analgesics to control pain may be helpful. Most mononeuropathies resolve over time.

Renal failure is one of the most ominous complications, accounting for up to 12% of all deaths in patients with diabetes—an estimated 3,000 annually. About one-fourth of all end-stage renal failure may be attributed to diabetic nephropathy. Although control of glycemia can prevent or reverse nephropathy early in the disease, once renal impairment has progressed beyond a certain point the process seems to become resistant to glycemic control measures. Early detection and treatment by control of glycemia is therefore essential. Microalbuminuria is an early sign of glomerular failure and is considered to be a predictor of future renal function decline.

Diabetic eye complications include retinopathy, cataract and corneal keratopathy. Retinopathy is now the leading cause of new cases of blindness in adults aged 20 to 70. The overall average incidence rate of retinopathy in populations of diabetics is 52%, and the condition increases in prevalence with increase in the duration of the underlying metabolic disorder.

A relationship has been found between glycemic control and development of retinopathy. Treatment of the condition is by ophthalmologic intervention and includes photocoagulation and laser therapy, and for restoration of vision, in some cases, vitrectomy.

Diabetes is a major factor in cataractogenesis, possibly because of the mediating role of aldose reductase in the accumulation of sugar alcohol (polyols) in the diabetic lens, a link established by Kinoshita and his colleagues in 1962 (see Chapter 2). Although surgery is the only treatment at present, recent data from animal studies suggest that "potent aldose reductase inhibitors . . . represent the only potential anticataract agents currently in development that may be effective in man."[306]

Keratopathy, a corneal complication following vitrectomy in diabetic patients, has in recent years declined substantially in incidence as a result of improved surgical technique.

Both IDDM and NIDDM are associated with an increased risk of atherosclerotic large vessel disease. An association between abnormal glucose tolerance and increased cardiovascular mortality has been reported.[324] No data exist documenting a benefit from glycemic control. Among the mechanisms proposed in the atherosclerotic process in diabetes are elevated lipoprotein, increased protein glycation, and polyols in blood vessels.

Diabetes is associated with a number of arthritic hand syndromes, notably Dupuytren's contracture and other finger joint contractures, often seen in young IDDM patients. This condition may be a marker for the microvascular late complications of diabetes. Although the mechanisms underlying the connective tissue changes characteristic of this syndrome are not known, improvement following treatment with an aldose reductase inhibitor has been reported.

Contents

Diabetes mellitus is characterized by hyperglycemia associated with long-term complications involving nerves, kidneys, eyes and blood vessels. Until the introduction of insulin in the treatment of diabetes mellitus more than 60 years ago, almost two out of three diabetic patients died in diabetic coma. After insulin, diabetic coma as a cause of death fell to 8% by 1936, and to 1% by 1968. It is the resulting increase of survival duration of diabetic persons that has gradually given rise to new and serious problems, the so-called late complications of diabetes: neuropathy; nephropathy; eye complications, including retinopathy, cataract and keratopathy; and an increased risk of atherosclerosis. Clinical expression and the development of diabetic complications depend on the duration of diabetes, and in many of these complications there is evidence linking hyperglycemia to their prevalence. The following chapter represents a review of literature on the complications of chronic diabetes in man in terms of prevalence, incidence, epidemiology, natural history, and response to treatment aimed at achieving glycemic control.

THE NERVES—DIABETIC NEUROPATHY

History

Knowledge of the association between diabetes mellitus and disease of the peripheral nervous system dates back almost two centuries. In 1798, John Rollo made reference to pain and paresthesia in the legs of patients with diabetes mellitus, but at that time, diabetes was believed to be secondary to a lesion of the nervous system rather than the reverse.[1] Marchal de Calvi (1864), in recording the occurrence of sciatic pain associated with peripheral sensory loss, is generally credited with defining the causal relationship between diabetes and nerve damage.[2] Clinical descriptions of nocturnal hyperesthesia (Pavy, 1855), of mononeuropathy of the cranial nerves (Althaus, 1866), of acute painful neuropathy (Althaus, 1883), and loss of the deep tendon reflexes (Bouchard, 1884) have appeared in the literature during the past 130 years.[2] It was not, however, until 1945[3] that diabetic autonomic neuropathy was described, and only within the last 13 years has the magnitude of the neuropathy problem with respect to the relative incidence of the disease in the diabetic population been appreciated.[4,5]

Incidence and epidemiology

The importance of diabetic neuropathy derives from its frequency and its clinical impact. Estimates of the incidence of peripheral diabetic neuropathy range broadly, depending on the diagnostic criteria considered.[2] When the presence of pain, muscle weakness and sensory loss are considered to be diagnostic criteria, the incidence is 40%.[6] When absence of deep tendon reflexes is used as the criterion, the incidence range is from 6% in diabetic patients under 29 years of age to 86% in patients 70 years of age or older.[7] Several investigators have found motor end plate changes, Wallerian degeneration, and segmental demyelinization in diabetic patients of all ages, regardless of date of onset, severity of diabetes, or degree of control.[8–11] If a reduction in nerve conduction velocity is used as the diagnostic criterion, then neuropathy occurs in virtually all diabetic patients, even in the absence of clinical symptoms or signs.

Regardless of the diagnostic criteria applied, the prevalence of diabetic neuropathy increases with age,[3,12,13] the duration of diabetes,[14] and with measures of glucose control.[14,15] The overall prevalence is similar in men and women, although some syndromes such as upper limb polyneuropathy, diabetic amyotrophy and diabetic neuropathic cachexia are more common in men.[5] Neuropathy occurs in both insulin-dependent diabetes mellitus (IDDM) and non-insulin-dependent diabetes mellitus (NIDDM). Differences in prevalence could well be ascribed to differences in age, duration and control of diabetes.[2] Certain neuropathic syndromes, however, may occur disparately. For example, mononeuropathies are uncommon in non-insulin-dependent diabetes, and diabetic amyotrophy is found particularly in men with NIDDM.[16] While clinical diabetic neuropathy is found uncommonly in children,[17–21] about 10% of them exhibited abnormalities in motor nerve conduction.[2]

Although peripheral somatic neuropathy is by far the most common clinical expression, autonomic neuropathy is quite common, with diverse manifestations. It may affect any part of the gastrointestinal and genitourinary tract, or the cardiovascular system. Diabetic autonomic neuropathy is more difficult to diagnose than somatic nerve dysfunction. Symptoms are often vague and nonspecific, and, with the exception of advanced cases, signs are difficult to detect on routine physical examination. Since specific tests of autonomic function are available but have generally not been applied in wide epidemiological investigations, the precise incidence of autonomic neuropathy in chronic diabetes is difficult to assess.[22] Measurement of supine respiratory rate (ŔR) variation during deep inspiration and during β-adrenergic blockade has been found to be a sensitive, quantitative and reproducible method to evaluate parasympathetic nervous activity in diabetic subjects. By this method, it has been found that cardiac parasympathetic activity may be diminished in diabetic subjects before clinical symptoms of autonomic neuropathy are evident.[23] Tests of autonomic function suggest that cardiac parasympathetic function becomes abnormal earlier than sympathetic function. Such tests make possible the detection of subclinical autonomic neuropathy and have established its prevalence in at least 20% of the diabetic population.[24]

Clinical features

Diabetic nerve disease is being increasingly implicated as a source of substantial morbidity in many persons with diabetes mellitus,[25] one which can cause severe disability and markedly curtail the performance of daily activities at work and at home.[26]

A simple and widely used clinical classification system is given in Table 1.[12]

Table 1. Classification of diabetic neuropathy.[12]

1. Polyneuropathy
- Distal symmetric sensorimotor polyneuropathy
- Autonomic neuropathy

2. Asymmetric neuropathy

Mononeuropathy and multiple mononeuropathy
- Cranial nerve lesions
- Peripheral nerve lesions

Diabetic amyotrophy

Polyneuropathy

Loss of peripheral nerve function can cause sensory disturbances, motor weakness and autonomic dysfunction.[27] The more commonly distressing clinical sequelae result from these two major classes of nerve dysfunction: sensorimotor polyneuropathy and autonomic neuropathy.[25–28]

Distal symmetric sensorimotor polyneuropathy

This is the most common form of diabetic neuropathy. As with other peripheral polyneuropathies, sensory disturbances may be considered as positive or negative symptoms.[29] Negative sensory symptoms involve diminution or loss of sensation and may include all sensory modalities: pain and temperature, touch-pressure, vibratory, two-point discrimination and joint position sense.[29] Negative sensory symptoms involve functional (or structural) loss of the involved afferent fibers.[30]

Positive sensory symptoms include paresthesia, dysesthesia, hyperesthesia (or hyperpathia) and pain.[29] Paresthesias are spontaneous aberrant sensations, such as pins and needles or tingling, and are a frequent accompaniment of a sensory or mixed sensorimotor neuropathy.[30,31] Dysesthesia is commonly used to describe an unpleasant sensation (such as burning) produced by an ordinarily painless stimulus (such as touch).[31] Similarly, hyperesthesia (or hyperpathia) is an excessive response to a sensory stimulus and generally refers to an unpleasant quality that has been added to cutaneous sensation.[31] Pain may occur, yet not all persons with these neuropathies have spontaneous pain.[30]

Diabetic sensorimotor polyneuropathy often presents clinically as a sensory loss in a stocking-glove distribution more common in the lower extremities[5,32]; occasionally, severe hyperesthesia to mild tactile sensation is seen. This may be associated with pain and/or paresthesia. The pain may be dull, aching, burning, lancinating or cramp-like and is characteristically accentuated during sleep. Sensations of numbness, coldness or tingling are commonly reported. Direct consequences of the impairment of sensation are painless trauma and/or burns in both the upper and lower extremities.[26,28] Neuropathic arthropathy is another result of repeated, painless joint trauma.[26,28]

Clinical exam may reveal motor involvement which, as with most chronic polyneuropathies, causes paresis of the affected muscles, principally of the hand, foot and lower leg.[30] Interosseous muscular atrophy may be noted, and the loss of strength can be sufficiently advanced to interfere with writing or walking.[26,28] Loss of tendon reflexes is also common in peripheral neuropathy and may be due to loss of afferent fibers from the muscle spindles as well as temporal dispersion of conduction.[30] Neuropathic ulcers, characteristically found on the plantar surface of the foot, result from loss of strength in the intrinsic foot musculature leading to a maldistribution of weight on the metatarsal heads.[28] Combined with the impaired sensation of pain, an ulcer commonly results. This may become infected, which, in the presence of impaired circulation and host-defense mechanisms (frequent concomitants in the diabetic person), may eventually lead to intractable osteomyelitis and amputation.[26,28]

Autonomic neuropathy

Symptoms and signs of autonomic neuropathy are rarely seen in patients without clinically apparent distal symmetrical polyneuropathy.[4,16,33] Consistent with its relationship to developed symptomatic sensorimotor neuropathy, symptomatic autonomic neuropathy usually is found only in long-standing diabetes.[34] Abnormalities in autonomic function are not evenly distributed, so that patients with clinical vasomotor disturbances may not necessarily have clinically evident gastrointestinal autonomic neuropathy.[35] Autonomic neuropathy is associated with a shortened life expectancy,[36] particularly when postural hypotension, hypoglycemic unawareness and gastric symptoms are present. Signs and symptoms of autonomic neuropathy, classified according to the involved body system, are given in Table 2.

Table 2. Signs and symptoms of autonomic neuropathy.[16]

Cardiovascular	Urogenital
• postural hypotension • resting tachycardia • abnormal beat-to-beat variation with respiration • abnormal valsalva ratio	• bladder atony • impotence • retrograde ejaculation • overflow incontinence
Gastrointestinal	**Sudomotor dysfunction**
• esophageal atony • gastric atony and dilatation • dilatation of the gallbladder • constipation • diarrhea	• heat intolerance • symmetric distal anhidrosis • gustatory sweating

Common clinical sequalae of diabetic autonomic dysfunction are urinary tract infections resulting from incomplete bladder emptying,[34,37] impotence and retrograde ejaculation,[4,34,37] and dizziness, faintness and syncope caused by orthostatic hypotension.[4,34,37]

The wide array of neuropathic somatic sensorimotor and autonomic symptoms and signs accompanying chronic diabetic polyneuropathy indicates involvement of all fiber types (large and small diameters as well as myelinated and unmyelinated) in diabetic neuropathy.[38–40] Therefore, while the clinical predominance of a certain symptom may reflect a certain fiber loss in an individual patient, more detailed examination is likely to reveal a variety of other clinical somatic sensorimotor and autonomic nerve abnormalities indicating a generalized multi-fiber-type involvement.

Asymmetric neuropathy

Mononeuropathies: cranial nerve lesions and isolated peripheral nerve lesions

Diabetic mononeuropathies involve one or more discrete cranial or peripheral nerves. They constitute roughly 15% of all diabetic neuropathies and are generally restricted to older diabetic patients.[4,16] The onset is usually acute and painful. The median, ulnar, deep peroneal, radial, femoral and sciatic nerves[12] are the most frequently affected peripheral nerves. Mononeuropathy may also involve single or multiple cranial nerves, usually those innervating the extraocular muscles and the facial nerve.[4,16]

Diabetic amyotrophy and neuropathic cachexia

Diabetic amyotrophy is an uncommon and poorly understood form of diabetic neuropathy seen more often in NIDDM. It is characterized by rapid onset with proximal muscle weakness followed by muscle atrophy.[41] The frequently unilateral symptoms tend to improve with time.[41] In combination with neuropathic cachexia, the syndrome begins with a weight loss (as much as 40% of initial body weight), depression, emotional lability, severe pains in the lower extremities, and progressive muscle wasting and weakness, most marked in the pelvic girdle and thigh. Patients are usually men in their fifties or sixties with relatively mild diabetes of recent onset. The syndrome progresses inexorably for about six months, then resolves (although not completely) over the succeeding one to two years.

Histopathological changes

Anatomy and physiology of the peripheral nervous system

The peripheral nervous system comprises those nerves that conduct sensory and motor impulses to and from the central nervous system. A typical peripheral nerve is composed of a group of nerve fibers. In cross-section, each nerve fiber consists of an axon generally surrounded by a Schwann cell, basement membrane, and the endoneurium[42,43] (Fig 1).

Peripheral nerves are usually composed of both myelinated and unmyelinated fibers bound together by connective tissue.[44] Axons over 1 micron in diameter are generally myelinated. Myelination involves the wrapping of the axon by a number of layers of the lipoprotein plasma membranes of Schwann cells. There may be

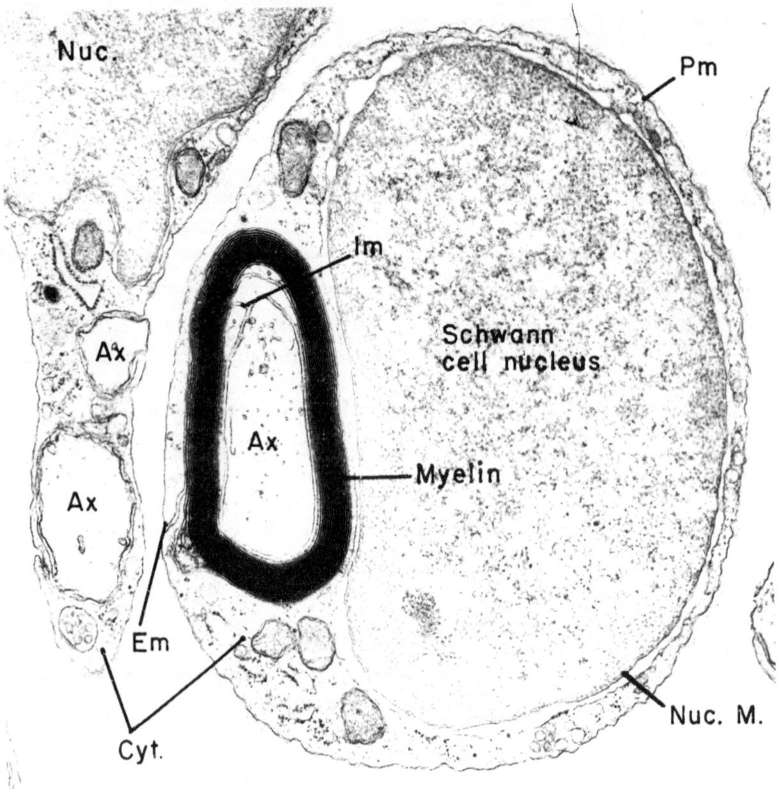

Figure 1. Peripheral nerve. (From Human Neuroanatomy, Williams & Wilkins, 1976)

from a few to 50 such layers in the myelin sheath.[45] At regular intervals along the axon, the myelin sheath of one Schwann cell abuts that of another at the nodes of Ranvier. The internodal distance varies in proportion to the diameter of the axon, and ranges from 50 to 1500 microns.[44] Unmyelinated fibers are generally smaller axons surrounded by a single layer of the Schwann cell's plasma membrane.[44] A single Schwann cell may surround up to 15 axons.[45]

The physiological role of the peripheral nervous system is to transfer information by propagating membrane depolarization.[44] Adequate depolarization generates an action potential. An adequate threshold stimulation follows the interaction of a neurotransmitter with receptor molecules or the stimulation of a sensory ending.[45]

Once initiated, the action potential propagates along the nerve fiber without decreasing in amplitude. This is accomplished by progressive depolarization of the axonal membrane and allows transfer of information over relatively long distances.[46] The energy to maintain the self-propagated action potential is supplied by the nerve fiber, maintaining the normal resting membrane potential by ion pumping and returning to its normal resting condition after the period of depolarization.[46] In myelinated fibers, the action potential skipping from node to node is referred to as saltatory conduction.[45] The conduction velocity of the nerve impulse corresponds to the internodal distance, which in turn correlates with the axonal diameter.[44] In an unmyelinated fiber, the nerve impulse moves along the entire axolemma as a self-propagating action potential, rather than jumping from node to node.[45] Unmyelinated fibers are, therefore, characterized by a relatively slow conduction velocity.[45]

Based principally upon conduction velocity and fiber diameter, three main types of peripheral nerve fibers have been identified. Myelinated "A" fibers have a large diameter (1 to 22 microns), are fast-conducting (5 to 120 meters/sec), and function as afferent fibers, for proprioception, vibration, touch and pressure, as well as somatic efferent fibers (innervating muscle). Myelinated "B" fibers have a smaller diameter (1 to 3 microns) and conduction velocity (3 to 15 meters/sec), and function as visceral afferent and preganglionic visceral efferent (autonomic) fibers. Unmyelinated "C" fibers have a small diameter (0.5 to 1.5 microns), are slow-conducting (0.6 to 2.0 meters/sec), and function as afferent fibers for pain and temperature, as well as postganglionic visceral efferent (autonomic) fibers.[44,45]

Regardless of the fiber diameter and conduction velocity, the ionic mechanisms of the action potential and its propagation are probably the same throughout the peripheral nervous system.[44]

Peripheral nervous system dysfunction

The most common disorders of the peripheral nervous system are the peripheral polyneuropathies in which degenerative changes cause sensory disturbances and/or motor weakness. There are many causes of peripheral polyneuropathy, including various toxins, nutritional deficiencies, and metabolic disorders such as diabetes mellitus.[45] Distal parts of the nerve are usually affected first, with symptoms starting in the hands or the feet.[45]

Diverse pathological changes have been described in the various peripheral polyneuropathies. Dyck[47] presents a classification based on the pathological findings: single or multiple nerve involvement (interstitial, ischemic or parenchymatous) and type of fiber degeneration (axonal degeneration/atrophy, segmental demyelination). The most common chronic peripheral neuropathies are associated with either distal axonal degeneration and/or segmental demyelination.[47] Axonal degeneration is the histologic consequence of events associated with the degeneration of the distal processes of neurons.[47] The term "segmental demyelination" implies disrupted myelin sheath with intact axon.[47] Axonal degeneration and segmental demyelination appear to be interrelated. The myelin irregularities and segmental demyelination are probably due to the axonal degeneration.[48]

In patients with diabetic neuropathy, histopathological changes have been described in the spinal cord, posterior roots and ganglia, peripheral nerves, the motor end plate, and muscle. Woltman and Wilder (1929) found the main pathology to be patchy loss of myelin. Their findings were corroborated by

Fagerberg (1959) and Dolman (1963), who found a similar degree of patchy demyelination in the peripheral nerves of 90% of the patients with severe diabetic neuropathy and, to a lesser extent, in diabetic patients without clinically evident diabetic neuropathy.[26] Changes were also found in the anterior horn cells of the lumbar spinal cord (Alderman, 1938; Bosanquet and Hensen, 1957) and in the dorsal root ganglia (Greenbaum et al, 1964; Olsson et al, 1968).

Thickening of the basement membrane of the Schwann cell was histologically identified as an early lesion in the peripheral nerves of diabetic patients, followed by segmental demyelination appearing before any changes in the axon or neuron.[49] The importance of segmental demyelination was later emphasized by Thomas and Lascelles (1965) when they examined individual teased single nerve fiber preparations. Their findings were confirmed by Chopra et al (1969), who reported that Wallerian and axonal degeneration were observed only in chronic, severe neuropathy, while discontinuous, segmental demyelination and remyelination appeared in the nerves of diabetics with or without severe clinical neuropathy. However, recent studies have suggested that the early morphologic abnormality in diabetic neuropathy is axonal degeneration.[50,51] Several groups of investigators suggest that the neuron is the primary target of the pathologic process, with the Schwann cell being secondary.[12,48] Electron microscopic examination of biopsied sural nerves from diabetics with neuropathy extend the controversy. Luse and Moon (1966) found the main ultrastructural pathology to be a loss of unmyelinated axons.[13] In a more extensive electron microscopic study, Bischoff (1967) observed myelin sheath disintegration to be the most prominent finding.[13] Qualitative electron microscopic analysis of sural nerves from patients with neuropathy associated with early diabetes showed a minor but distinct single nerve fiber abnormality consistent with primary axonal degeneration (Bischoff, 1973), and in the investigation of biopsied sural nerves from eight juvenile diabetics, seven of short duration, definite changes were found in every nerve preparation, with the ultrastructural feature corresponding to abnormalities consistent with primary axonal degeneration.[13]

Electron microscopic studies of the peripheral nerves of animal models appear to support the concept that neuronal damage occurs early in the course of diabetic neuropathy and is followed by axonal degeneration and segmental demyelination and remyelination of the surviving axons. In the nerves of young rats with short-term streptozocin-induced diabetes, the earliest morphologic change found was a decrease in the calibre of the myelinated fibers with no decrease in the total number of nerve fibers.[52–55] This was accompanied by a slight widening of the nodes of Ranvier and swelling of the paranodal bulbs in the teased nerve fibers, although no segmental demyelination was detected.[55] The findings were not corroborated in streptozocin-diabetic older rats since myelinated fiber diameter did not alter, nor did the relationship between myelin sheath thickness and axon circumference.[56,57] The various neuropathologic results found in experimental diabetic rats were attributed to age-related differences in the effects of prolonged hyperglycemia on the peripheral nerve.[52]

Evidence supporting axonal damage as the earliest manifestation of diabetic neuropathy has been obtained in diabetic Chinese hamsters.[58] Axonal dwindling without evidence of segmental demyelination was also reported in genetically diabetic mice (db/db).[59]

Autonomic nervous system dysfunction

There is very little histopathological information on autonomic neuropathy. Widespread degenerative changes in sympathetic, preganglionic communicating rami, with destruction of both axons and myelin sheaths have been reported.[59–64]

Associated vascular changes

Evidence of vascular changes associated with diabetic neuropathy was entertained by Pryce[65] in 1893. Woltman and Wilder[66] furthered this supposition, and the theory that diabetic polyneuropathy is the consequence of an ischemic lesion caused by atherosclerosis of the neural vessels was widely held for the next 30 years. Successive electron microscopic studies of biopsied nerves from diabetic patients both with and without clinical polyneuropathy have generally failed to confirm that endothelial hyperplasia and intimal thickening is a consistent finding in diabetic polyneuropathy.[67,68]

There is now abundant evidence, however, that diabetic mononeuropathies are a direct consequence of ischemic events.[37] In a single case study of the nerves of a patient with diabetic mononeuropathy multiplex cited by Fagerberg,[69] Raff and Asbury demonstrated multiple small infarcts in affected nerves. In histologic examination of two cases of diabetic mononeuropathy affecting the third cranial nerve, thickening and hyalinization of the arteriolar and capillary walls and narrowing of the lumina of the major nutrient vessels were observed as well as discrete ischemic lesions in the central portion of the nerve, though the peripheral fibers were spared.[70,71]

Recent application of electron microscopic and morphometric techniques have underscored structural and functional changes in endoneurial capillaries of the retina and golmeruli. According to Bischoff,[13] the classic morphologic abnormalities found in diabetic endoneurial vessels consist of endothelial hyperplasia, thickening and reduplication of the capillary basement membrane, and expansion of the collagen-rich pericapillary space. Other investigators have found that the endoneurial capillaries are frequently obstructed by fibrin or aggregated platelets, particularly following periods of severe metabolic imbalance.[72–74] Asbury and Johnson[41] have speculated that such structural alterations in endoneurial capillaries could render them excessively permeable, subject to leakage resulting in a toxic effect on the structure and function of the cells. Early animal studies suggested leakage of toxins into the endoneurial space in animals with experimental diabetes,[75] but more recent studies have indicated that the blood-nerve and perineurial barriers of such animals are intact.[76,77]

Summary

It is evident that the chronic polyneuropathy of diabetes is associated with a broad array of histopathological changes in the peripheral nerve, including both axonal degeneration and segmental demyelination. The axonal changes involve large- and small-diameter as well as myelinated and unmyelinated nerve fibers.[49–58] The preponderance of evidence supports the view that the segmental demyelination may be secondary to axonal degeneration and that both morphological findings may reflect the same underlying nerve dysfunction. This peripheral nerve dysfunction is manifested by a wide range of clinical symptoms and signs as well as electrophysiological disturbances.

Electrophysiological changes

Electrophysiological techniques of increasing sophistication have been developed, primarily in the last 40 years, for the in vivo evaluation of nerve function.[78,79] While many new and promising techniques are under development, including microneuronography[80] and determination of the distribution of conduction velocities,[81] conventional nerve conduction values have been shown to assess nerve function sensitively and specifically. Nerve conduction studies assess peripheral motor and sensory nerve function by recording the evoked response to electrical stimulation of the peripheral nerve.[78,79] Nerve conduction involves stimulating the peripheral nerve at an accessible point, usually with skin surface electrodes, and recording the compound action potential, again using skin surface electrodes, at another point along the nerve (for sensory nerve conduction) or at a muscle innervated by the nerve (for motor nerve conduction).[79] Sensory nerve conduction may be performed either orthodromically (stimulating a cutaneous nerve and recording over a mixed sensorimotor nerve) or antidromically (stimulating a mixed sensorimotor nerve and recording over a cutaneous nerve).[78] The time between the instant of stimulation and that time at which a recorded response begins is called the latency period.[79] Stimulation (or recording) at two or more points at measurable distances along a given nerve enables nerve conduction velocity to be calculated from the difference between proximal and distal latencies, divided by the distance.[44] Because conduction velocity increases with myelination and nerve fiber size, conventional nerve conduction velocities directly measure the velocity in the largest-diameter myelinated fibers.[78,79] Standard studies of motor nerve conduction involve the ulnar and median nerves in the upper extremities and the tibial and peroneal nerves in the lower extremities.[78] Standard sensory nerve conduction studies may involve the ulnar, median, radial, plantar and sural nerves.[78] By carefully considering and removing possible sources of interference and error (such as variation in limb temperature and position),[81] conventional nerve conduction studies offer a sensitive in vivo index of nerve function.

Neurophysiology in diabetic neuropathy

The pattern of electrophysiological abnormalities seen in diabetic neuropathy reflects both axonal degeneration and segmental demyelination.[78]

Numerous studies measuring motor and sensory nerve conduction as well as electromyography have shown electrophysiological abnormalities to be present, even in diabetes of early onset. The early stage of diabetic neuropathy is marked by reduction of sensory nerve conduction velocity and decreased amplitude of the compound nerve action potential.[82] Sensory perception thresholds may be impaired shortly after the onset of diabetes and may be a sensitive index of peripheral neuropathy.[83] Motor nerve conduction velocity is definitely reduced in patients with established clinical neuropathy, but the mean velocity is also reduced in diabetics without clinical neuropathy when compared with normal subjects.[84–86]

Nerve conduction changes in diabetic patients can be demonstrated in both motor and sensory nerves.[16] The conduction velocity in peroneal nerve may be slowed already upon diagnosis of diabetes.[87]

A proximal-distal gradient of the decrease in conduction velocity shown to occur in diabetic neuropathy indicates greater impairment in the more distal parts of the nerve.[88] These observations, which agree with neuropathological findings, suggest the greater susceptibility of the longest and thinnest nerve fibers to diabetic neuropathies.[16]

The fact that the sensory action potentials in the peripheral nerve of the diabetic are abnormally resistant to ischemia[89–91] underscores the importance of alterations in metabolism as related to nerve function. There is currently no proven explanation of this resistance, which is seen, regardless of the clinical state of the nerve and the initial conduction velocity in the non-ischemic state. The phenomenon is also occurring in patients with uremia and liver failure.[26] Seneviratne and Peiris[92] suggest that in the normal nerve, ischemia changes ion transport across membranes and postulate that if these membranes are damaged, ionic movement is affected to a lesser degree. Low et al[93] attribute the resistance to ischemic conduction block in experimental diabetic neuropathy to the ability of diabetic nerves to maintain a higher level of anaerobic glycolysis for a longer time than normal nerves. While it was initially not clear that function was related to morphology, a recent study of nerve biopsies by Dyck et al showed a very good correlation between pathological findings and tests of sensory function and nerve conduction velocity.[94]

Relationship of diabetic polyneuropathy to the duration of disease and glycemic control

The incidence, prevalence and severity of chronic diabetic polyneuropathy increase with the duration of diabetes and with the degree of hyperglycemia. These associations are supported regardless of whether clinical or electrophysiological assessments of nerve function are employed. Therefore, both the clinical and electrophysiological alterations of diabetic polyneuropathy are related to the degree of hyperglycemia and duration of diabetes.

Relationship of clinical measures

Numerous reports have established a direct relationship between the clinical assessment of diabetic neuropathy and the glycemic control and duration of diabetes mellitus. In a prospective study of diabetic patients started in 1947, Pirart[14,95] collected clinical and biochemical data annually from 4,398 cases; 2,796 of them were treated from the time of diagnosis and followed continuously for up to 25 years. Annual ratings for the degree of glycemic control were assigned, based on the degree of glycosuria reported during the day, postprandial blood sugar levels, fasting blood sugar levels, and the presence or absence of ketotic and hyperglycemic symptoms.

> A diagnosis of diabetic neuropathy was made in cases of loss of Achilles and/or patellar reflexes, possibly combined with a clear diminution of vibratory sensation. Also considered as diabetic neuropathy was a more dramatic polyneuropathy or mono- or multineuropathy on the conditions that (1) they comprised objective, clinical signs; (2) a thorough neurological examination could not detect any other cause; and (3) any associated alcoholism clearly played only a minor role. Cases were not so diagnosed if they showed total loss of tendon reflexes at any age without symptoms or other signs of neuropathy; isolated bilateral Achilles reflex loss and/or slight diminution of vibratory sensation after age 65; or acute idiopathic paralysis of a cranial nerve without other sign of peripheral neuropathy.[95]

Using these criteria, Pirart reported a positive correlation between the incidence and prevalence of clinical neuropathy and the duration of diabetes. The prevalence of clinical neuropathy rose from less than 10% at the onset of diabetes to 50% after a duration of 25 years. This increasing prevalence of clinical neuropathy as a function of the known duration of diabetes was noted regardless of the age of onset of diabetes. The increasing prevalence of clinical neuropathy as a function of the known duration of diabetes varied as a function of the degree of glycemic control. Although the rate of neuropathy increased in the "good" control group, it rose much more steeply in the "poor" control group. After 25 years of diabetes, the prevalence of clinical neuropathy was about 10% to 20% in the "good" control group compared with 60% to 70% in the "poor" control group.

Nielson and Lund[96] also noted a positive correlation between clinical neuropathic parameters (reduced corneal sensitivity, decreased vibratory perception, and the presence of areflexia) and the duration of diabetes in 100 diabetic patients. Using an assessment of vibration sensory threshold as a measure of clinical neuropathy, Hillson et al[97] found that threshold values were associated with the mean fasting blood glucose in 71 patients with NIDDM. When 41 diabetic patients with symptomatic neuropathy were compared to diabetic subjects without neuropathy, the neuropathy group had higher levels of glycosylated hemoglobin and mean blood glucose, confirming an inverse relationship between symptomatic neuropathy and glycemic control.[98] In a study of 20 diabetic patients, it was found that the presence and type of fiber abnormalities (segmental demyelination, remyelination and axonal degeneration) in sural nerve biopsies could be related to the duration of diabetes and to neuropathic symptoms.[29] In reviewing diabetic neuropathy, Brown and Asbury[99] stated the following:

> The presence and extent of polyneuropathy generally parallels the duration and severity of diabetes, even when diabetes is secondary to acquired pancreatic disease. There is no evidence that the neuropathic complications of Type 1 and Type 2 diabetes differ. Although neuropathic signs have been elicited within months of onset in Type 1 diabetes, clinical neuropathy usually does not appear in diabetics until after 5 or 10 years of hyperglycemia.

Relationship between electrophysiologic measurements and glycemic control

Numerous reports have suggested a positive correlation between poor glycemic control, duration of diabetes mellitus, and reduced motor nerve conduction.

Based on obtained results in 145 diabetic subjects, Gregersen[100] concluded that mean motor conduction velocity decreased with increasing duration of diabetes and was slower in poorly-controlled than in well-controlled patients. Subsequently, Gregersen[89] found that repeat measurements of motor conduction velocity in 14 previously untreated diabetic patients showed improved nerve function velocity after the institution of glycemic control by insulin treatment. Ward et al[101] measured motor conduction velocity in the median and lateral peroneal nerves in 39 newly diagnosed diabetics at the time of diagnosis and again after six weeks and six months of treatment. Following treatment, the motor conduction velocity was significantly improved. Fraser et al[87] examined peripheral nerve function in six insulin-treated newly diagnosed male diabetics. There was significant impairment of motor conduction velocity in the peroneal nerve, with improvement over the six months following initiation of insulin treatment.

Hansen and Ballantyne[102] found a significant negative correlation between motor nerve conduction velocities and the duration of diabetes. Similarly, in a study of 56 patients with diabetic neuropathy, Braddom et al[103] noted that the number of abnormal nerve conduction parameters in each patient was a function of the duration of diabetes. In studying sequential motor and sensory nerve conduction determinations of 108 diabetic children, Eng et al[104] also found a clear correlation between the duration of diabetes and the presence of abnormal motor and sensory nerve conduction velocities.

Graf et al[105] reported that glycosylated hemoglobin levels were directly correlated with slowing of motor nerve conduction velocity but not sensory nerve conduction in 20 patients with untreated diabetes mellitus. In studying variables of glycemic control and motor and sensory nerve conduction velocity in a group of 18 NIDDM subjects before and after institution of diabetes therapy, Graf et al[106] found that improvement in median, peroneal and tibial motor nerve conduction velocity was related to the reduction of hyperglycemia. Canal and Comi[107] detected in 51 diabetic children a significant correlation between glycosylated hemoglobin levels and both peroneal motor and median sensory nerve conduction velocity.

Halar et al[108] investigated the relationship between nerve conduction velocity and hyperglycemia at the time of diagnosis and following treatment in 25 Type 2 diabetic patients. Median, peroneal and tibial motor nerve conduction velocities significantly correlated with the level of hyperglycemia at the time of diagnosis. Following treatment, the improvement in median motor nerve conduction velocities after three and 12 months, and peroneal motor nerve conduction velocity after three months, directly correlated with the decreased fasting plasma glucose levels.

Normalization of glycemic control through continuous subcutaneous insulin infusion (CSII) has produced significant changes in motor nerve conduction velocity. Following near normalization of glycemic control in ten patients for six weeks using continuous subcutaneous insulin infusion, Pietri et al[109] noted a statistically significant increase in motor nerve conduction velocity in both the median and peroneal nerves but not in the ulnar motor nerve or in any of the sensory nerves tested. No changes occurred in five patients while on a conventional insulin regimen. In nine patients with painful diabetic neuropathy, Boulton et al[110] reported a significant improvement in motor nerve conduction velocity during a four-month period of improved glycemic control with CSII. Gambardella et al[111] showed significantly improved motor conduction velocity in the peroneal and median nerves following one to three months of glycemic control by CSII. Similarly, Troni et al[112] reported that prominent improvement in motor nerve conduction velocity occurred in 12 patients with IDDM treated with CSII for six months.

In 79 teenage diabetic patients, Young et al[113] reported that both motor and sensory peripheral nerve conduction abnormalities were related to poor glycemic control and duration of diabetes. Hoffman et al[114] found that duration of diabetes and diabetes control each had a significant and independent effect on the prevalence of delayed ulnar and peroneal nerve conduction. Chiasson et al[115] presented evidence that regardless of the insulin regimen used, improved metabolic control was associated with increased nerve conduction velocities in 12 patients with IDDM.

Summary

A substantial body of evidence has established that both clinical and neuroelectrophysiological assessments reflect the nerve dysfunction of chronic diabetic neuropathy, which is related to the duration of diabetes and degree of glycemic control. Motor nerve conduction velocity often correlates with glycemia and improves with treatment. Sensory nerve conduction velocity is abnormal but usually does not correlate with glycemia and may not improve with treatment.

Treatment

Current therapy of the diabetic neuropathies is nonspecific,[25,27] because presently there is no drug available that would interfere with the toxic effects of hyperglycemia.[25,27] The administration of an aldose reductase inhibitor has been shown to ameliorate the diabetes-related changes in nerve sorbitol and myoinositol and improve nerve conduction velocities in rats[116] and humans[117] with an apparent beneficial effect in painful diabetic neuropathy.[118,119] However, long-term prospective studies are needed to evaluate the potential role of aldose reductase inhibitors on the progression of early diabetic nephropathy. A discussion of the commonly employed symptomatic treatments of the diabetic neuropathies, and their limitations, follows.

Polyneuropathy

Distal symmetric sensorimotor polyneuropathy

Since a great deal of evidence suggests that hyperglycemia contributes to diabetic neuropathy, treatment of distal symmetrical polyneuropathy is aimed primarily at achieving the best glycemic control.[4,120] Improvement in nerve function and accompanying clinical symptomatology may occur with the attainment of near-normal glycemic control.[25,27,109,121,122] However, improvement with better glycemic control is not universal,[25,27] and the achievement of markedly improved blood glucose control is often quite difficult.[25,27] In IDDM, intensified insulin treatment to improve blood glucose control necessitates both[95] frequent insulin administration throughout the day (or continuously via a mechanical device)[14] and home blood glucose monitoring and patient adherence to a prescribed dietary program.[25,123] The required high degree of patient motivation is, however, not always present. In NIDDM, improved blood glucose control involves either weight loss[25,124] or therapy with oral hypoglycemic drugs or insulin.

In painful neuropathy, several symptomatic and supportive measures may be undertaken, although the pain encountered is frequently of a recalcitrant nature.[4,120] Relief of the neuropathic symptoms usually requires the administration of analgesics, varying in potency from aspirin to the narcotics.[25] In addition, other drugs have been used, though with varying reports of efficacy: diphenylhydantoin,[25] carbamazepine,[25,125] and amitryptiline and fluphenazine.[25,126,127] Their use is also often limited by adverse reactions or toxicity.[25]

When a neuropathic ulcer does occur, local antisepsis and devices to avoid weight bearing or trauma are prescribed until healing occurs.[4]

Autonomic neuropathy

Treatment of the various forms of diabetic autonomic neuropathy is also nonspecific.[4,128] As with sensorimotor neuropathy, control of the blood glucose is attempted.

Postural hypotension is treated variously with elastic stockings, ephedrine, indomethacin, monoamine oxidase inhibitors and pindolol, a beta-blocker with intrinsic β-adrenergic activity. Currently, fludrocortisone seems to be the treatment of choice.[129]

Bladder dysfunction and urinary retention are treated by encouraging patients to void every three to four hours during the day. Antibiotics are used for urinary tract infection.[130] Depending on the clinical presentation, cholinergic drugs, indwelling catheters, or a transurethral resection of the bladder neck may be needed.[130]

Impotence is difficult to treat. While psychological and sexual counseling have offered some help to patients, androgenic hormone therapy has not usually been helpful.[131] There are some anecdotal reports of aldose reductase inhibitors leading to an improvement in sexual function.[118]

Sweating may be excessive because of loss of much of the usual sweating surface. This can be helped with anticholinergic drugs.[132]

Alimentary system disorders such as symptomatic gastric atony have been helped somewhat by metoclopramide and by domperidone.[133,134] Broad-spectrum antibiotics are sometimes useful in the treatment of diabetic diarrhea,[135] but narcotics may be necessary.

Summary

Current treatment programs designed to ameliorate the symptoms caused by the diabetic polyneuropathies generally offer nonspecific relief because of the lack of any pharmacologically active compound specifically interfering with the pathophysiology of the disorder.

Mononeuropathy and multiple mononeuropathy

Cranial nerve lesions

Cranial mononeuropathies are presumed to be the result of vascular occlusion. It is assumed, therefore, that they will resolve spontaneously. Treatment consists of efforts to avoid recurrent thrombosis, together with analgesics to control pain.[4]

Peripheral nerve lesions

Mononeuropathies of peripheral nerves are persistent, frequently painful, and often lead to muscle atrophy. Most will resolve if recurrent trauma is avoided. Peripheral mononeuropathies may not respond well to analgesics, but radiculopathies, femoral neuropathies, and meralgia paresthetica can be treated with local nerve blocks if necessary.[4]

Diabetic amyotrophy

Diabetic amyotrophy and neuropathic cachexia generally get better over time, but this may be prolonged and is quite variable. There are no specific treatments, but antidepressants have been used.[4,120]

THE KIDNEY AND RENAL TRACT—DIABETIC NEPHROPATHY

History

In 1836, Richard Bright, a Guy's Hospital physician, described albumin in the urine as a sign of serious kidney disease.[136] This observation, reinforced by the even earlier reports of Cotunnius in 1770[137] and Rollo in 1798[138] that the urine of some diabetics contained proteins, led Rayer to postulate[139] that diabetes might cause a form of "Bright's disease." In 1912, Van Noorden[140] demonstrated sporadic instances of albumin in the urine of as many as 21.5% of diabetic patients examined. Finally, in 1936, Kimmelstiel and Wilson's description[141] of spherical hyaline masses in the glomeruli of diabetic patients who died of renal failure led to establishing the concept of a specific diabetic renal complication.[142] Clinically, the illness described was characterized by albuminuria, nephrotic edema and progressive renal failure. Susequently, in 1942, autopsies of diabetic persons demonstrated diffuse glomerular lesions as well as nodular lesions[143] and hyaline arteriolosclerosis.[144] The natural history of diabetic renal disease was described in 1949 by Mann and colleagues.[145] They noted that death from renal failure most commonly occurred in insulin-dependent diabetes of long duration. The concept of diabetic nephropathy as one of the specific diabetic complications has now been well established.[146]

Incidence and epidemiology

Renal failure is one of the most ominous complications of diabetes mellitus. As with other complications of diabetes, there is a wide range in the severity and type of kidney damage experienced.[147] Knowles has reported that, depending upon accepted diagnostic criteria, the prevalence of diabetic glomerulosclerosis varies from 8% to 78%. Once diagnosed clinically, the course of diabetic renal disease is generally progressive, with the eventual occurrence of renal failure. Overall, approximately 25% of reported end-stage renal failure occurs in patients with diabetes.[148] Renal disease accounts for 5.3% to 12% of deaths among all patients with diabetes mellitus.[149] Knowles has estimated that at least 3,200 diabetic patients die each year in the U.S. from renal disease.[149]

The onset of proteinuria is the earliest and best characterized clinical sign of diabetic nephropathy. Recent studies indicate that approximately 30% to 40% of young, insulin-dependent diabetics will develop persistent proteinuria[149,150] and progressive renal failure in an average of 15 to 20 years after onset.[150] White found that 50% of insulin-dependent diabetic patients (IDDM) surviving for 20 years or more have some form of renal disease.[151] Survival after the onset of clinically evident renal disease was found to be variable but generally poor, with the mean interval between onset of proteinuria and death being approximately seven years, and only two to five years after the sustained elevation of serum creatinine was noted.[152]

Renal failure due to diabetic nephropathy is the single major cause of death (30%) in IDDM patients.[149,150] While patients having NIDDM also develop kidney disease, it contributes to a relatively small degree to the excess mortality in this group[153] possibly due to earlier death from other causes.

The age of onset of diabetes appears to be a factor in the development of renal disease, with the risk being significantly higher in patients with onset at less than ten years of age.[152]

In a large population study of 973 subjects, West and colleagues[154] found an impressive relationship between plasma glucose levels at the time of examination and frequency of both nephropathy and retinopathy. In fact, the prevalence of diabetic nephropathy is frequently coincident with known retinopathy. In a study of 111 diabetic patients with duration of diabetes of 20 years or more, 95% were found to have background or proliferative retinopathy, and undetected, significant nephropathy was found to be present in a substantial number of these patients.[155] Evidence supporting the correlation between glycemic control and the onset of diabetic nephropathy is afforded by the large prospective study of Pirart,[95] which concludes as follows:

> 1. Poor [glycemic] control assessed cumulatively over the years is definitely related to a higher prevalence and incidence of neuropathy and microangiopathy, particularly severe retinopathy. This highly significant correlation has been found in the total population, in the inception cohort, and in every group and subgroup so far studied.
>
> 2. The annual incidence of neuropathy, retinopathy, and nephropathy is also

clearly and separately related to the glycemic control achieved during the year preceding the annual examination, whatever the prior degree of control.

In addition to the level of plasma glucose and possibly the age of onset of diabetes, recent evidence supports a direct influence of arterial blood pressure on the progression of diabetic nephropathy.[156–159]

Despite the presence of these risk factors, however, some patients with IDDM appear to be spared, even after a very long duration of diabetes. In a comparison of two age- and sex-matched groups of patients with IDDM who received uniform treatment from the onset of the disease, Deckert and Poulsen[160] found that one group developed severe diabetic nephropathy after 14.5 ± 3.3 years (mean ± SD), while the other showed no evidence of nephropathy after more than 32 years of disease. In fact, while the risk of developing diabetic nephropathy may be as high as 30% to 50% in young IDDM patients, for unknown reasons, 50% to 70% of these will never develop nephropathy in spite of a long duration of diabetes.[151,152] The nature of the factors protecting many diabetics against the deleterious effects of diabetes on renal function are unknown; however, several investigators have speculated that they may be of genetic or immunological origin.[160,161]

Natural history

Diabetic kidney disease progresses in three stages. The first stage, or latency period, is characterized by definite functional and pathological changes, including hypertension, nephromegaly and microproteinuria.[162] Some of the functional abnormalities can be reversed with tight diabetic control during the latency period.[161,162] During the second stage, intermittent proteinuria, detectable by the usual laboratory methods, appears and becomes constant.[161] There is a progression of the structural changes first noted during the latency period, including thickening of the basement membrane, mesangial expansion and glomerular arteriolar alteration.[162] Throughout the second stage, strict metabolic control and treatment of some of the complications, particularly the arterial hypertension, has been reported to retard progress to the next stage.[159,163] The third stage is the period of clinical renal insufficiency leading to renal failure. It is characterized by proteinuria, high blood pressure, a decline in glomerular function and the progressive onset of irreversible renal failure.[162]

The natural history of diabetic nephropathy in patients with NIDDM is less well known, probably because of the difficulty of identifying the precise onset of diabetes, the frequent presence of confounding concurrent disease and concomitant medication, and the problems associated with a 20-plus-year follow-up of an older population.

The natural history of diabetic nephropathy is considered so predictable that adult diabetic patients with proteinuria are presumed to have diabetic nephropathy. However, in some diabetic patients, proteinuria may be the result of a concurrent renal lesion superimposed on diabetic nephropathy or of an unrelated disorder.[164] Thus, Kasinath and associates[164] found renal disorders other than diabetic nephropathy in ten of 122 diabetic patients who underwent renal biopsy, including lupus glomerulonephritis, acute glomerulonephritis, focal glomerulosclerosis, idiopathic membrane nephropathy, and nonspecific immune complex glomerulonephritides. The appearance of urinary abnormalities or deterioration in renal function inconsistent with the natural history of diabetic nephropathy should lead to a more detailed evaluation, since some non-diabetic renal diseases may be amenable to treatment.

Much has been written recently about the latency period of nephropathy in IDDM. Shortly after the onset of diabetes, there is a 25% expansion of renal tissue mass.[165,166] To determine whether the enlargement affected glomerular structures, Østerby and Gundersen[167] conducted a morphometric study of glomeruli in kidney biopsies taken from young diabetics one to six years after onset. They found mean glomerular volume and capillary lumen per glomerulus enlarged to twice the normal size. Their findings were confirmed by Kroustrup et al[168] who demonstrated an 80% increase in glomerular filtration area in patients with early diabetes. These findings agree with the elevation of glomerular filtration rate (GFR) in newly diagnosed insulin-dependent diabetics.[169] Such an increase in glomerular filtration rate is found in insulin-dependent diabetics of all ages.[170–172] Several groups have demonstrated that the enlargement of the kidneys was approximately of the same magnitude as the increase in GFR,[166,169,173] and one group found that GFR remained elevated for more than 15 years after the diagnosis of diabetes, until the onset of proteinuria.[173] In experimental animals, increased kidney volume is associated with increased protein synthesis.[174]

Opinions differ on whether the early alterations in GFR and renal size, including mesangial mass, remain amenable to normalization with improved diabetic control during the latency period.[161,165,175] Mogensen and Anderson have shown that nephromegaly can be reduced in man by improved blood glucose control,[165,169] and Mogensen[176] has demonstrated that with good diabetic control, both increased GFR and kidney size decrease to normal. In contrast, Christiansen et al found that improvement of metabolic control in patients with IDDM for one week induced a 10% to 20% reduction in elevated GFR, while kidney size and enlarged glomerular filtration surface area remained unchanged.[177] Recently, Wiseman et al[178] observed that in patients with IDDM, strict glycemic control normalizes GFR, although kidneys remain enlarged. Findings concerning renal plasma flow (RPF) in diabetic patients have also been conflicting, with one group reporting these values unchanged with metabolic control[176] and the other group reporting increased values.[166]

A number of investigators have suggested that the elevated GFR in young, uncontrolled IDDM patients may be related in part to hypersecretion of growth hormone.[179] Abnormal growth hormone levels appear to correlate with the degree of poor metabolic control and are restored to normal after strict glycemic control.[180]

Hyperglycemia per se might contribute to the elevated GFR in diabetics, since in strictly-controlled insulin-dependent diabetics, when blood glucose levels were raised from 4.6 ± 0.2 to 16.0 ± 0.6 mmol/L, GRF and RPF were increased,[181] though not by lack of insulin.[182]

In addition to alterations in GFR and RPF, an early defect in protein excretion develops during the latency period. Keen and Chlouverakis[183] demonstrated in 1963 that in diabetic patients an increased urinary albumin excretion rate (AER) precedes the appearance of clinical proteinuria.[161,184] Elevation in AER has been characterized as microalbuminuria and is defined as excretion of less than 250 mg/day of albumin. AER levels three- to four-fold above normal have been found in newly detected NIDDM subjects.[185] Elevated AER levels have also been found in newly diagnosed IDDM patients[186] and in short-term IDDM patients whose control was deliberately worsened by the brief withdrawal of insulin.[187] In conventionally treated insulin-dependent patients with diabetes of six months' to 39 years' duration, albumin and IgG excretion rates were raised in approximately 30% to 45% of subjects, with a higher proportion in patients with a duration of diabetes of ten to 20 years.[188,189]

Early alterations in AER are amenable to normalization with improved diabetic control. Near normalization of glycemia obtained by continuous subcutaneous insulin infusion (CSII) led to a prompt fall of microalbuminuria in a group of insulin-dependent diabetic patients.[189,190] In another group, exercise-induced increase in AER was also corrected by CSII.[191]

Glomerular basement membrane (GBM) thickness is normal at the onset of insulin-dependent diabetes and increases with time, a slight thickening appearing after two years, a 35% increase, after five years, a more rapid progress occurring in less well-controlled patients[192] (Fig 2). After ten to 20 years, GBM thickening or arteriolar lesion may lead to complete closure of many glomeruli.[193,194]

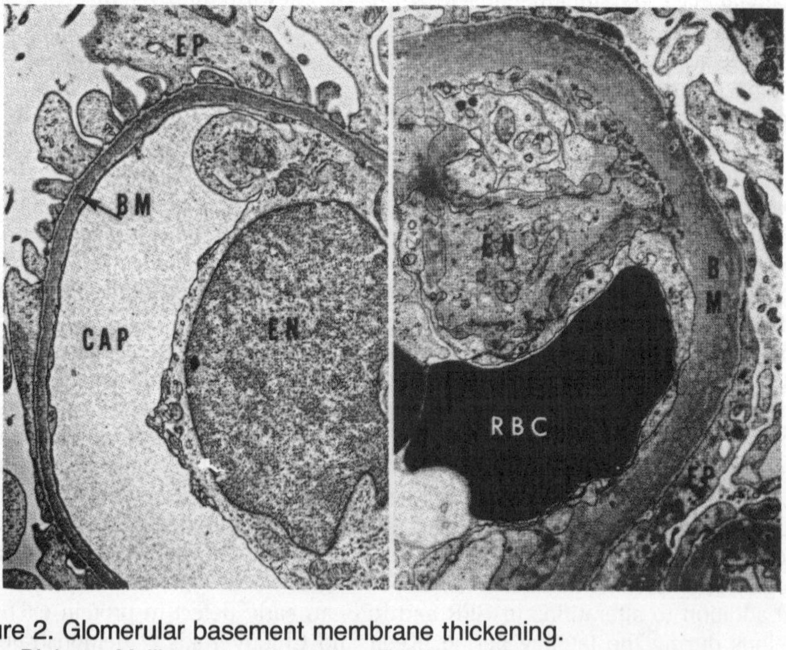

Figure 2. Glomerular basement membrane thickening.
(From Diabetes Mellitus, seventh edition, Eli Lilly and Company, 1969, page 184)

The clinically-evident period of diabetic nephropathy is characterized in its early stage by intermittent proteinuria, detectable by the usual clinical methods, and later by increasing urinary albumin excretion, during both day and night.[161] Clinically evident nephropathy begins to occur after eight to 17 years of diabetes.[195,196] Onset of constant clinical proteinuria is variable, but usually does not occur in patients with insulin-dependent diabetes after fewer than 15 to 20 years' duration, and often with the accompanying complication of retinopathy.[147–161]

Progression through the clinically-evident phase with increasing proteinuria occurs with a markedly variable time course.[197,198] Generally, significant proteinuria inaugurates the phase leading to progressive decline of renal function and end-stage renal failure.[199] GFR may be normal or even raised at the onset of significant proteinuria, but then will proceed relentlessly to fall,[156,196,200] with a rate of decline ranging from 1.0 mL/min/month to 2.4 mL/min/month (mean 1.2 mL/min/month), in a pattern strikingly linear with time.[199]

In some patients with significant proteinuria and renal impairment, long-term antihypertensive treatment has been shown to slow the rate of decline in renal function in diabetic nephropathy.[159,163] In a small study of six diabetic men treated for moderate hypertension and studied for a mean of 73 months for the effect on the progression of nephropathy, Mogensen reported that monthly decline in GFR fell from −1.23 mL/min/month to −0.49 mL/min/month with treatment; and in all patients, the mean yearly increase in albumin clearance (expressed as a percentage of the GFR) fell from 107% before treatment to 5% during treatment.[159]

During the final phase of diabetic kidney disease, there is considerable variability among patients in the progression toward renal failure; in each patient, however, the progression is constant.[201] In a 1976 report from the Joslin Clinic, early renal failure appeared two years after onset of significant proteinuria, and severe renal failure, four years after the onset of proteinuria. Mean duration of life after the onset of severe renal failure was six months with a mortality of 53% of the patients, with 59% of the deaths due to renal failure and 36% due to cardiovascular disease. Jones et al reported that the interval between the diagnosis of diabetes and the onset of end-stage renal failure varies between 12 and 32 years (mean 21 years).[201]

Terminal uremia occurs in diabetic nephropathy when serum creatinine is above 8 mg/dL and creatinine clearance is below 20% of normal. At this stage, many patients have coronary artery disease or peripheral vascular disease and medial vascular calcification. Severe neuropathy is also common,[202] perhaps complicated by uremia as an etiology. Typically, there is fluid overload, with the cerebral complications of hypertension.[161]

Patients with advanced diabetic nephropathy often have other diabetic complications. Almost all have retinopathy; 80% suffer from proliferative retinopathy, and about 25% are blind.

Prediction and prevention

In an attempt to identify those diabetic patients at high risk for developing serious renal disease, several groups have undertaken long-term studies which correlate albumin excretion rate (AER) with degree of risk in both IDDM and NIDDM patients. In 1966–1967, Viberti and colleagues[197] measured the overnight AER of 87 patients with IDDM; they obtained information on 63 patients of the original group 14 years later. Only two of 55 patients with AER below 30 μg/min developed clinical proteinuria during this 14-year period, while clinical proteinuria developed in seven of eight patients with AER between 30 and 140 μg/min. Thus, the risk of clinical diabetic nephropathy in the latter group was 24 times higher than in the former. Additionally, 9.1% of patients with AER below 30 μg/min had died, as compared with 37.5% with higher AER. They concluded that elevated AER strongly predicts the development of diabetic nephropathy and suggested that since AER is potentially reversible, early detection could, perhaps, lead to prevention.

The results of Parving et al[198] confirm these conclusions. In a six-year study of 15 females and eight males with long-term IDDM and without clinical proteinuria, five females and three males had elevated AER at screening. The five patients with the highest AER developed persistent albuminuria, elevated serum creatinine and raised blood pressure during the six-year observation period. Of the 15 patients with normal AER at screening, intermittent proteinuria developed in only two patients, while all values were virtually unchanged in the remaining 13 patients.

The results of several recent studies[157,203,204] reconfirm the above findings. However, each author defined a different upper limit associated with low risk. From an investigation conducted over a 14-year period of 44 patients with IDDM of at least seven years' duration, Mogensen and Christensen[203] concluded that microalbuminuria predicts the development of diabetic nephropathy and that elevated GFR and increased blood pressure may also contribute to this progression. Of the 14 patients with initial AER at or above 15 μg/min, 12 had clinically detected proteinuria upon restudy; of the 29 patients with initial AER below 15 μg/min, none had clinically detected proteinuria upon later examination. Those patients whose condition had progressed to clinically overt proteinuria had elevated GFR and higher blood pressures at the initial exam compared with those in whom proteinuria did not develop.

Mathiesen et al[204] conducted two investigations to define those patients with IDDM without proteinuria who would later be at risk of nephropathy. Of the 71 patients studied longitudinally for six years, seven patients with initial AER of more than 70 μg/min developed persistent proteinuria, while only three of the remaining 64 patients with AER at or below 70 μg/min developed clinical proteinuria. They concluded, therefore, that patients with AER of more than 70 μg/min are at risk and designated this stage as incipient nephropathy. In the cross-sectional study of 227 patients, Mathiesen and his colleagues[204] further characterized patients with incipient nephropathy as having increased systolic and diastolic blood pressure and elevated GFR compared to normal patients.

In a study of 28 patients with IDDM with different degrees of microalbuminuria, Wiseman and colleagues[157] assessed the role of plasma glucose levels and arterial pressure in identifying those diabetic patients at increased risk of nephropathy. Both low and high microalbuminuria groups were found to have significantly higher glycosylated hemoglobin levels and mean plasma glucose concentrations during a 24-hour profile than their respective control subjects. Moreover, a significant correlation between glycosylated hemoglobin level and AER was found in the whole study group ($r = 0.48$; $p < 0.001$). Arterial pressure was significantly higher in the high microalbuminuria groups, and a significant correlation was found between arterial pressure and AER in the whole study population ($r = 0.49$; $p < 0.001$), as well as in the pooled microalbuminuria group ($r = 0.43$; $p < 0.05$). Multiple regression analysis showed that glycosylated hemoglobin and arterial pressure levels were independently correlated with AER. It was seen that diabetic patients with microalbuminuria have worse glycemic control than those without it and that higher levels of arterial pressure are associated with microalbuminuria predictive of development of proteinuria. Thus, Wiseman and colleagues[157] concluded that high plasma glucose and high arterial pressure characterize diabetic patients at increased risk of nephropathy but observed that these indices of risk are potentially reversible.

Elevated AER in patients with NIDDM has also been shown to predict the later development of proteinuria and early mortality.[205] In a nine-year study, 76 NIDDM patients between the ages of 50 and 75 years with an initial albuminuria of 30 μg/mL to 140 μg/mL were compared with diabetic patients with lower albuminuria and 28 diabetic patients with higher albuminuria. After nine years, the group with albuminuria concentrations of 30 μg/mL to 140 μg/mL was more likely to have clinically detectable proteinuria (> 400 μg/mL) than were the groups with lower initial concentrations. Moreover, mortality was 148% higher in this group than in the normal controls.

Relation to plasma glucose control

The mechanisms underlying the development of diabetic nephropathy are still obscure. However, several recent reviews suggest that control of diabetes alters the development of diabetic nephropathy.[95,206–208] Two independent groups[95,150] following patients with long-standing diabetes have observed that patients with better glycemic control had fewer complications than those controlled less well. Normal kidneys will develop angiopathy when transplanted to diabetic patients,[209,210] thus supporting metabolic abnormalities as a prime cause of diabetic nephropathy. Studies of biopsy specimens of kidney and quadriceps muscle from seven pairs of identical twins who were discordant for IDDM have helped to distinguish metabolic from genetic factors in the development of diabetic microangiopathy.[211] Of the diabetic patients, five had normal renal function and only minor clinical indications of complications, and two had clinical diabetic nephropathy, including hypertension, marked albuminuria, and a substantially reduced creatinine clearance. All the normal twins had normal glomerular BM widths and normal volumes of the mesangium. Glomerular and tubular BM width and mesangial volume in each diabetic twin exceeded values in respective siblings ($p \leq 0.0035$) even in instances where the diabetic twin lay within established normal ranges. Values for muscle capillary BM widths in the diabetic twins did not differ from those in their siblings ($p = 0.5$). According to Steffes et al,[211] these observations suggest that "the metabolic abnormalities of diabetes are necessary, if not sufficient, for the development of glomerular abnormalities." But the question of whether hyperglycemia influences the microvascular complications of diabetes is still debated.[212]

In man as well as in animals, some early characteristics of nephropathy have been seen to respond to glycemic control. Early abnormalities of hyperfiltration, microalbuminuria, and possibly nephromegaly have been shown to improve by strict glycemic control.[176,188,213] Wiseman et al investigated the relation between blood glucose control, GFR, and enlarged kidneys in patients with IDDM. After one year, patients treated with CSII showed significantly improved glycemic control ($p < 0.001$) and a corresponding, significant fall in GFR ($p < 0.001$), which became normal in four of the six patients. There was, however, no change in kidney volume.[178]

Steffes and Mauer[214] state that the many observations of rapid and significant changes occurring in the kidneys of patients with recent onset of IDDM emphasize the fact that "diabetic microangiopathy occurs as a result of diabetes and not because of another coinherited pathophysiological process." Significant morphologic changes, such as enlargement of the BM surface area and increased thickness of the glomerular BM,[215] the presence of glomerular arteriolar thickening,[210] and the disposition of immunoglobulins in all extracellular renal membranes[216] occur within two to four years of the onset of diabetes. They point out that renal hypertrophy and a coincident increase in GFR, filtration fraction, and exercise-induced urinary albumin excretion occur within weeks after the onset of diabetes.[214] Moreover, elevated levels of each of these return toward normal with strict glycemic control.[176]

Mauer et al[210,216] observed the development of diabetic nephropathy in normal kidneys taken from donors with no evidence of nephropathy and no preordained genetic cause of diabetic microangiopathy, upon transplantation into diabetic recipients. They concluded that diabetic glomerulopathy may develop in any kidney exposed to the abnormal metabolic environment of diabetes mellitus. In a reverse study, two diabetic kidneys with glomerulosclerosis and capillary BM thickening transplanted into non-diabetic recipients resulted in a major improvement of the pathologic findings after seven months.[217]

In patients with persistent proteinuria due to diabetic nephropathy, antihypertensives have been effective in reducing AER. Twelve patients with IDDM and persistent proteinuria >0.5g/day, diastolic blood pressure ≥ 95 mm Hg were treated with metoprolol, hydralazine and furosemide or thiazide. During the 12-month treatment period, blood pressure decreased from 151/104 mm Hg to 133/85 mm Hg ($p < 0.001$), the AER diminished from 1447 μg/min to 613 μg/min ($p < 0.005$), and GFR declined from 96 to 89 mL/min/1.73 m^2 ($p < 0.01$), indicating that early and aggressive treatment of arterial hypertension in IDDM patients decreases albuminuria, probably due to reduced intraglomerular filtration pressure.[218]

Unfortunately, late-stage nephropathy shows little responsiveness to intensive efforts of glycemic control. Bending and associates[219] observed that renal failure has complex metabolic consequences which alter insulin metabolism and affect daily insulin requirements. Thus, while strict glycemic control with CSII was difficult to achieve in these patients, the control was superior to that achieved in a matched group with conventional insulin treatment. The authors concluded that difficulty in controlling blood glucose concentrations in diabetic patients with persistent proteinuria may contribute to the failure of intensified insulin regimens to influence the progression of diabetic renal disease. Tamborlane et al[220] found no evidence that intensive insulin therapy reversed retinopathy or nephropathy in insulin-dependent diabetics. With respect to stable NIDDM, it was concluded that insulin treatment is not better than diet alone in altering the course of vascular complications after a ten-year study in which fasting glucose levels in the treated group were approximately 110 mg/dL during the first five years and 120 mg/dL after ten years.[221]

The findings of Viberti and colleagues[222] demonstrate that by the time glomerular function has begun to fail in diabetic nephropathy, the process culminating in end-stage renal failure may well be self-perpetuating and little influenced by degree of metabolic control. In six insulin-dependent diabetics with proteinuria due to nephropathy, CSII for up to 24 months greatly improved metabolic control, but had no significant effect on decline of GFR, on increase of plasma creatinine concentrations, or on progressive rise of fractional clearance of albumin, indicating a progression of glomerular damage. While continuing deterioration of advanced nephropathy is the rule, even in response to metabolic correction, exceptions may still exist.[222] Thus, in the Viberti study, one patient did improve. The rate of fall of filtration fraction and rise of plasma creatinine concentration slowed considerably, and there was no evidence of renal disease, even on biopsy.

In assessing the relation of diabetic control to renal damage, and particularly, in attempting to determine the reasons for the failure of near normal control to deter further renal damage in advanced diabetic nephropathy, there are a number of factors which must be taken into account:

1. the degree of glycemic control achieved by such intensive measures as CSII may be improved, but may not be sufficient;[222]
2. the treatment periods may not have been of adequate duration;
3. once renal function has deteriorated markedly, the nephropathic process may have become self-perpetuating and independent of the diabetic metabolic abnormalities which initiated it.[220,223]

Viberti and others speculate that there may be "a point of no return for the kidney" in diabetic nephropathy as there is for the eye in diabetic retinopathy.[220,222,223] Strong experimental evidence indicates that the compensatory hyperfiltration process in surviving nephrons occurring after major nephron loss is ultimately self-destructive.[158] Thus the major problem in establishing a treatment for diabetic nephropathy may well involve the quantifying of renal damage before the loss of renal function and early treatment of those patients targeted to be susceptible. For early detection, Viberti and his colleagues consider albuminuria as the indicator of diabetic glomerular damage[188] and suggest a new definition of incipient clinical diabetic nephropathy (urinary AER between 50 mg/24 hr and 200 mg/24 hr) to identify patients responsive to therapeutic intervention.[197]

Summary

Diabetic nephropathy occurs frequently in both IDDM and NIDDM patients. It can lead to progressive renal failure and is a major cause of diabetic mortality, particularly in IDDM. Microalbuminuria is an early finding and appears to be a predictor of future morbidity. Glycemic control may reverse progression early on, but as the disorder progresses, other factors, such as hypertension, contribute importantly to the rate of decompensation, which seems to become independent of glycemic regulation and therapeutic intervention.

THE EYE—RETINOPATHY, CATARACT, KERATOPATHY

Retinopathy

Estimates made in 1978 by the National Society to Prevent Blindness list diabetic retinopathy as the fifth leading cause of blindness, accounting at that time for approximately 4,700 new cases and an estimated 32,600 existing cases.[224] Diabetic retinopathy is now the leading cause of new cases of blindness among persons aged 20 to 74 years.[225] In England and Wales diabetic retinopathy is the most common cause of blindness in the 30- to 65-year-old age group and the most common cause of the newly registered blind for the years 1963 to 1968.[226] Diabetic subjects are at risk for visual loss due to diabetic retinopathy, glaucoma and cataracts. Among the eye complications of diabetes, retinopathy is the cause of about 84% of blindness in diabetic patients.[227] Approximately 2% of all diabetic subjects are blind from retinopathy, which is a prevalence ten times greater than that of blindness from all causes in the general population.[228]

Natural history

Diabetic retinopathy is divided into three different types: nonproliferative (background), pre-proliferative, and proliferative (Fig 3). Nonproliferative diabetic retinopathy is characterized by microvascular changes in the retinal capillary bed[229,230] and the formation of microaneurysms, exudates, and small intraretinal hemorrhages.[231] All these changes are intraretinal and the main pathogenetic mechanisms are vascular leakage and occlusion.[232–234] Edema and/or ischemia of the macula are thought to be the main cause of reduced visual acuity.[235,236] At some point, the capillary endothelium may begin to proliferate, typically at the periphery of zones of retinal ischemia.[237] This more florid and advanced phase of background retinopathy, referred to as pre-proliferative retinopathy, is characterized by soft exudates (cotton-wool spots), multiple large blot hemorrhages, venous beading, and intraretinal microvascular abnormalities.[238,239] In proliferative diabetic retinopathy, neovascularization in the optic disk area and elsewhere in the retina is in evidence.[238] The proliferative lesions pass through three well-defined states: fine, naked new blood vessels; vasoproliferation accompanied by connective tissue formation; and regression of new vessels with contraction of the connective tissue component. If the proliferative lesions have penetrated the internal limiting

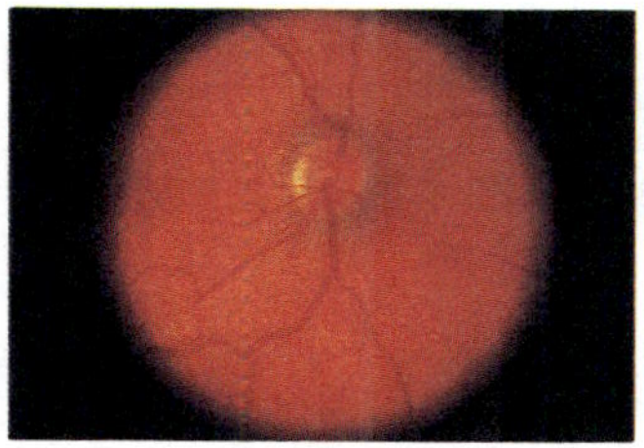

Stage I — Nonproliferative

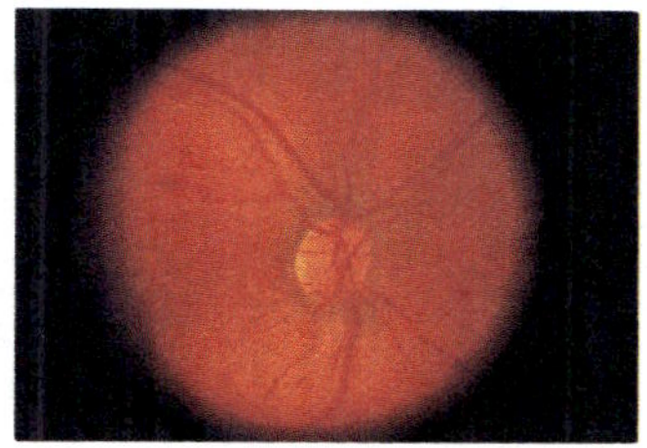

Stage II — Pre-proliferative

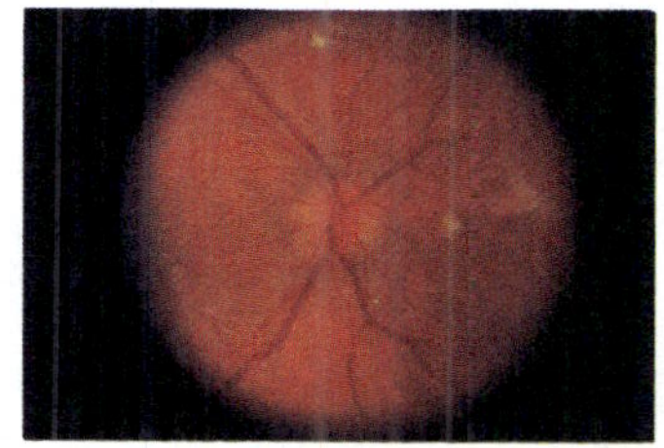

Stage III — Proliferative

Figure 3. Diabetic retinopathy stages.

Stage I: An example of very early diabetic retinopathy characterized by dilated and tortuous veins and microaneurysms.

Stage II: The pathological changes include multiple dilated and tortuous veins in addition to dilated capillary beds. Multiple flame-shaped hemorrhages are seen in the presence of hard and soft exudates.

Stage III: Advanced disease is demonstrated by an area of neovascular growth extending diagonally across the vein at 1.5mm superior-nasal to the optic disc. Intraretinal microvascular abnormalities are present near the twelve o'clock margin. The veins are dilated and tortuous and there are areas of soft exudates in the retina.

(Illustrations courtesy of Stephen S. Feman, M.D., Professor of Ophthalmology and Director of Retina Services, Vanderbilt University, School of Medicine.)

membrane of the retina and entered the vitreous cavity, major hemorrhage may result from the traction of the adherent vitreous gel as the connective tissue component contracts. Traction also leads to retinal detachment with severe visual loss.[231,238]

Epidemiology

Wide variations are apparent in the incidence and prevalence reported for retinopathy among the different diabetic populations of the world.[240,241] L'Esperance and colleagues estimate an overall average incidence rate among diabetic populations of 52%,[241] based on considerations of four large population studies (Table 3).

Recently, Mitchell[240] reported the diabetic retinopathy prevalence rates among Australians (Table 4).

Table 3. Diabetic retinopathy incidence among different diabetic populations of the world.

Investigator and Ref. No.	Population	Number of Patients	Incidence
Lundbaek (242)	Danish	——	77%
Kornerup (243)	Swedish	1,000	47%
Kojima (244)	Japanese	4,875	33%
Cullen (245)	British	5,147	50%

Table 4. Diabetic retinopathy prevalence rates (Australian Caucasian Studies).[240]

Ophthalmoscopic Retinopathy		Vision-Threatening Retinopathy		
Newcastle Study		**Retinopathy**	**Maculopathy**	**Total**
Clinic 1977–78 n = 1210	49%	7%	5% (10)	13%
Rural n = 99	36%	3%	7% (8)	10%
W. Aust. Study				
1978–81 n = 1238	28%	3%	10%	13%

Numbers in parentheses indicate total maculopathy.

In a prospective study of 4,400 patients observed for 25 years, Pirart reported that the prevalence of retinopathy, especially in its serious form, increases as a function of the duration of diabetes, reaching a plateau toward the 15th to 20th year.[95] Over the course of 25 years, the annual incidence for retinopathy increased from 3% to 13%. After 20 to 25 years, the whole population showed retinopathy in about 55% of cases. The prevalence of retinopathy was positively correlated with chronically poor control.

Regarding the prevalence rate of diabetic retinopathy in the general population of the United States, the Framingham Eye Study cites a prevalence rate of about 2% at the age of 52 to 65 years, rising to about 3% at age 65 to 74 years, and 7% at age 75 to 85 years.[246] Palmberg and associates[247] report that prevalence reaches 50% at just over seven years' duration in IDDM and approaches 90% at 17 to 50 years. The prevalence of proliferative retinopathy is reported to be 26% at 26 to 50 years. The Wisconsin epidemiologic study cites a prevalence which varies from 17% to 97.5% in persons with diabetes for less than five and 15 or more years' duration, respectively.[248] Proliferative retinopathy varied from 1.2% to 67% in persons with diabetes for less than ten and more than 35 years, respectively.[248] Among 1,370 patients diagnosed as diabetic at age 30 or older, the prevalence of diabetic retinopathy varied from 28.8% in persons with diabetes for less than five years to 77.8% in persons with diabetes for 15 or more years.[249] Rate of proliferative retinopathy varied from 2.0% in persons who had diabetes for less than five years to 15.5% in persons with diabetes for 15 or more years.[249]

L'Esperance observes[241] that there is evidence of an increasing frequency of retinopathy over the past several decades, which seems to coincide with the general increase in frequency of diabetes. He cites Wagener's findings in three series of diabetic patients, each series observed a decade apart since 1921,[250] in which there is a rising frequency of retinopathy from 8.3% in 1921, to 17.7% in 1934, and 30.6% in 1945. Frequency of proliferative retinopathy has also increased concurrently with the increased frequency of diabetes and retinopathy in general, especially since insulin has increased the life expectancy of diabetic patients.[241] The Wagener series[250] showed an increase in proliferative as well as nonproliferative retinopathy from 0 in 1921 to 10.7% in 1934 and to 13.4% in 1945. Root et al[251] reported a 30% incidence of proliferative retinopathy during the period from 1946 to 1956, with a 58.4% incidence among juvenile diabetics who survived for 25 to 35 years after the onset of diabetes.

Both the frequency and severity of retinopathy are influenced by the duration and the age at onset of diabetes.[95,226,241,248,249,252] In the Wisconsin study, the severity of retinopathy for persons under 30 years of age with diabetes of ten years' duration or less was related to duration, age at the time of examination, and levels of glycosylated hemoglobin.[248] After ten years, severity was related to duration, level of glycosylated hemoglobin, presence of proteinuria, diastolic blood pressure, and the male sex.[248] In diabetic patients of age 30 or older, risk factors determining severity of retinopathy were duration of diabetes, age at diagnosis, glycosylated hemoglobin levels, systolic blood pressure, use of insulin, presence of proteinuria, and body mass.[249] In the Pirart Study,[95] the prevalence of retinopathy increased as a function of duration of diabetes, plateauing toward the 15th to 20th year. The annual incidence for retinopathy increased from 3% to 13% over the course of 25 years.[95] Younger patients whose diabetes is diagnosed prior to age 30 show relatively longer durations of diabetes before retinopathy appears,[241] with the frequency rising from 50% after ten to 12 years of diabetes to 75% or more after 20 years. In patients older than 30 years at the diagnosis of diabetes, after 20 years there is a reported frequency of 75% to 80%.[241] The frequency of retinopathy increases with duration of diabetes up to 20 to 30 years; thereafter, it may decline to approximately 60% among patients surviving for 30 or more years.[253] This decline is probably accounted for by the selective effects of mortality when examining 30-plus-year survivors of diabetes.[241]

The relative importance of duration of diabetes before and after 13 years of age as a risk factor for retinopathy was investigated through the use of data from 200 persons who were younger than 26 years of age. Retinopathy was found in 9% of persons who were younger than 13 years and in 34% of persons who were 13 years or older and had been diagnosed at or after 13 years. Presence of retinopathy was more strongly associated with duration of diabetes in persons 13 years old or older.[254]

Diabetic retinopathy shows variations in frequency with sex as well as age and duration. The frequency in both sexes rises with age, with a peak frequency between 50 and 70 years, followed by a decline.[241] It predominates among men younger than 45, then among women older than 45.[241] Bodansky and associates[226] also found a marked excess of men (ratio 2:1) with severe retinopathy in a population of IDDM patients. In a study of 568 patients it was found that men who develop retinopathy may be at greater risk than women of proliferative disease.[255] In the sample group, 41.7% of men had proliferative diabetic retinopathy, as compared with 26.4% of women ($p < 0.05$ significance).[255]

In the diabetic population, there is a wide range in frequency of proliferative versus nonproliferative retinopathy. Among the diabetics with established retinopathy, the reported frequency of proliferative retinopathy was 6%,[256] 8%,[242] and 20%.[251] Palmberg and associates[247] report a 26% prevalence rate for proliferative retinopathy at 26 to 50 years' duration of diabetes. L'Esperance calculates that 8% to 10% is probably a reasonable estimate of the frequency of proliferative retinopathy among representative groups of diabetics with established retinopathy of all types.[241]

The prognosis for patients with proliferative retinopathy is considerably worse than that for nonproliferative retinopathy patients. There appears to be general agreement that in patients with proliferative retinopathy, the risk of blindness is approximately 50% within five years, with younger patients generally faring better than older.[241] When Deckert and colleagues[257] followed up 51 patients with proliferative retinopathy from two to 18 years, they found that 50% were blind (20/200 or less) in both eyes after five years, and after ten years, virtually all were blind in at least one eye. Reporting on the visual status of 33 patients with proliferative retinopathy followed for five years, Dobree[258] found that 76% were blind; and Caird and colleagues found that 50% of 22 patients with proliferative retinopathy were blind after five years.[259] In Beetham's series of 1,149 proliferative retinopathy patients followed for 20 years, a 40% rate of blindness (20/200 or worse) was noted in maturity onset diabetic patients during an 11-year period and a 25% rate among juvenile-onset diabetics.[260] The findings of Deckert and his co-workers that patients with onset of proliferative retinopathy before age 35 appeared to fare better than did patients with onset after 35 were similar to those of the Beetham study, indicating that proliferative retinopathy follows a more malignant course among older or older onset patients with diabetes.[257] Visual prognosis appears to be worse if neovascular changes involve the optic disk or if proteinuria is present. In the Deckert study, the onset of proteinuria signaled a worsened visual prognosis, with 50% of these patients becoming blind in both eyes in two years.[257] In patients with disk neovascularization, after ten years 100% were blind in one eye and 90% were blind in both eyes.[257] In a study of 44 eyes with proliferative changes on the optic disk, Kohner and associates observed that within six months, 18% of these eyes developed extensive fibrous proliferation or vitreous hemorrhage, and that at four years, 66% had suffered similar changes.[261] The visual acuity deteriorated significantly in 57% of these eyes, and 34% became blind.[261]

The Diabetic Retinopathy Study[262] Research Group has identified the following four retinopathy factors that increase the two-year risk of developing severe visual loss:

1. presence of vitreous or preretinal hemorrhage
2. presence of new vessels
3. location of new vessels on or near the optic disk
4. severity of new vessels.[261]

The severity of retinopathy may be of prognostic significance in determining the severity of generalized microvascular disease and survival of the diabetic patient.[241] In a study of mortality rates among diabetics with retinopathy, Caird observed that in comparison with diabetics without retinopathy, diabetics with hemorrhages and exudates have five-fold greater mortality, and diabetics with proliferative retinopathy have seven-fold greater mortality.[228,263] A retrospective evaluation of hospital records of 907 diabetic patients attending an ophthalmic diabetic clinic showed that the presence and type of retinopathy are closely associated with a prognosis of survival.[264] Patients with proliferative retinopathy had the poorest survival rates as a group, the cumulative observed five-year survival rate being 86% for females and 79% for males, versus a survival rate approximating 100% for patients with no retinopathy, and an intermediate position for those patients with nonproliferative retinopathy.[264] Among the blind diabetic patients, mortality rates average 15% per year for all ages.[263] The major causes of death among a large group of patients with proliferative retinopathy were found to be nephropathy (45%) and arteriosclerotic heart disease (37%).[251] The key study to determine risk is the Diabetic Retinopathy Study (DRS) in which a large group of diabetic patients was followed prospectively for mortality for an average of four and a half years. Of the 1,742 patients enrolled in the DRS, the majority of whom had proliferative diabetic retinopathy, 409 died.[265] The one-year and five-year cumulative mortality rates were 3.0% and 22.6% respectively, and the annual mortality rate was approximately 5%.[265]

Summary

There are wide variations in the incidence and prevalence reported for diabetic retinopathy worldwide, with an estimated overall average incidence rate of 52% among diabetic populations. Prevalence of retinopathy increases as a function of the duration of diabetes, with a reported range of 50% at just over seven years' duration in IDDM and approaching 90% at 17 to 50 years. There is also evidence of an increasing frequency of retinopathy over the past several decades, which seems to coincide with the general increase in frequency of diabetes. A wide range in frequency of proliferative versus nonproliferative retinopathy is reported in the diabetic population, with a reasonable estimate of the frequency of proliferative retinopathy being 8% to 10% among representative groups of diabetics with established retinopathy of all types.

Classification of diabetic retinopathy

Eight elements are generally recognized as contributing to the diagnosis of diabetic retinopathy: venous abnormalities, microaneurysms, hemorrhages, edema, exudates, new vessel formation, glial proliferation, and vitreo-retinal traction.[266] These elements are seen in various combinations; each consists of a continuum progressing from lesser to more severe defects (Fig 4).

Relation to glycemic control

Pathologically, diabetic retinopathy is a disease of the microvasculature. Changes in the retinal capillaries eventually lead to proliferation of new vessels extending from the retina into the vitreous, with secondary hemorrhages, retinal detachment, and eventual loss of vision. Investigations to date have proposed various metabolic, endocrine and hematological abnormalities as pathophysiologically important.[267]

The original basis for the belief that good control of blood glucose lessens the likelihood of diabetic retinopathy is the retrospective analysis of the clinical records of patients from large clinics.[268] One such example is the Joslin Clinic report of 360 juvenile diabetic patients studied after 20 to 40 years of diabetes, in which among patients judged to have "good" control only 7% were found to have marked or extreme retinopathy, while in 82 patients with "fair" control, 19% fell into these categories, and in 166 patients with "poor" control, the figure rose to 43%.[269] The Pirart study of 4,400 patients[95] concluded the following: "Poor control assessed cumulatively over the years is definitely related to a higher prevalence and incidence of neuropathy and microangiopathy, particularly of severe retinopathy. This highly significant correlation has been found in the total population, in the inception cohort, and in every group and subgroup so far studied."

A large number of studies have looked at various aspects of the relationship between control and retinopathy. Several studies have demonstrated the reversal of ocular functional abnormalities with improved control.[270–272] Functional improvements included correction of diabetes-related electroretinogram (ERG) changes and diabetes-related abnormalities in fluorophotometry. A relationship between these functional disturbances and diabetic retinopathy has not been proven. Other studies have investigated the relationship between glucose control and the progression of established retinopathy. Job[273] and Eschwege[274] showed that in

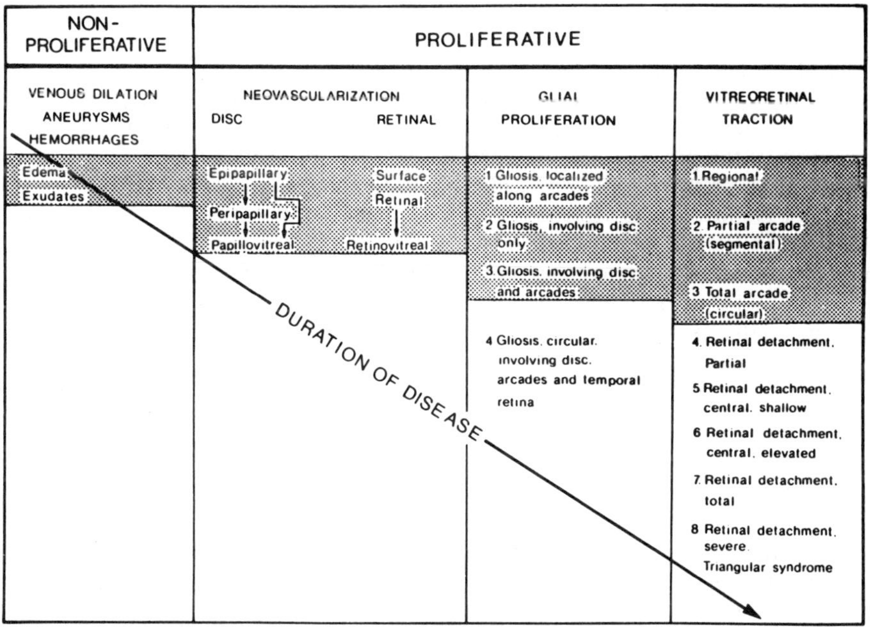

Classification for nonproliferative and proliferative diabetic retinopathy involving gradation of the type of nonproliferative changes as well as the type of neovascularization, glial proliferation, and vitreoretinal traction for proliferative diabetic retinopathy. Shaded zones indicate the type and severity of those retinal abnormalities that can be considered for photocoagulation treatment. Duration of the diabetic state is directly related to the progression of the diabetic retinopathy from the nonproliferative to the proliferative phase.

Figure 4. Diabetic retinopathy continuum scale.[266]

subjects receiving multiple daily insulin injections, there is less progression of retinopathy than in those receiving a single injection. In a group of teenaged, insulin-dependent diabetics, a high correlation was found between the degree of metabolic control as assessed by glycosylated hemoglobin level, and the presence of early retinopathy changes as defined by angiography.[275]

While some benefit has been suggested in non-randomized trials, Tamborlane's[220] one- to two-year study of insulin-dependent diabetic patients given continuous subcutaneous insulin infusion (CSII) therapy suggested that the established diabetic microvascular complications were not reversed.

Several studies have indicated that the rapid lowering of blood glucose by means of both CSII and multiple insulin injections may in fact promote rapid, perhaps transient deterioration of retinopathy.[276–280] In one study the eyes of four poorly controlled patients with moderate-to-severe background retinopathy were reported to deteriorate rapidly within three to six months after the initiation of CSII, with progression to florid proliferative retinopathy.[281] Precipitous development of retinopathy occurred in a 31-year-old woman in whom the institution of glycemic control through CSII followed years of inadequate treatment.[279] The apparent frequency of deterioration in patients with background retinopathy and undergoing CSII[270,282] suggests that very tight glycemic control after years of inadequate control may trigger the process by which proliferative retinopathy develops.[279]

However, recently reported results indicate that longer periods of improved glycemic control may not have long-term adverse effects on diabetic retinopathy. In the KROC Collaborative Study, it was observed that glycemic normalization, which initially provoked the appearance of specific retinopathy lesions, was followed by regression of these lesions with continued treatment for a second year. The group concluded that there is no evidence that intensified insulin treatment has long-term adverse effects on mild to moderate diabetic retinopathy.[283]

Treatment

Efforts should be made to diagnose proliferative diabetic retinopathy (PDR) as early as possible, as the finding of advanced fundus abnormalities on initial examination results in poor visual prognosis.[284] Panretinal photocoagulation has been proven to delay the progression of moderate to severe PDR. Recent data suggest that application of laser therapy is indicated in mild and possibly in pre-proliferative retinopathy. For selected patients with established vitreous hemorrhage, vitrectomy has been proven beneficial in the restoration of vision.[266] The Diabetic Retinopathy Study[285-287] reported that photocoagulation therapy reduced the risk of severe visual loss in proliferative retinopathy by 50% or more after two and three years of treatment in eyes with mild and severe proliferative retinopathy, respectively. The National Eye Institute is sponsoring the Early Treatment Diabetic Retinopathy Study (ETDRS), currently underway, to determine whether photocoagulation should be used early in the course of diabetic retinopathy or deferred until high-risk characteristics develop, to evaluate the effects of photocoagulation in eyes with diabetic macular edema, and also to determine the effect of aspirin.[288] Results to date indicate that treatment of macular edema should be undertaken early. Retinopathy patients should be counseled to avoid traumatic physical activity and encouraged to control their blood glucose level as well as possible. Women should be apprised of the possible adverse effects of pregnancy.

When the diagnosis of Type I or Type II diabetes mellitus is established, the patient should be referred to an ophthalmologist for a baseline assessment, regardless of the presence or absence of retinopathic changes noted by the primary care physician. Subsequent ophthalmological follow-up on a regular basis (annually or more frequently as indicated by progressive changes) is mandatory in order that interventive therapy (e.g., photocoagulation) may be administered before irreversible, visually-threatening pathology develops.

Summary

Diabetic retinopathy is the leading cause of new cases of blindness among persons aged 20 to 74 years. Classified into three types, nonproliferative (background), pre-proliferative, and proliferative, diabetic retinopathy has a frequency and severity that are influenced by the duration and age at onset of diabetes. For patients with proliferative retinopathy, the risk of blindness is approximately 50% within five years. The severity of retinopathy itself may bc of prognostic significance in assessing the severity of generalized microvascular disease and survival of the diabetic patient. A large number of studies have indicated a relationship between glycemic control and retinopathy. Early diagnosis and treatment can delay the progression of moderate to severe PDR.

Cataract

The crystalline lens of the eye is located directly behind the iris. It focuses incoming light on the photoreceptors of the retina. When the lens loses its normal transparency, either focally or diffusely, and there is interference with the passage of light through the lens, a cataract is present. Visual impairment is determined by the location, size and density of the lens opacity. The only currently available treatment for cataracts is surgical removal of the lens, with eyeglasses, contacts or intraocular lenses being used to compensate for the lost focusing due to lens removal.[289] (Fig 5)

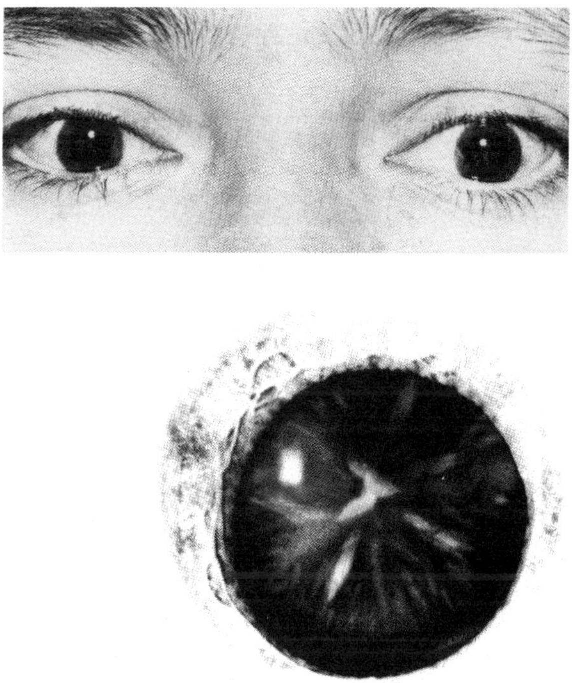

Figure 5. Diabetic cataract.
(From: Ophthalmology, Year Book Medical Publishers, 1979, page 115)

Epidemiology

Diabetes is frequently cited among the risk factors for cataractogenesis (Tables 5 and 6). Many prevalence studies have shown an association of lens opacities and cataract with diabetes.[246,290–295] It has been suggested that the prevalence of cataracts is not increased in diabetics but that diabetic patients are more likely to be referred to ophthalmologists and therefore to have cataracts removed.[296] However, when this hypothesis was tested with the data from two population surveys, the HANES Group[291] and the Framingham Eye Study,[246,290,291] a marked

Table 5. Factors showing statistically significant differences between cataract and control populations by univariate analysis.[297]

Variable	In patients
Diabetes	More
Serious infective bacterial illness	Less
Cardiovascular	More
Psychiatric illness	More
Major tranquillizers	More
Antibiotics	Less
Diuretics	More
Alcohol	More total abstainers and heavy drinkers
Tobacco	More
Reproductive history (female)	Prevalence of cataract increases with no. of children
Blood pressure	Higher
Glaucoma	More
Uveitis	More
Macular degeneration	Less
Physical injury	More
Topically applied ophthalmic drugs	More

Table 6. Possible risk factors for cataracts from the National Advisory Eye Council on Vision Research.[298]

1. Ultraviolet light long wavelength UV (UVL)
   a. Sunlight
   b. Occupational exposure
2. Ionizing radiation
3. Radiofrequency and microwave radiation
4. Toxic drugs and chemicals
5. Diabetes
6. Blood pressure
7. Family history
8. Biochemical agents

excess prevalence of senile cataract was observed in diabetic patients less than 65 years old.[293] Hiller and Kahn reported that diabetes substantially increases the probability of cataract extraction in the age group from 40 to 49, approximately doubles or triples this probability for age 50 to 69, and has little effect as a risk factor only at age 70 and beyond.[294] Ederer et al[293] have found that diabetic subjects between the ages of 55 and 64 years have a three-fold greater risk of developing cataracts than non-diabetics. Cotlier[297] has also reported that diabetes accelerates senile cataract formation, finding a difference of 9.6 years in age in a comparative analysis of diabetic and non-diabetic patients from whom cataracts of equal severity were removed.

In the Framingham Eye Study,[246,290,291] senile lens change was more common in diabetic than in non-diabetic subjects for each five year age group up to age 69, and thereafter lens changes appeared with equal frequency in both groups. In the HANES Group,[291] lens change was more common in diabetic than in non-diabetic subjects for all ages except the group aged 60 to 64, for whom lens changes were slightly more common in the non-diabetic group. Both studies showed a marked excess prevalence of senile cataract in diabetic persons under 65, particularly in the 50 to 64 year age group. In a Danish study, an excess prevalence of diabetes was found in the cataractous population below 70 years of age.[300] In cataract-extracted males and females below age 40, the prevalence in diabetic patients was 15 to 25 times that of the general population, and higher among females than males. When a review was made of 1,485 cataract extractions carried out in the Oxford Eye Hospital in the years 1957 to 1962, it was reported that in the 50 to 69 year age group, cataract extraction was over seven times as common in diabetic patients as in non-diabetics.[295] A retrospective analysis of 388 records of patients undergoing surgery for cataracts between 1968 and 1978 revealed that about 13.7% of patients admitted were diabetic, with a striking excess of diabetic women over men with cataracts.[301] The analysis also revealed that diabetic patients required surgery earlier than non-diabetics and that myopes were more likely to require surgery than nonmyopes.[301] Review of available epidemiological data and clinical investigations supports the position that diabetes mellitus accelerates the development of senile cataracts in man.

A single cause of senile cataract formation most likely does not exist. In fact, research to date has suggested that there are many mechanisms of cataract formation in man. Of these mechanisms, only the aldose reductase involvement in sugar cataract formation has actually been identified.[302]

In her classic review of the galactose cataract, Van Heyningen reports that the production of cataract in rats fed a high galactose diet was first described in 1935 and not until ten years later was it observed as a complication of galactosemia in human infants (Mellinkoff, Roth and Mac Laggen, 1945; Bruck and Rapoport, 1945).[303] At first it was not known whether galactose exerted its harmful effect directly or indirectly on the lens. The early morphological changes shown by Friedenwald and Rytel in 1955 suggested that osmotic swelling occurred within the lens fibers, which became swollen and eventually ruptured.[303] The work of Van Heyningen (1959, 1962) established that the metabolic reaction in the lens common to sugars to produce cataract is mediated by the enzyme aldose reductase.

But it was Kinoshita, Merola and Dikmark (1962) who realized that the non-metabolized sugar alcohol formed in the lens accumulates and exerts a strong osmotic effect which gradually leads to cataract formation. For a discussion of the pathogenesis of sugar cataracts, see Chapter 2.

The relation between age and susceptibility to galactose cataract has been demonstrated in experimental animals. Kinoshita has shown that in the older rat, accumulation of dulcitol is compensated by a lower volume of water than in the young rat. As the lens ages, the fibers become more and more tightly compressed, and the lens, more resistive to the uptake of water. Thus old lenses are less susceptible to galactose cataract than young, because they are less elastic and less permeable.[303]

Classification

The widely accepted classification system for cataracts currently in use is based on the stereoscopic method of lens photography developed by Chylack.[304] The system evolved from the need of lens scientists, particularly those who form the Cooperative Cataract Research Group (CCRG) established in the late 1970s, to classify excised human cataracts.[304,305] The classification system, which was adopted by the CCRG in 1978, places all cataracts into one of three types, based on separate and independent photographic documentation of opacification and nuclear color: Hypermature, Mature, or Immature.[305]

Treatment

Most ophthalmologists are in agreement that no medical treatment of cataract other than surgery currently exists.[306] Kador has reviewed the many agents presently available that claim to prevent, delay or even reverse cataracts associated with aging (senile cataracts), radiation exposure or diabetes.[306] Kador observes that "in most cases the apparent rationale for these agents is not consistent with present knowledge of lens biochemistry and physiology," and that "evaluation of their efficacy has been generally superficial and highly subjective."[306] The sole exception is in aldose reductase inhibitors in experimental diabetic cataract. Their efficacy in animals suggests that "potent aldose reductase inhibitors . . . represent the only potential anticataract agents currently in development that may be effective in man."

Summary

Many prevalence studies have established diabetes as a significant risk factor for cataractogenesis, in particular the HANES Group, Framingham Eye Study, and the Hiller and Kahn Study which reported that diabetes substantially increases the probability of cataract extraction in the age group from 40 to 49 and approximately doubles or triples the probability of cataract extraction in the age group from 50 to 69. No single cause of cataract formation is likely to exist; to date, only aldose reductase involvement in sugar cataract formation has been identified as a formative mechanism in man. The relation between age and the susceptibility to galactose cataract has been demonstrated in experimental animals.

Keratopathy

History

Diabetic keratopathy has been defined by Cobo[307] as "a broad clinical term applied to changes seen in the diabetic cornea ranging from trivial punctate epithelial erosions, seen in approximately 50% of diabetic patients,[308] to vision-threatening neurotrophic (noninfectious) corneal ulcerations."[309] While keratopathy is an infrequent cause of permanent visual loss in diabetic patients when compared with diabetic retinopathy, it is, nonetheless, a clinically significant problem,[307] which has been recognized only within the last decade as a complication of long-standing diabetes.[310] A diabetic keratopathy is shown in Fig 6.

The first clinical abnormality reported in diabetic cornea was decreased sensation.[310] It has been demonstrated that only 30% of diabetic patients reacted to a 6-cm length of filament on the Cochet-Bonnet esthesiometer, whereas 90% of normal individuals reacted to this stimulus.[311] Nielson and Lund reported significantly reduced corneal sensitivity in 100 diabetic patients, which correlated well to age, duration of diabetes above 15 years, and diabetic retinopathy.[96] These subjects also showed a significant reduction in vibratory sensation and increasing

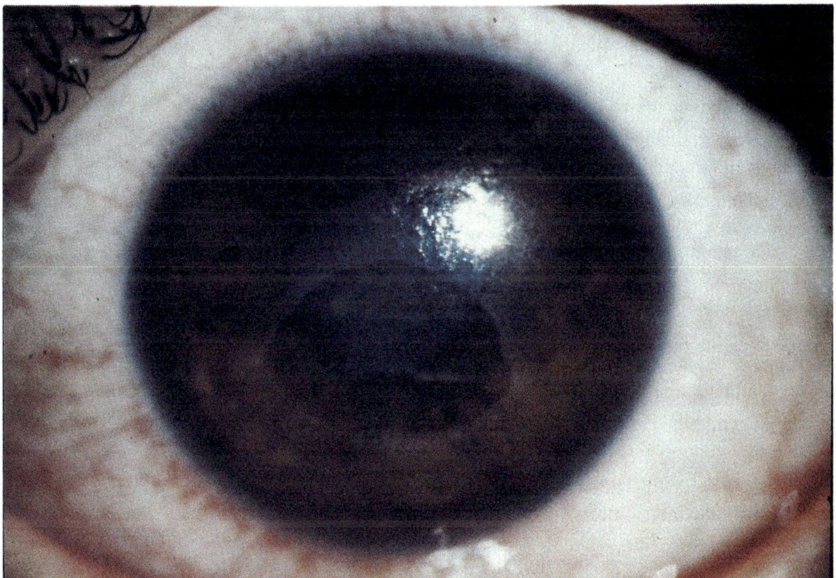

Figure 6. Diabetic keratopathy, characterized by a well-demarcated central disciform epithelial defect. Note adjacent edematous, irregular epithelium highlighted by the light reflex. The patient is a 21-year-old IDDM patient.

areflexia, suggesting that the reduced corneal touch threshold forms part of polyneuropathy in diabetes.[96] In 1977, Hyndiuk and associates[309] reported the occurrence of sterile ulcers in the corneas of diabetic patients, which they thought might be neurotrophic.

When vitrectomy became a frequently performed surgical procedure, diabetic corneal changes became clinically significant.[312–314] In the early days of vitrectomy, it was observed that following the insertion of the vitrectomy instrument into the eye, the corneal epithelium of diabetic patients often became cloudy and had to be removed to permit visualization of the posterior segment of the eye.[315–317] In two clinical studies of patients undergoing vitrectomy, 57% of the diabetic patients required such epithelial removal, as compared with only 13% among non-diabetic subjects.[313,314] Postoperatively, 65% of the diabetic patients developed corneal epithelial problems, as compared with 10% among the non-diabetic subjects,[313,314] including superficial corneal ulcers, recurrent and persistent epithelial defects, and vascularization.[312–314] There is also a higher than normal incidence of endothelial failure as evidenced by persistent stromal edema occurring in approximately 25% of diabetic and only 10% of non-diabetic vitrectomy patients.[313]

Constant washing by the infusion solution during corneal vitrectomy and abrasion by lenticular or other particulate material can cause, in rare cases, irreversible epithelial damage with permanent corneal clouding. One such case was reported in a 45-year-old diabetic woman after pars plana vitrectomy.[318]

During the 1980s, the incidence of corneal complications following vitrectomy has decreased substantially, due to improved surgical techniques.[319] Still, the increased vulnerability of the diabetic cornea is indicative of abnormalities of both the epithelium and the endothelium associated with long-term diabetes.[310] Even presumably trivial stress, such as that caused by contact lenses[320] and ocular manipulation during retinal photocoagulation,[317,321] is less well tolerated by the diabetic cornea.

Treatment

The corneal complications frequently seen in diabetic patients after eye surgery are best averted by short operating times, careful handling of the cornea, avoidance of epithelial scraping or the use of irrigating solutions designed to coddle the endothelium.[310] Postoperatively, healing can be facilitated by the use of thin, extended-wear contact lenses for several months, concurrent with topical, broad-spectrum antibiotic therapy.[310] Stromal edema has been successfully treated with topical and systemic steroids to reduce intraocular inflammation.[310]

Based on the demonstrated presence of aldose reductase (AR) in corneal and conjunctival epithelium by the immunoperoxidase method,[322] the aldose reductase inhibitor sorbinil was used in a case of corneal keratopathy in a 24-year-old diabetic woman in poor glycemic control.[307] The reported beneficial effects may be related to studies of surgically debrided epithelia that have shown detectable levels of sorbitol and fructose in diabetic patients, but not in normal controls.[307,316]

Summary

Keratopathy is a clinically significant problem, which has been recognized only within the last ten years as a complication of long-standing diabetes. It was first observed when vitrectomy became a frequently performed surgical procedure; however, during the 1980s improved surgical techniques have substantially decreased the incidence of corneal complications following vitrectomy.

LARGE VESSELS—ATHEROSCLEROSIS

There is an increased prevalence of atherosclerotic large vessel disease in both IDDM and NIDDM. The development of atherosclerosis in diabetes is multifactorial. Such factors include lipid and lipoprotein abnormalities, smoking, obesity, hypertension, microangiopathy, neuropathy and hyperviscosity.[323] Nevertheless, a relationship between abnormal glucose tolerance and increased mortality from cardiovascular disease has recently been reported by Jarrett and associates.[324] The fact that diabetic patients can survive for long periods of time without developing vascular complications and that a low incidence of atherosclerosis is reported among the diabetic population in some parts of the world[325] suggests an important role for environmental factors.

Clinical studies suggest that people with diabetes have an unusually high prevalence of atherosclerosis.[326] The relationship between diabetes and atherosclerosis is complicated, however, by the problems of describing a high prevalence of one common disease in the presence of another[327] and of establishing whether this relationship is independent of the other "risk factors" common to one or the other. In this case, the "risk factors" for atherosclerosis are commonly found also in diabetes, namely, obesity, hyperlipidemia and hypertension. Several epidemiological studies in unselected population groups have helped somewhat to resolve these problems.

Epidemiology

The reported prevalence of coronary artery disease (CAD) in diabetic patients ranges from 9.5% to 55%,[328–333] while prevalences of 1.6% and 4.1% are reported for the general population.[334,335] Autopsy studies of diabetic patients have shown prevalence rates of CAD ranging from 18% to 75%,[336–345] which is from 1.2 to 6.5 times the prevalence found in non-diabetics. While CAD is reported to be the most common cause of death in NIDDM, it is also found frequently in patients with IDDM.[346–348]

Large-scale prospective studies have helped to define the cardiovascular risk in the diabetic population. In the Framingham study,[349] a cohort was followed for 16 years, and comparisons were made of both cardiovascular morbidity and mortality in subjects aged 30 to 62 years at the entry of the study. Diabetic men and women showed a considerable increase in incidence of coronary, cerebral and peripheral vascular disease, as compared with rates from the population as a whole, with the incidence of claudication being particularly high in diabetics. The mortality rate from cardiovascular disease in diabetic subjects was almost three times that in the general population. The impact of diabetes on coronary heart disease was most significant in women,[350] especially those treated with insulin, indicating a unique effect of diabetes, not explained by the associated cardiovascular risk factors.

Two other prevalence studies have reported an association of diabetes and vascular disease in unselected population groups. In the Bedford study[325] a standardized cardiovascular survey was performed in three population groups classified as normal, borderline or diabetic on the basis of sugar level two hours after ingestion of 50 g of glucose. The frequency of cardiovascular disease was highest in the diabetic group, intermediate in the borderline group, and lowest in the normal. The trend toward increasing frequency with increasing blood sugar values was greater in women than in men, and more marked in those over age 50. In a second prevalence study,[351] diabetic subjects at every age category had more vascular disease than in the population as a whole, and conversely, hyperglycemia was considerably more frequent in subjects with cardiovascular disease than in the general population. Hyperglycemia was an independent risk factor for coronary heart disease[352] and was seen to be at least as significant as either hypertension or hypercholesterolemia.

Similarly, in a group of 370 diabetic males in an industrial population followed for ten years,[353] the death rate of diabetics was reported to be 2.6 times higher than in non-diabetics, with excessive mortality highest in the group under 45 years of age. The most striking difference was in the incidence of coronary heart disease, which caused the deaths of nearly three times as many diabetic subjects as non-diabetics.

The incidence of myocardial infarction (MI) is increased in diabetic patients, accounting perhaps for as many as 20% of deaths within the diabetic population.[354] In a study of MI in diabetics reported from Birmingham,[355] a mortality rate of 39.7% was recorded for those admitted to the hospital, a total approximately twice as high as for non-diabetics.

The prevalence of coronary heart disease (CHD), left ventricular failure, and hypertension was found to be higher in a representative group of 133 newly diagnosed subjects with NIDDM, aged 45 to 64 years, than in a group of age-matched non-diabetic control subjects.[356] The prevalence of previous MI was increased 1.7-fold in male diabetic and 4.4-fold in female diabetic subjects than in the respective non-diabetic groups. The use of digitalis was 3.3 times more frequent in male diabetic subjects ($p = 0.006$) and 3.9 times more frequent in female diabetic subjects ($p = 0.001$) than in the respective non-diabetic subjects. The prevalence of hypertension, based on elevated blood pressure levels and/or current use of antihypertensive drugs, was increased 1.6- to 1.7-fold among the diabetic subjects.

When the prevalence rates of diabetes, asymptomatic hyperglycemia, and cardiovascular risk factors were examined in an employed population of 28,895 whites and 2,607 blacks, aged 25 to 64, persons with diabetes or hyperglycemia in both races had age-adjusted death rates over 50% higher than normoglycemic persons, with about one half of the deaths in this cohort attributable to cardiovascular causes.[357]

Perhaps the most important epidemiological information regarding the association of diabetes and atherosclerosis derives from the recent publication of a number of previously unexamined relationships between cardiovascular risk factors and vascular disease in diabetes from the multinational WHO study,[358] which evaluated CAD, peripheral vascular disease (PVD) and cerebrovascular disease in diverse populations of diabetics of different ethnic origin living in 14 nations.[153] The study reported marked differences in frequency of macrovascular complications of diabetes, which strongly implies that macrovascular disease need not be an inevitable accompaniment to diabetes.[359] Studies of Asian diabetic subjects who have moved from Japan to Hawaii show a previously low CAD incidence increasing in conjunction with change in diet and lifestyle, thus emphasizing the interaction of diabetes with environmental factors.[360] The WHO study confirmed plasma-lipids as risk factors for atherosclerosis in diabetic persons.[153] In particular, plasma triglycerides showed a strong correlation with CAD, independent of other risk factors. Plasma cholesterol levels were also associated with CAD, although less strongly than were plasma triglycerides.

While the risk of developing cardiovascular disease is high in the diabetic population in general, all diabetic persons are not equally at risk. Risk varies substantially with age, sex, and with the level of associated cardiovascular risk factors.[361] The relative impact of diabetes on the risk of cardiovascular sequelae is substantially greater for women than men.[361] In the Framingham study, morbidity and mortality from each of the cardiovascular diseases was higher for diabetic women than for non-diabetic men.[362] The annual incidence of cardiovascular disease increases with age in the diabetic as in the non-diabetic population; however, the relative risk, when comparing diabetic populations with non-diabetic, tends to decrease with age, particularly in women. Diabetic persons develop cardiovascular disease at the rate of non-diabetics 20 years their senior.[361]

Not only the incidence but the extent of coronary artery involvement is greater in diabetic persons than in non-diabetics. A large, multinational pathological study of coronary arteries in diabetic and non-diabetic subjects and controls showed that diabetes was associated with an increased incidence of fatty streaks and atherosclerotic lesions as well as an increased prevalence of advanced lesions (fibrous plaques, complicated lesions, calcified lesions and coronary stenosis).[363] These findings were substantiated by coronary angiography.[364,365]

Summary

Atherosclerosis is the same in diabetic as in non-diabetic individuals. However, diabetes is a risk factor that accelerates the progress and therefore raises the likelihood of atherosclerotic large vessel disease. Since great variety exists in different diabetic populations, other factors must be critical. Moreover, relation to glycemic control has not been well demonstrated, probably because other risk factors are so important. There are at present no studies showing the benefits of control. The following mechanisms have been postulated as playing a role in atherosclerosis: elevated lipoprotein, glycation and polyols in vessels.

LIMITED JOINT MOBILITY SYNDROME

The fact that diabetes mellitus may be accompanied by a variety of rheumatic hand syndromes has been recognized for more than a century.[366] Dupuytren's contracture was first described in association with diabetes in 1883,[367] and in recent history (1957), Lundbaek[368] described stiffness of the hands associated with increased skin thickness in long-term diabetes. Contractures of the finger joints were again reported by Rosenbloom and Frias in 1974[369] and by Grgic et al in 1976.[370] Subsequently, several larger studies in insulin-dependent diabetic children have confirmed Grgic's findings.[371,372] From their study of 460 diabetic patients with nonpainful contractures of finger joints and/or palmar fascia, Lawson and associates[373] observed that Dupuytren's contracture and limited joint mobility accounted for 99% of the clinical manifestations of diabetic hand abnormalities. Although hand abnormalities are the most striking manifestation of the limited joint mobility syndrome, larger joints, such as elbow and ankle, may also be involved.[374]

Prevalence

The overall prevalence of joint contractures in the reported studies[368–372] varied from 9% to 42%. Dupuytren's contracture is known to occur more frequently in diabetic persons than in the normal population.[375] The relationship of limited joint mobility to onset, duration, and control of diabetes mellitus, and to the presence of microvascular disease, has not been definitely established,[374] although it appears that patients with these abnormalities have an increased frequency of microvascular complications.[372,373,376] Hand abnormalities in association with diabetic neuropathy have also been observed.[377,378] Severity of joint limitation was also shown to correlate with definite pathological changes in the kidney, namely, with basement membrane thickening or duplication, and with arteriolar hyalinization and mural hyperplasia.[379] Limited joint mobility could, therefore, act as a marker for microvascular complications in long-standing diabetes.[372,379,380] Early systematic examination by goniometry appears to be a sensitive, quantitative, and inexpensive procedure to detect joint stiffness at an early stage of diabetes.[381]

In a study of 254 young diabetic subjects and 110 controls, a generalized reduction in joint mobility was present in diabetics of all ages two years after diagnosis.[374] Diabetic patients diagnosed before puberty were more severely affected than those with postpubertal onset, independent of duration of diabetes. Finger joint contractures were a significant feature of long-standing diabetes (nine years or more duration) only. Lower overall joint mobility was observed in poorly-controlled diabetic patients, indicating that hyperglycemia per se is implicated in the generation of limited joint mobility.

Rosenbloom and associates detected limited joint mobility of small and large joints in 92 (30%) patients with diabetes who were one to 28 years old.[372] Among those patients who had diabetes for more than 4.5 years' duration, 82 of 169 had limited joint mobility, and 41 of the 82 also had microvascular complications, while only ten of the 87 patients without joint limitation showed evidence of the microvascular complications. Life-table methods used to estimate the risk of complications in the two groups indicated an 83% risk for microvascular complications after 16 years of diabetes if joint limitation was present, but only a 25% risk if limited joint mobility was absent.

Lawson et al reported a close correlation between limited joint mobility and diabetic retinopathy.[373] In a study of the hands of 299 diabetic patients with retinopathy and 161 without, limited joint mobility and Dupuytren's contractures occurred in 48% and 36%, respectively, of those patients with retinopathy, and in 24% and 16%, respectively, of those patients without retinopathy. The differences were statistically significant ($p < 0.001$). The higher prevalence and greater severity of limited joint mobility in the retinopathy group mainly affected those with severe proliferative retinopathy. There was no difference observed between patients with background retinopathy and those without retinopathy. Dupuytren's contracture was less clearly related to severe retinopathy.

Pathophysiology and treatment

The mechanisms mediating the connective tissue changes characteristic of limited joint mobility and Dupuytren's contactures are not understood. Recognized abnormalities in collagen metabolism in diabetic patients[382,383] may be implicated.[367] There has been an anecdotal report of a reduction in skin thickness in three diabetic patients controlled by insulin infusion pump.[384] Moreover, recently a clinically successful response to this incapacitating hand syndrome was reported: Eaton et al achieved improvement in range of motion and in strength of digital flexion and extension in three patients with Type 1 (insulin-dependent) diabetes who were treated with the aldose reductase inhibitor sorbinil.[367] Prompted by their finding, Eaton et al have postulated that the syndrome was caused by osmotic swelling due to collagen hydration produced by sorbitol accumulation. The collagen constituents of periarticular tissues of the hands have thus been added to the list of tissues known or suspected to be vulnerable to polyol accumulation, hence controllable by treatment with aldose reductase inhibitors.

References

1. Martin MM: Diabetic neuropathy: A clinical study of 150 cases. *Brain* 1953;76: 594–624.
2. Thomas PK, Ward JD: Diabetic neuropathy, in Keen H, Jarrett J (eds): *Complications of Diabetes.* Chicago, Year Book Medical Publishers, Inc., 1975.
3. Rundles RW: Diabetic neuropathy: General review with report of 125 cases. *Medicine* 1945;24:110–160.
4. Clements RS, Bell DSH: Diagnostic, pathogenetic, and therapeutic aspects of diabetic neuropathy. *Special Topics in Endocrinol and Metab* 1982;3:1–43.
5. Clements RS, Bell DSH: Diabetic neuropathy: Peripheral and autonomic syndromes. *Postgrad Med* 1982;71:50–67.
6. Rundles RW: Diabetic neuropathy. *Medicine* 1954;24:111–160.

7. Mayne N: Neuropathy in diabetic and nondiabetic populations. *Lancet* 1965;2: 1313–1316.
8. Chopra JS, Hurwitz LJ, Montgomery DAD: The pathogenesis of sural nerve changes in diabetes mellitus. *Brain* 1969;92:391–418.
9. Awad EA: Motor-point biopsies in diabetic neuropathy. *Arch Phys Med Rehabil* 1970;51:418–422.
10. Ward JD: Improvement in motor nerve conduction following treatment in newly diagnosed diabetes. *Adv Metab Disord* 1973;1(suppl):596–573.
11. Lundbaek K: Recent contributions to the study of diabetic angiopathy and neuropathy. *Adv Metab Disord* 1972;6:99–129.
12. Thomas PK, Elaissin S: Diabetic neuropathy, in Dyke P, Thomas PK, Lambert E (eds). *Peripheral neuropathy.* Philadelphia, WB Saunders, 1975, pp 956–981.
13. Bischoff A: Morphology of diabetic neuropathy. *Horm Metab Res* 1980;9(suppl): 18–28.
14. Pirart J: Diabetic neuropathy: A metabolic or a vascular disease? *Diabetes* 1965;14: 1–9.
15. Palumbo PJ, Elveback LR, Whisnant JP: Neurologic complications of diabetes mellitus: Transient ischaemic attack, stroke, and peripheral neuropathy, in Shoenberg BS (ed): *Advances in Neurology,* vol 19. New York, Raven Press, 1978, pp 593–599.
16. Matikainen E, Juntunen J: Diabetic neuropathy: Epidemiological, pathogenetic, and clinical aspects with special emphasis on type 2 diabetes mellitus. *Acta Endocrinol* 1984;262(suppl):89–94.
17. Jordan WR: Neuritic manifestations in diabetes mellitus. *Arch Intern Med* 1936;57: 307–366.
18. Rudy A, Epstein SH: Review of 100 cases of 'diabetic neuropathy' followed from one to ten years. *J Clin Endocrinol Metab* 1945;5:92–98.
19. Martin MM: Diabetic neuropathy: A clinical study of 150 cases. *Brain* 1953a;76:594–624.
20. Hoffman J: Peripheral neuropathy in children with diabetes mellitus. *Acta Neurol Scand* 1964;40(suppl 8):1–65.
21. Eeg-Olofsson O, Petersen I: Childhood diabetic neuropathy: A clinical and neurophysiological study. *Acta Paediatr Scand* 1966;55:163–176.
22. Viniki AI, Glowniak JV: Hormonal secretion in diabetic autonomic neuropathy. *NY State J of Med* 1982;May:871–886.
23. Pfeifer MA, Cook D, Brodsky J, et al: Quantitative evaluation of cardiac parasympathetic activity in normal and diabetic man. *Diabetes* 1982;31:339–345.
24. Clarke BF, Ewing DJ: Cardiovascular reflex tests. *NY State J Med* 1982;82:903–908.
25. Porte D, Halter JB: The Endocrine Pancreas and Diabetes Mellitus, in Williams RH (ed): *Textbook of Endocrinology.* Philadelphia, WB Saunders, 1981, pp 716–843.
26. Ward JD: Diabetic neuropathy. *J Clin Endocrinol Metab* 1972;1:809–826.
27. Levin ME, Boniuk I, Anderson CB, Avioli LV: Prevention and treatment of diabetic complications. *Arch Intern Med* 1980;140(5):691–696.
28. Ellenberg M: Diabetic neuropathy: Clinical aspects. *Metabolism* 1976;25:1627–1655.
29. Dyck PJ, Sherman WR, Hallcher LM, et al: Human diabetic endoneurial sorbitol, fructose, and myoinositol related to sural nerve morphometry. *Ann Neurol* 1980;8:590–596.
30. Thomas PK: Clinical features and differential diagnosis, in Dyck P, Thomas PK, Lambert E (eds):. *Peripheral Neuropathy,* vol 1. Philadelphia, WB Saunders, 1975, Chap 24.
31. Schaumberg HH: Diseases of the peripheral nervous system, in Wyngaaner JB, Smith LH (eds): *Cecil Textbook of Medicine.* Philadelphia, WB Saunders, 1985, pp 2188–2189.

32. Busswinger PJ: Neuropathic and vascular complications occurring in diabetes. *Postgrad Med* 1976;59:169–174.
33. Ewing DJ, Burt AA, Williams IR, Campbell IW, Clarke BF: Peripheral motor nerve function in diabetic autonomic neuropathy. *J Neurol Neurosurg Psychiatry* 1976;39:453–460.
34. Clarke BF, Ewing DJ, Campbell IW: Diabetic autonomic neuropathy. *Diabetologia* 1979;17:195–212.
35. Hosking D, Bennett T, Hampton J: Diabetic autonomic neuropathy. *Diabetes* 1978;27:1043–1054.
36. Ewing DJ, Campbell IW, Clarke BF: The natural history of diabetic autonomic neuropathy. *Q J Med* 1980;49:95–108.
37. Clements RS: Review—Diabetic neuropathy—New concepts of its etiology. *Diabetes* 1979;28:604–611.
38. Thomas PK: Diabetic neuropathy, in Brodoff BN, Bleicher SJ (eds). *Diabetes Mellitus and Obesity.* Baltimore, Williams and Wilkins, 1982, pp 687–696.
39. Evans RW, Harati Y: What's new: Review of clinical presentations, pathophysiology, and treatment of diabetic neuropathies. *Tex Med* 1983;79:50–54.
40. Young RJ, Prescott RJ, Ewing DJ, et al: Variations in neurophysiology and type of diabetic peripheral neuropathy. Abstract, Peripheral Neuropathy Association of America, Keystone, Colorado, June 18–22, 1984.
41. Asbury AK, Johnson PC: Diabetic neuropathies, in Bennington JL (ed): *Pathology of Peripheral Nerve.* Philadelphia, WB Saunders, 1978, pp 96–102.
42. Greep RO, Weiss L: *Histology,* ed 3. New York, McGraw- Hill Book Company, 1973, pp 264, 270.
43. Carpenter MB, Sutin J: *Human Neuroanatomy.* Baltimore, Williams & Wilkins, 1983, pp 107–108, 114.
44. Smorto MP, Basmajian JV (eds): *Electrodiagnosis: A Handbook for Neurologists.* Maryland, Harper and Row, 1977, pp 73–90.
45. Barr ML: Peripheral nervous system, in *The Human Nervous System: An Anatomical Viewpoint,* ed 2. Maryland, Harper & Row, 1974, pp 27–43.
46. Goodgold J, Eberstein A (eds): *Electrodiagnosis of Neuromuscular Diseases,* ed 3. Baltimore, Williams & Wilkins, 1983, pp 10–44.
47. Dyck PJ: Pathologic alterations of the peripheral nervous system of man, in Dyck PJ, Thomas PK, Lambert EH (eds): *Peripheral Neuropathy.* Philadelphia, WB Saunders, 1975, vol 1, Chap 15.
48. Dyke PJ, Johnson WJ, Lambert EH, O'Brien PC: Segmental demyelination secondary to axonal degeneration in uremic neuropathy. *Mayo Clin Proc* 1971;46:400–431.
49. Anderson JW: Metabolic abnormalities contributing to diabetic complications. II. Peripheral nerves. *Amer J Clin Nutr* 1976;29:402–408.
50. Behse F, Buchthal F, Carlsen F: Nerve biopsies and conduction studies in diabetic neuropathy. *J Neurol Neurosurg Psychiatry* 1977;40:1072–1082.
51. Bischoff A: Ultrastructural pathology of peripheral nervous system in early diabetes, in Camerini-Davalos RA, Cole HS (eds): *Vascular and Neurological Changes in Early Diabetes.* New York, Academic Press, 1977, pp 441–449.
52. Jakobsen J: Peripheral nerves in early experimental diabetes: Expansion of the endoneurial space as a cause of increased water content. *Diabetologia* 1978; 14:113–119.
53. Jakobsen J, Lundback K: Neuropathy in experimental diabetes: An animal model. *Br Med J* 1976;2:278–279.
54. Jakobsen J: Axonal dwindling in early experimental diabetes I. A study of cross sectioned nerves. *Diabetologia* 1976;12:539–546.

55. Jakobsen J: Axonal dwindling in early experimental diabetes II. A study of isolated nerve fibers. *Diabetologia* 1976;12:547–553.
56. Sharma AK, Thomas PK, Demolina AF: Peripheral nerve fiber size in experimental diabetes. *Diabetes* 1977;26:689–692.
57. Hildebrand J, Joffoy A, Graff G, et al: Neuromuscular changes with alloxan hyperglycemia. Electrophysiological, biochemical and histological studies in rats. *Arch Neurol* 1968;18:633–641.
58. Schlaepfer WW, Gerritsen GC, Dulin WE: Segmental demyelination in the distal peripheral nerves of chronically diabetic chinese hamsters. *Diabetologia* 1974;10:541–548.
59. Sima AAF, Robertson DM: Peripheral neuropathy in the mutant diabetic mouse [C57BL/Ks(db/db)]. *Acta Neurol Pathol* 1978;41:85–89.
60. Olsson Y, Sourander P: Changes in the sympathetic nervous system of diabetes mellitus. A preliminary report. *J Neurovisc Rel* 1968;31:86–95.
61. Olsson Y, Save-Soderbergh J, Sourander P, Angervall P: A pathoanatomical study of the central and peripheral nervous system in diabetes of early onset and long duration. *Pathol Europ* 1968;3:62–79.
62. Budzilovich GN: Peripheral sympathetic nervous system in diabetes mellitus, in Proc. VIth Internat. Congr. Neuropath. Paris, Masson, 1970, pp 725–729.
63. Appenzeller O, Richardson EP, Jr: The sympathetic chain in patients with diabetic and alcoholic polyneuropathy. *Neurology* 1966;16:1205–1209.
64. Hensley GT, Soergel KH: Neuropathologic findings in diabetic diarrhea. *Arch Pathol* 1968;85:587–597.
65. Pryce TD: On diabetic neuritis, with a clinical and pathological description of diabetic pseudo-tabes. *Brain* 1893;16:416–424.
66. Woltman HW, Wilder RM: Diabetes mellitus: Pathologic changes in the spinal cord and peripheral nerves. *Arch Intern Med* 1929;44:576–603.
67. Dolman CL: The morbid anatomy of diabetic neuropathy. *Neurology* 1963; 13:135–142.
68. Greenbaum DA, Brown MA, Braunstein SN, et al: Comparison of clinical course and sequential electrophysiological tests in patients with symptomatic polyneuropathy and its implications for clinical trials. *Diabetes* 1981;30:139–147.
69. Fagerberg SE: Diabetic neuropathy: A clinical and histological study on the significance of vascular affections. *Acta Med Scand* 1959;164(suppl 354):1–9.
70. Asbury AK, Aldredge H, Hershberg R, et al: Oculomotor palsy in diabetes mellitus; a clinicopathological study. *Brain* 1970;93:555–566.
71. Dreyfus PM, Hakim S, Adams RD: Diabetic ophthalmoplegia: Report of a case with postmortem study and comments on vascular supply of human oculomotor nerve. *Arch Neurol Psychiatry* 1957;77:337–349.
72. Timperley WR: Vascular and coagulation abnormalities in diabetic neuropathy and encephalopathy. *Horm Metab Res* 1980;9(suppl):43–49.
73. Timperley WR, Ward JD, Preston FE, Duckworth T, O'Malley BG: Clinical and histological studies in diabetic neuropathy: A reassessment of vascular factors in relation to vascular coagulation. *Diabetologia* 1976;12:237–243.
74. Williams E, Timperley WR, Ward JD, Duckworth T: Electron microscopic studies of vessels in diabetic peripheral neuropathy. *J Clin Pathol* 1980;33:462–470.
75. Seneviratne KN: Permeability of blood nerve barriers in the diabetic rat. *J Neurol Neurosurg Psychiatry* 1972;35:156–162.
76. Jakobsen J, Malmgren L, Olsson Y: Permeability of the blood-nerve barrier in the streptozotocin-diabetic rat. *Exp Neurol* 1978;60:277–285.
77. Sima AAF, Robertson DM: The perineurial and blood-nerve barriers in experimental diabetes. *Acta Neuropathol* 1978;44:189–195.

78. Daube JR: Nerve conduction studies, in Aminoff MJ (ed): *Electrodiagnosis in Clinical Neurology.* New York, Churchill Livingstone, 1980, pp 229–264.
79. Warmolts JR: Electrodiagnosis in neuromuscular disorders. *Ann Intern Med* 1981;95:599–608.
80. Vallbo AB, Hagbarth KE, Torebjork HE: Somatosensory proprioceptive and sympathetic activity in human peripheral nerves. *Physiol Rev* 1979;59:919–957.
81. Cummins KL, Dorfman LJ: Nerve fiber conduction velocity distributions: Studies of normal and diabetic human nerves. *Ann of Neurol* 1981;9:67–74.
82. Lamontagne A, Buchthal F: Electrophysiological studies in diabetic neuropathy. *J Neurol Neurosurg Psychiatry* 1970;33:442–452.
83. Chochinov RH, Ullyot GLE, Moorhouse JA: Sensory perception thresholds in diabetic subjects and their close relatives. *Diabetes* 1971;20(suppl 1):330–331.
84. Mulder DW, Lambert EH, Bartron JA, Sprague RG: The neuropathies associated with diabetes mellitus: A clinical and electromyographic study of 103 unselected diabetic patients. *Neurology* 1961;11:275–284.
85. Lawrence DG, Locke S: Motor nerve conduction velocity in diabetes. *Arch Neurol* 1961;5:483–489.
86. Skillman TG, Johnson EW, Hamwi GJ, Driskill HJ: Motor nerve conduction velocity in diabetes mellitus. *Diabetes* 1961;10:46–51.
87. Fraser DM, Campbell IW, Ewing DJ, et al: Peripheral and autonomic nerve function in newly diagnosed diabetes mellitus. *Diabetes* 1977;26:546–550.
88. Troni W: Analysis of conduction velocity in the H pathway. *J Neurol Sci* 1981; 751:235–246.
89. Gregersen G: Variations in motor conduction velocity produced by acute changes in the metabolic state in diabetic patients. *Diabetologia* 1968;4:273–277.
90. Castaigne P et al: Les réponses de nerfs et des muscles à des stimulations électriques an cours d'une epreuve de garrot ischémique chez l'homme normal et chez le diabétique. *Rev Neurol* 1966;115:61–66.
91. Seneviratne KN, Peiris OA: Effects of ischaemia on the excitability of sensory nerves in diabetes mellitus. *J Neurol Neurosurg Psychiatry* 1968;31:348–353.
92. Seneviratne KN, Peiris OA: Peripheral nerve function in chronic liver disease. *J Neurol Neurosurg Psychiatry* 1970:33:609–614.
93. Low PA, Ward K, Schmelzer JD, Brimijoin S: Ischemic conduction failure and energy metabolism in experimental diabetic neuropathy. *Am J Physiol* 1985;248 (Endocrinol. Metab. II):E457–E462.
94. Dyck PJ, Karnes JL, Daube J, et al: Clinical and neuropathological criteria for the diagnosis and staging of diabetic polyneuropathy. *Brain* 1985;108:861–880.
95. Pirart J: Diabetes mellitus and its degenerative complications: a prospective study of 4,400 patients observed between 1947 and 1973. *Diabetes Care* 1978;1:168–188.
96. Nielson NV, Lund FS: Diabetic polyneuropathy: Corneal sensitivity, vibratory perception and Achilles tendon reflex in diabetics. *Acta Neurol Scand* 1979;59:15–22.
97. Hillson RM, Hockaday TDR, Newton DJ: Hyperglycemia is one correlate of deterioration in vibration sense during the 5 years after diagnosis of Type 2 (noninsulin dependent) diabetes. *Diabetologia* 1984;26:122–126.
98. Boulton AJM, Worth RC, Drury J, et al: Genetic and metabolic studies in diabetic neuropathy. *Diabetologia* 1984;26:15–19.
99. Brown MJ, Asbury AK: Diabetic neuropathy. *Ann Neurol* 1984;15:2–12.
100. Gregersen G: Diabetic neuropathy: Influence of age, sex, metabolic control, and duration of diabetes on motor conduction velocity. *Neurology* 1967;17:972–980.
101. Ward JD, Fisher DJ, Barnes CG, Jessop JD, Baker RWR: Improvement in nerve conduction following treatment in newly diagnosed diabetics. *Lancet* 1971;1:428–431.

102. Hansen S, Ballantyne JP: Axonal dysfunction in the neuropathology of diabetes mellitus. *J Neurol Neurosurg Psychiatry* 1977;40:555–564.
103. Braddom RL, Hollis JB, Castell DO: Diabetic peripheral neuropathy: A correlation of nerve conduction studies and clinical findings. *Arch Phys Med Rehabil* 1977;58: 308–313.
104. Eng GD, Hung W, August GP, et al: Nerve conduction velocity determinations in juvenile diabetes: Continuing study of 190 patients. *Arch Phys Med Rehabil* 1976; 57:1–5.
105. Graf RJ, Halter JB, Halar E, Porte D Jr: Nerve conduction abnormalities in untreated maturity-onset diabetes: Relation to levels of fasting plasma glucose and glycosylated hemoglobin. *Ann Intern Med* 1979;90:298–303.
106. Graf RJ, Halter JB, Pfeifer MA, et al: Glycemic control and nerve conduction abnormalities in noninsulin-dependent diabetic subjects. *Ann Intern Med* 1981;94:307–311.
107. Canal N, Comi G: Peripheral nerve abnormalities in newly diagnosed diabetic children. Abstract, Peripheral Neuropathy Association of America, Keystone, Colorado, June 18–22, 1984.
108. Halar EM, Graf RJ, Halter JB, et al: Diabetic neuropathy: A clinical laboratory and electrodiagnostic study. *Arch Phys Med Rehabil* 1982;63:298–303.
109. Pietri A, Ehle AL, Raskin P: Changes in nerve conduction velocity after six weeks of glucoregulation with portable insulin infusion pumps. *Diabetes* 1980;29(8):668–671.
110. Boulton AJM, Drury J, Clarke B, et al: Continuous subcutaneous insulin infusion in the management of painful diabetic neuropathy. *Diabetes Care* 1982; 5(4):386–390.
111. Gambardella S, Napoli A, Spallone V, et al: Influence of glucoregulation with continuous subcutaneous insulin infusion on nerve conduction velocity and beat to beat variation in diabetics. *J Endocrinol Invest* 1983;6(5):363–367.
112. Troni W, Carta Q, Cantello R, et al: Peripheral nerve function and metabolic control in diabetes mellitus. *Ann Neurol* 1984;16:178–183.
113. Young RJ, Ewing DJ, Clarke BF: Nerve function and metabolic control in teenage diabetics. *Diabetes* 1983;32:142–147.
114. Hoffman WH, Hart ZH, Frank RN: Correlates of delayed motor nerve conduction and retinopathy in juvenile-onset diabetes mellitus. *J Pediatr* 1983;102:351–356.
115. Chiasson JL, Ducros F, Poliquin-Hamet M, et al: Continuous subcutaneous insulin infusion (Mill-Hill Infuser) versus multiple injections (Medic-Jector) in the treatment of insulin-dependent diabetes mellitus and the effect of metabolic control on microangiopathy. *Diabetes Care* 1984;7:331–337.
116. Greene DA, Lattimer SA: Action of sorbinil in diabetic peripheral nerve: Relationship of polyol (sorbitol) pathway inhibition to a myo-inositol-mediated defect in sodium-potassium ATPase activity. *Diabetes* 1984;33:712–716.
117. Judzewitsch RG, Jaspan JB, Polonsky KS, et al: Aldose reductase inhibition improves nerve conduction velocity in diabetic patients. *N Engl J Med* 1983;308:119–125.
118. Jaspan J, Herold K, Maselli R, Bartkus C: Treatment of severely painful diabetic neuropathy with an aldose reductase inhibitor: relief on pain and improved somatic and autonomic nerve function. *Lancet* 1983;2:758–762.
119. Young RJ, Ewing DJ, Clarke BF: A controlled trial of sorbinil, an aldose reductase inhibitor in chronic painful diabetic neuropathy. *Diabetes* 1983;32:938–942.
120. Kozak GP, Yoo J, Ganz K: Diabetic neuropathies. *Am Fam Physician* 1977; 15:112–122.
121. Boulton AJM, Drury J, Ward JD: Use of continuous subcutaneous insulin infusion (CSII) in the treatment of painful and ulcerative diabetic neuropathy. *Diabetes* 1981;30(suppl 1):91A.

122. White NH, Waltman SR, Krupin T, Santiago JV: Reversal of neuropathic and gastrointestinal complications related to diabetes mellitus in adolescents with improved metabolic control. *J Pediatr* 1981;99(1):41–45.
123. Skyler JS, Seigler DE, Reeves ML: Optimizing pumped insulin delivery. *Diabetes Care* 1982;5(2):135–139.
124. Felig P: The endocrine pancreas: Diabetes mellitus, in Felig P, Baxter JD, Broadus AE, Frohman LA (eds). *Endocrinology and Metabolism.* New York, McGraw-Hill, 1981, pp 761–868.
125. Rull JA, Quibrera R, Gonzalez Millan H, et al: Symptomatic treatment of peripheral diabetic neuropathy and carbamazepine [Tegretol]: Double-blind crossover trial. *Diabetologia* 1969;5:215–218.
126. Davis JI, Lewis SB, Gerich JE, et al: Peripheral diabetic neuropathy treated with amitryptiline and fluphenazine. *JAMA* 1977;238(21):2291–2292.
127. Battla H, Silverblatt CW: Clinical trial of amitryptiline and fluphenazine in diabetic peripheral neuropathy. *South Med J* 1981;74(4):417–418.
128. Williams JG: Autonomic neuropathy in diabetes: A review. *J Royal Soc Med* 1983;76:502–507.
129. Moskowitz MA, in Landsberg L (ed): *Clinics in Endocrinology and Metabolism,* vol 3. Philadelphia, WB Saunders, 1977, pp 735–768.
130. Frimodt-Møller C, Mortesen S: Treatment of diabetic cystopathy. *Ann Intern Med* 1980;92:327–328.
131. Ellenberg M: Impotence in diabetes: The neurologic factor. *Ann Intern Med* 1971;75:213–219.
132. Watkins PJ: Facial sweating after food: A new sign of diabetic autonomic neuropathy. *Br J Med* 1973;1:583–587.
133. Gordon SJ, Joseph RE: Diabetic gastroparesis and colonic dilation treated with domperidone. *Lancet* 1981;1:390.
134. Snape WJ, Battle WM, Schwartz SS, et al: Metoclopramide to treat gastroparesis due to diabetes mellitus. *Ann Intern Med* 1982;96:444–446.
135. Ewing DJ, Clarke BF: Diagnosis and management of diabetic autonomic neuropathy. *Br Med J* 1982;285:916–918.
136. Bright R: Cases and observations illustrative of renal disease accompanied with the secretion of abulminous urine. *Guy's Hosp Rep* 1836;1:338–400.
137. Cotunnius D: *De Ischiade Nervosa.* Vienna, 1770.
138. Rollo J: *Cases of the Diabetes Mellitus,* ed 2. London, Dilly, 1798.
139. Rayer P, in Baillere, Tindall, Cox (eds): *Traite des Maladies du Rein,* vol 2. Paris, 1840.
140. Van Noorden C: *Die Zuckerkrankheit und ihre Behandlung,* ed 6. Berlin, 1912, p 133.
141. Kimmilstiel P, Wilson C: Intercapillary lesions in glomeruli of kidney. *Am J Path* 1936;12:83–97.
142. Cameron JS, Ireland JT, Watkins PJ: The kidney and renal tract, in Keen H, Jarret J (eds): *Complications of Diabetes.* Chicago, Year Book Medical Publishers, Inc., 1975, pp 99–150.
143. Fahr T: Ueber Glomerulosklerose. *Virchows Archiv fur Pathologische Anatomie und Physiologie und fur klinische Medizin.* 1942;309:16.
144. Bell ET: Renal lesions in diabetes mellitus (abstract). *Amer J Pathol* 1942;18:744–745.
145. Mann GV, Gardner C, Root HF: Clinical manifestations of intercapillary glomerulosclerosis in diabetes mellitus. *Am J Med* 1949;7:3–14.
146. Lundbaek K: Diabetic angiopathy: A specific vascular disease. *Lancet* 1954; 1:377–379.
147. Merkel FK, Straus AK, Armbruster KRW, Lewis EJ: The diabetic kidney. *Compr Ther* 1975;1:40–48.

148. Wyngaarden JB, Smith LH Jr: Cecil Textbook of Medicine, vol 2. Philadelphia, WB Saunders, 1985, pp 1320–1341.
149. Knowles HC Jr: Magnitude of the renal failure problem in diabetic patients. *Kidney Intl* 1974;6(suppl 1):2–7.
150. Deckert T, Poulsen JE, Larsen M: Prognosis of diabetics with diabetes onset before the age of thirty-one. I. Survival, causes of death, and complications. *Diabetologia* 1978; 14:363–370.
151. White P: Natural course and prognosis of juvenile diabetes. *Diabetes* 1956;5:445.
152. Deckert T, Anderson AR, Christiansen JS, Anderson JA: Course of diabetic nephropathy. Factors related to development. *Acta Endocrinol* 1981;1981(suppl 242):14–15.
153. WHO Expert Committee on Diabetes Mellitus. Second Report. Technical Report Series 646. WHO, Geneva, 1980, pp 1–80.
154. West KM, Eredreich LJ, Stober JA: A detailed study of risk factors for retinopathy and nephropathy in diabetes. *Diabetes* 1980;29:501–508.
155. Feldman JN, Beyer MM, Hirsh S, et al: Prevalence of diabetic nephropathy coincident with known retinopathy. *Kidney Intl* 1981;19:125.
156. Parving HH, Smidt UM, Friisberg B, Bonnevie-Nielson V, Anderson AR: A prospective study of glomerular filtration rate and arterial blood pressure in insulin-dependent diabetics with diabetic nephropathy. *Diabetologia* 1981;20:457–461.
157. Wiseman M, Viberti G, Mackintosh D, Jarrett RJ, Keen H: Glycaemia, arterial pressure and micro-albuminuria in Type I (insulin-dependent) diabetes mellitus. *Diabetologia* 1984;26:401–405.
158. Hostetter TH, Rennke HG, Brenner BM: The case for intrarenal hypertension in the initiation and progression of diabetic and other glomerulopathies. *Am J Med* 1982;72:375–380.
159. Mogensen CE: Long-term antihypertensive treatment inhibiting progression of diabetic nephropathy. *Br Med J* 1982;285:685–688.
160. Deckert T, Poulsen JE: Diabetic nephropathy: Fault or destiny? *Diabetologia* 1981;21:178–183.
161. Wajchenberg BL, Sabbaga E, Fonseca JA: The natural history of diabetic nephropathy in type I diabetes and the role of metabolic control in its prevention, reversibility and clinical course. *Acta Diabetol Lat* 1983;20:1–18.
162. Keen H, Viberti GC: Genesis and evolution of diabetic nephropathy. *J Clin Pathol* 1981;34:1261–1266.
163. Mogensen CE: Antihypertensive treatment inhibiting the progression of diabetic nephropathy. *Acta Endocrinol* 1980;94(suppl 238):103–111.
164. Kasinath BS, Mujais SK, Spargo BH, Katz AI: Nondiabetic renal disease in patients with diabetes mellitus. *Am J Med* 1983;75:613–617.
165. Mogensen CE, Anderson MJF: Increased kidney size and glomerular filtration rate in untreated juvenile diabetes: Normalization by insulin treatment. *Diabetologia* 1975;11:221–224.
166. Christiansen JS, Gammelgaard J, Frandsen M, Parving HH: Increased kidney size, glomerular filtration rate and renal plasma flow in short-term insulin-dependent diabetics. *Diabetologia* 1981;20:451–456.
167. Østerby R, Gundersen HJG: Glomerular size and structure in diabetes mellitus. I. Early abnormalities. *Diabetologia* 1975;11:225–229.
168. Kroustrup JP, Gundersen HJG, Østerby R: Glomerular size and structure in diabetes mellitus. III. Early enlargement of the capillary surface. *Diabetologia* 1977; 13:207–210.

169. Mogensen CE, Anderson MJF: Increased kidney size and glomerular filtration rate in early juvenile diabetes. *Diabetes* 1973;22:706–712.
170. Stalder G, Schmid R: Severe functional disorders of glomerular capillaries and renal hemodynamics in treated diabetes mellitus during childhood. *Ann Pediatr* 1959;193:129–134.
171. Ditzel J, Junker K: Abnormal glomerular filtration rate, renal plasma flow and renal protein excretion in recent and short-term diabetics. *Br Med J* 1972;2:9–13.
172. Mogensen CE: Glomerular filtration rate and renal plasma flow in short-term and long-term juvenile diabetes mellitus. *Scan J Clin Lab Invest* 1971;28:91–100.
173. Mogensen CE, Østerby R, Gundersen HJG: Early functional and morphologic vascular renal consequences of the diabetic state. *Diabetologia* 1979;17:71–76.
174. Seyer-Hansen K: Renal hypertrophy in streptozotocin-diabetic rats. *Clin Sci Molec Med* 1976;51:551–555.
175. Mogensen CE, Steffes MW, Deckert T, Christiansen JS: Functional and morphological renal manifestations in diabetes mellitus. *Diabetologia* 1981;21:89–93.
176. Mogensen CE: Renal function changes in diabetes. *Diabetes* 1976;25(suppl 2):872–879.
177. Christiansen JS, Gammelgaard J, Tronier B, Svedsen PA, Parving HH: Kidney function and size in diabetics before and during initial insulin treatment. *Kidney Intl* 1982;21:683–688.
178. Wiseman MJ, Saunders AJ, Keen H, Viberti GC: Effect of blood glucose control on increased glomerular filtration rate and kidney size in insulin-dependent diabetes. *N Engl J Med* 1985;312:617–621.
179. Hayford JT, Danney MM, Hendrix JA, Thompson RG: Integrated concentration of growth hormone in juvenile-onset diabetes. *Diabetes* 1980;29:391–398.
180. Hansen AP: Normalization of growth hyper-response to exercise in juvenile diabetics after "normalization" of blood sugar. *J Clin Invest* 1981;50:1806–1811.
181. Christiansen JS, Frandsen M, Parving H-H: Effect of intravenous glucose infusion on renal function in normal man and in insulin-dependent diabetics. *Diabetologia* 1981;21:368–373.
182. Christiansen JS, Frandsen M, Parving H-H: The effect of intravenous insulin infusion on kidney function in insulin-dependent diabetes mellitus. *Diabetologia* 1981;20:199–204.
183. Keen H, Chlouverakis C: An immunoassay method for urinary albumin at low concentrations. *Lancet* 1963;2:913–916.
184. Bogusky RT: Diabetic nephropathy. *Postgrad Med* 1983;74:339–349.
185. Keen H, Chlouverakis C, Fuller JH, Jarrett RJ: The concomitants of raised blood sugar: Studies in newly detected hyperglycaemias. II. Urinary albumin excretion, blood pressure and their relation to blood sugar levels. *Guy's Hosp Rep* 1969;118:247–252.
186. Mogensen CE: Urinary albumin excretion in early and long-term juvenile diabetes. *Scan J Clin Lab Invest* 1971;28:101–109.
187. Parving H-H, Noer I, Deckert T, et al: The effect of metabolic regulation on microvascular permeability to small and large molecules in short-term diabetes. *Diabetologia* 1976;12:161–166.
188. Viberti GC, Mackintosh D, Bilous RW, Pickup JC, Keen H: Proteinuria in diabetes mellitus: Role of spontaneous and experimental variation of glycaemia. *Kidney Intl* 1982;21:714–720.
189. Viberti GC, Pickup JC, Jarrett RJ, Keen H: Effect of control of blood glucose on urinary excretion of albumin and B-2-microglobulin in insulin-dependent diabetes. *New Engl J Med* 1979;300:638–641.

190. Pickup JC, Keen H, Viberti GC, et al: Continuous subcutaneous insulin infusion in the treatment of diabetes mellitus. *Diabetes Care* 1980;3:290–300.
191. Viberti GC, Pickup JC, Bilous RW, Keen H, Mackintosh D: Correction of exercise-induced microalbuminuria in insulin-dependent diabetics after 3 weeks of subcutaneous insulin infusion. *Diabetes* 1981;30:818–823.
192. Østerby R: Morphometric studies of the peripheral glomerular basement membrane in early juvenile diabetes. *Diabetologia* 1972;8:84–92.
193. Gundersen HJG, Mogensen CE, Seyer-Hansen K, Østerby R, Lundbaek K: Early and late changes in the diabetic kidney. *Adv Nephrop* 1979;8:43–62.
194. Gundersen HJG, Østerby R: Glomerular size and structure in diabetes mellitus. II. Late abnormalities. *Diabetologia* 1977;13:43–48.
195. Deckert T, Poulsen JE: Prognosis for juvenile diabetics with late diabetic manifestations. *Acta Med Scand* 1968;183:351–356.
196. Mogensen CE: Progression of nephropathy in long-term diabetics with proteinuria and effect of initial antihypertensive treatment. *Scand J Clin Lab Invest* 1976; 36:383–388.
197. Viberti GC, Hill RD, Jarrett RJ, et al: Microalbuminuria as a predictor of clinical nephropathy in insulin-dependent diabetes mellitus. *Lancet* 1982;1:1430–1432.
198. Parving HH, Oxenboll B, Svendsen PA, Christiansen JS, Anderson AR: Early detection of patients at risk of developing diabetic nephropathy: A longitudinal study of urinary albumin excretion. *Acta Endocrinol* 1982;100:550–555.
199. Viberti G, Keen H: The patterns of proteinuria in diabetes mellitus: Relevance to pathogenesis and prevention of diabetic nephropathy. *Diabetes* 1984;33:686–692.
200. Kalant N: Diabetic glomerulosclerosis: Current status. *Can Med Assoc J* 1978; 119:146–153.
201. Jones RH, Hayakawa H, Mackay JD, Parsons V, Watkins PJ: Progression of diabetic nephropathy. *Lancet* 1979;1:1105–1106.
202. Watkins P: Nephropathy. *Br Med J* 1982;285:627–629.
203. Mogensen CE, Christensen CK: Predicting diabetic nephropathy in insulin-dependent patients. *N Eng J Med* 1984;311:89–93.
204. Mathiesen ER, Oxenboll B, Johansen K, Svendsen PA, Deckert T: Incipient nephropathy in Type I (insulin-dependent) diabetes. *Diabetologia* 1984;26:406–410.
205. Mogensen CE: Microalbuminuria predicts clinical proteinuria and early mortality in maturity-onset diabetes. *N Engl J Med* 1984;310:356–360.
206. Cahill GF: Current concepts of diabetic complications with emphasis on hereditary factors: A brief review. *Prog Clin Biol Res* 1979;32:113–125.
207. Steffes MW, Brown DM, Mauer SM: Diabetic glomerulopathy: A dynamic process produced by the diabetic environment. *Adv Exp Med Biol* 1979;124:157–166.
208. Job D, Eschwege E, Guyot-Argenton C, Aubrey JP, Tchoubroutsky G: Effect of multiple daily insulin injections on the course of diabetic retinopathy. *Diabetes* 1976; 25:463–469.
209. Mauer SM, Steffes MW, Michael AF, Brown DM: Studies of diabetic nephropathy in animals and man. *Diabetes* 1976;25(suppl 2):850–857.
210. Mauer SM, Barbosa J, Vernier RL, et al: Development of diabetic vascular lesions in normal kidneys transplanted into patients with diabetes mellitus. *N Engl J Med* 1976;295:916–920.
211. Steffes MW, Sutherland DER, Goetz FC, Rich SS, Mauer SM: Study of kidney and muscle biopsy specimens from identical twins discordant for Type I diabetes mellitus. *N Engl J Med* 1985;312:1282–1287.
212. Siperstein MD: Diabetic microangiopathy and the control of blood glucose. *N Eng J Med* 1983;309:1577–1579.

213. Sandahl-Christiansen J, Gammelgaard J, Tronier B, Svendsen PA, Parving HH: Kidney function and size in diabetics before and during initial insulin treatment. *Kidney Intl* 1982;21:683–688.
214. Steffes MW, Mauer SM: Diabetes and nephropathy: Progression, regression, and the effect of therapy. *Compr Ther* 1984;10:59–62.
215. Østerby R: Early phases in the development of diabetic glomerulopathy: A quantitative electron microscopic study. *Acta Med Scand* 1975;574(suppl):1–80.
216. Mauer SM, Miller K, Goetz FC, et al: Immunopathology of renal extracellular membranes in kidneys transplanted into patients with diabetes mellitus. *Diabetes* 1976;25:709–712.
217. Abouna GM, Al-Adnani MS, Kremer GD, et al: Reversal of diabetic nephropathy in human cadaveric kidneys after transplantation into non-diabetic recipients. *Lancet* 1983:1274–1276.
218. Parving HH, Anderson AR, Smidt UM, et al: Reduced albuminuria during early and aggressive antihypertensive treatment of insulin-dependent diabetic patients with diabetic nephropathy. *Diabetes Care* 1981;4(4):459–463.
219. Bending JJ, Pickup JC, Viberti GC, Keen H: Glycemic control in diabetic nephropathy. *Br Med J* 1984;228:1187–1191.
220. Tamborlane WV, Puklin JE, Bergman M, et al: Long-term improvement of metabolic control with the insulin pump does not reverse diabetic microangiopathy. *Diabetes Care* 1982;5:58–64.
221. Knatterud GL, Klimt CR, Goldner MG, et al: Effects of hypoglycemic agents on vascular complications in patients with adult-onset diabetes. VIII. Evaluation of insulin therapy: final report. *Diabetes* 1982;31 (suppl 5):1–26.
222. Viberti GC, Bilous RW, Mackintosh D, Bending JJ, Keen H: Long-term correction of hyperglycemia and progression of renal failure in insulin dependent diabetes. *Br Med J* 1983;286:598–602.
223. Lawson P, White M, Rosenstock J, Kohner E: Failure of continuous subcutaneous insulin infusion as a therapeutic tool in severe forms of diabetic retinopathy. Abstract, *Diabetologia* 1981;21:510.
224. *Vision Problems in the U.S.* New York, National Society to Prevent Blindness, 1980.
225. Kahn HA, Hiller R: Blindness caused by diabetic retinopathy. *Am J Ophthalmol* 1974;78:58–67.
226. Bodansky JH, Cudworth AG, Drury PL, Kohner EM: Risk factors associated with severe proliferative retinopathy in insulin-dependent diabetes mellitus. *Diabetes Care* 1982;5:97–100.
227. Kahn HA, Bradley RF: Prevalence of diabetic retinopathy: Age, sex, and duration of diabetes. *Br J Ophthalmol* 1975;59:345–349.
228. Caird FI, Pirie A, Ramsell TG: *Diabetes and the Eye.* Oxford, Blackwell Scientific Publications, 1969, pp 1–7.
229. Cogan DG, Kuwabara T: Capillary shunts in the pathogenesis of diabetic retinopathy. *Diabetes* 1963;12:293–300.
230. Cogan DG, Toussaint D, Kuwabara T: Retinal vascular patterns: IV Diabetic retinopathy. *Arch Ophthalmol* 1961;66:366–378.
231. Liang JC, Goldberg MF: Treatment of diabetic retinopathy. *Diabetes* 1980;29:841–851.
232. Kohner EM, Dollery CT: The natural history of diabetic retinopathy, in Goldberg MF, Fine SL (eds): *Symposium on the Treatment of Diabetic Retinopathy.* Washington, D C, Public Health Service Publication No. 1890, 2969, pp 65–79.
233. Kohner EM, Dollery CT: Fluorescein angiography of the fundus in diabetic retinopathy. *Br Med Bull* 1970;26:166–170.

234. Scott DJ, Dollery CT, Hill DW, et al: Fluorescein studies of diabetic retinopathy. *Br Med J* 1964;1:811–814.
235. Ticho U, Patz A: The role of capillary perfusion in the management of diabetic edema. *Am J Ophthalmol* 1973;76:880–886.
236. Schatz H, Patz A: Cystoid maculopathy in diabetes. *Arch Ophthalmol* 1976; 94:761–768.
237. Ashton N: Studies of the retinal capillaries in relation to diabetic and other retinopathies. *Br J Ophthalmol* 1963;47:521–538.
238. Patz A: Retinal vascular disease. *N Eng J Med* 1978;298(no. 26):1451–1454.
239. Watkins PJ: Diabetic complications: Retinopathy. *Br Med J* 1982;285:425–427.
240. Mitchell P: Diabetic retinopathy: Population studies and implications, in Baba S, Gould MK, Zimmit P (eds). *Diabetes Mellitus.* New York, Academic Press, 1984, pp 201–205.
241. L'Esperance FA, James WA Jr: The problem of diabetic retinopathy, in Little HL, Jack RL, Patz A, Forsham PH (eds): *Diabetic Retinopathy.* New York, Thieme-Stratton, Inc., 1983, pp 11–20.
242. Lundbaek K: *Long-term Diabetes: The Clinical Picture in Diabetes Mellitus of 5–25 Years Duration With a Follow-up of a Regional Series of Cases.* Copenhagen, Einar Munksgaard, 1955.
243. Kornerup, T: Studies in diabetic retinopathy. An investigation of 1,000 cases of diabetes. *Acta Med Scand* 1955;CLIII:81–101.
244. Kojima K, Numi K, Watanabe S: Diabetic retinopathy, in Tsuji S, Wada M (eds). *Diabetes Mellitus in Asia, 1970.* Amsterdam, Excerpta Medica, 1971.
245. Cullen JF: Diabetic retinopathy: Hope or despair? *Trans Ophthalmol Soc UK* 1972;92:59–68.
246. Kahn HA, Leibowitz HM, Ganley JP, et al: The Framingham Eye Study. I. Outline and major prevalence findings. *Am J Epidemiol* 1977;106:17–32.
247. Palmberg P, Smith M, Waltman S, et al: The natural history of retinopathy in insulin-dependent juvenile-onset diabetes. *Ophthalmology* 1981;88:613–618.
248. Klein R, Klein BEK, Moss SE, Davis MD, De Mets DL: The Wisconsin epidemiologic study of diabetic retinopathy. II. Prevalence and risk of diabetic retinopathy when age at diagnosis is less than 30 years. *Arch Ophthalmol* 1984;102:520–526.
249. Klein R, Klein BEK, Moss SE, Davis MD, De Mets DL: The Wisconsin epidemiologic study of diabetic retinopathy. III. Prevalence and risk of diabetic retinopathy when age at diagnosis is 30 or more years. *Arch Ophthalmol* 1984;102:527–532.
250. Wagener HP: Retinopathy in diabetes mellitus. *Proc Am Diabetes Assoc* 1945;5:203–216.
251. Root HF, Mirsky S, Ditzel J: Proliferative retinopathy in diabetes mellitus, review of eight hundred forty-seven cases. *JAMA* 1959;169:903–909.
252. Frank RN, Hoffman WH, Podgor MG, Joondepth HC, et al: Retinopathy in juvenile-onset type I diabetes of short duration. *Diabetes* 1982;31:874–882.
253. Oakley WG, Pyke DA, Tattersall RB, Watkins PJ: Long-term diabetes. *Q J Med* 1974;43:145–156.
254. Klein R, Klein BEK, Moss SE, Davis MD, De Mets DL: Retinopathy in young-onset diabetic patients. *Diabetes Care* 1985;8:311–315.
255. Aiello LM, Rand LI, Briones JC, Weiss JN, Wafai MZ: Nonocular clinical risk factors in the progression of diabetic retinopahty, in Little LL, Jack RL, Patz A, Forsham PH (eds): *Diabetic Retinopathy*. New York, Thieme-Stratton, 1983, pp 21–32.
256. Burditt AF, Caird FI, Draper GJ: The natural history of diabetic retinopathy. *Q J Med* 1968;37:303–317.

257. Deckert T, Simonsen SE, Poulsen JE: Prognosis of proliferative retinopathy in juvenile diabetes. *Diabetes* 1967;16:728–733.
258. Dobree JH: Evolution of lesions in proliferative diabetic retinopathy: An eight-year perotographic survey, in Goldberg MJ, Fine SL (eds): *Symposium on the Treatment of Diabetic Retinopathy.* USPHS Pub No. 1890. Washington, DC, 1968.
259. Caird FI, Burditt AF, Draper GJ: Diabetic retinopathy, a further study of prognosis for vision. *Diabetes* 1968;17:121–123.
260. Beetham WP: Visual prognosis of proliferating diabetic retinopathy. *Br J Ophthalmol* 1963;47:611–619.
261. Kohner EM, Panissett A, Cheng H, Fraser TR: Diabetic retinopathy: new vessels arising from the optic disc. I. Grading system and natural history. *Diabetes* 1971: 20:816–823.
262. The Diabetic Retinopathy Study Research Group. Four risk factors for severe visual loss in diabetic retinopathy: The third report from the Diabetic Retinopathy Study. *Arch Ophthalmol* 1979;97:654–655.
263. Caird FI: Epidemiology of diabetic retinopathy, in Lynn JR, Snyder WB, Vaiser A (eds): *Diabetic Retinopathy.* New York, Grune & Stratton, Inc., 1974.
264. Sharma NK, Archer DB, Hadden DR, Merrett JD, Maguire CJF: Morbidity and mortality in patients with diabetic retinopathy. *Trans Ophthalmol Soc UK* 1980;100:83–89.
265. Knatterud GL: Mortality experience in the Diabetic Retinopathy Study. *Isr J Med Sci* 1983;19:424–428.
266. L'Esperance FA, James WA Jr: The eye and diabetes mellitus, in Ellenberg M, Rifkin H (eds): *Diabetes Mellitus: Theory and Practice,* ed 3. New York, Medical Examination Publishing Co., 1983.
267. Buzney SM, Weiter JJ: Pathogenesis of diabetic retinal angiopathy: proposed mechanisms and current research. *Intl Ophthalmol Clin* 1984;24(4):1–12.
268. Prout TE: The role of diabetic control in diabetic retinopathy. *Intl Ophthalmol Clin* 1978;18:73–89.
269. Bradley RF, Ramos E: The eye and diabetes, in Marble A, White P, Bradley RF, et al (eds): *Joslin's Diabetes Mellitus.* Philadelphia, Lea & Febiger, 1971.
270. Lauritzen T, Larsen HW, Frost-Larsen K, Deckert T, the Steno Study Group: Effect of 1 year of near-normal blood glucose levels on retinopathy in insulin-dependent diabetics. *Lancet* 1983;1:200–204.
271. Frost-Larsen K, Christiansen JS, Parving HH: The effect of strict short-term metabolic control on retinal nervous system abnormalities in newly diagnosed type 1 (insulin-dependent) diabetic patients. *Diabetologia* 1983;24:207–209.
272. Waltman SR, Oestrich C, Krupin T, et al: Quantitative vitreous fluorophotometry; a sensitive technique for measuring early breakdown of the blood-retinal barrier in young diabetic patients. *Diabetes* 1978;27:85–87.
273. Job D, Eschwege E, Guyot-Argenton C, et al: Effect of multiple daily insulin injections on the course of diabetic retinopathy. *Diabetes* 1976;25:463–469.
274. Eschwege E, Job D, Guyot-Argenton C, et al: Delayed progression of diabetic retinopathy by divided insulin administration: a further follow-up. *Diabetologia* 1979:16:13–15.
275. Doft BH, Kingsley LA, Orchard TJ, et al: The association between long-term diabetic control and early retinopathy. *Ophthalmology* 1984;91:763–769.
276. Dahl-Jorgensen K, Hanssen KF, Smeland E, et al: Long term strict control in type 1 (insulin-dependent) diabetes mellitus: Effect on late diabetic complications. *Diabetologia* 1983;25:149.

277. Dahl-Jorgensen K, Brinchmann-Hansen O, Sandvik L, Hansen KF, Aker Diabetes Group: Rapid lowering of blood glucose may lead to cotton wool exudates in the retina: studies in Type 1 (insulin-dependent) diabetic patients treated with continuous subcutaneous insulin infusion and multiple insulin injections. *Diabetologia* 1984;27:266A.
278. Dahl-Jorgensen K, Brinchmann-Hansen O, Hanssen KF, Sandvik L, Aaginaes O, Aker Diabetes Group: Rapid tightening of blood glucose control leads to transient deterioration of retinopathy in insulin-dependent diabetes mellitus: the Oseo study. *Br Med J* 1985;290:811–815.
279. Dandona P, Bolger JP, Boag F, Fonesca V, Abrams JD: Rapid development and progression of proliferative retinopathy after strict diabetic control. *Br Med J* 1985;290:895–896.
280. Malone JI, Grizzard WS, Espinoza LR, Achenbach KE, Van Cader TC: Risk factors for diabetic retinopathy in youth. *Pediatrics* 1984;73:756–761.
281. Ballegooie E Van, Hooymans J MM, Timmerman Z, et al: Rapid deterioration of diabetic retinopathy during treatment with continuous subcutaneous insulin infusion. *Diabetes Care* 1984;7:236–242.
282. Lawson PM, Champion MC, Canny C, et al: Continuous subcutaneous insulin infusion (CSII) does not prevent progression of proliferative and preproliferative retinopathy. *Br J Ophthalmol* 1982;66:762–766.
283. The KROC Collaborative Study Group: The KROC Study Patients at two years: A report on further retinal changes. Abstract 156. *Diabetes* 1985;34(suppl 1): 39A.
284. Valone J Jr: Proliferative diabetic retinopathy and patient age: Presentation, prognosis, and management. *Int Ophthalmol Clin* 1984;24(4):71–82.
285. The Diabetic Retinopathy Study Research Group: Preliminary report on effects of photocoagulation therapy. *Am J Ophthalmol* 1976;81:383–396.
286. The Diabetic Retinopathy Study Research Group: Photocoagulation treatment of proliferative diabetic retinopathy: The second report of diabetic retinopathy study findings. *Ophthalmology* 1978;85:82–106.
287. The Diabetic Retinopathy Study Research Group. Photocoagulation treatment of proliferative diabetic retinopathy: Clinical application of diabetic retinopathy study (DRS) findings, DRS Report Number 8. *Ophthalmology* 1981;88:538–600.
288. Rice TA: The Early Treatment Diabetic Retinopathy Study. *Trans Pa Acad Ophthalmol Otolaryngol* 1982 (Spring);35(1):24–30.
289. Leske MC, Sperduto RD: The epidemiology of senile cataracts: A review. *Am J Epidemiol* 1983;118:152–165.
290. Kahn HA, Leibowitz HM, Ganley JP, et al: The Framingham Eye Study. II. Association of Ophthalmic pathology with single variables previously measured in the Framingham heart study. *Am J Epidemiol* 1977;106:33–41.
291. Leibowitz HM, Krueger DE, Maunder LR, et al: The Framingham Eye Study monograph. *Surv Ophthalmol* 1980;24(suppl):335–610.
292. National Health and Nutrition Examination Survey: Ophthalmology Examination Protocol. Hyattsville, Md, Welfare, National Center for Health Statistics, 1972.
293. Ederer F, Hiller R, Taylor HR: Senile lens changes and diabetes: Two population studies. *Am J Ophthalmol* 1981:91:381–395.
294. Hiller R, Kahn HA: Senile cataract extraction and diabetes. *Br J Ophthalmol* 1976;60:283–286.
295. Caird FI, Hutchinson M, Pirie A: Cataract and diabetes. *Br Med J* 1974;2:665–667.
296. Sommer A: Cataracts as an epidemiologic problem. *Am J Ophthalmol* 1977; 83:334–339.

297. Cotlier E: Senile cataracts: Evidence for acceleration by diabetes and deceleration by salicylate. *Can J Ophthalmol* 1981;16:113–118.
298. Claton RM, Cuthbert J, Seth J, et al: Epidemiological and other studies in the assessment of factors contributing to cataractogenesis, symposium. *Human Cataract Formation* 1984;106:25–47.
299. National Advisory Eye Council. Vision Research; A National Plan 1983–1987, vol 2, pt 3: Report of the Cataract Panel. Bethesda, Md, US Department of Health and Human Services (NIH Publication No. 82-3473) 1983:51–59.
300. Bernth-Peterson P, Bach E: Epidemiologic aspects of cataract surgery. III: Frequencies of diabetes and glaucoma in a cataract population. *Acta Ophthalmol* 1983;61:406–416.
301. Perkins ES: Cataract: Refractive error, diabetes, and morphology. *Br J Ophthalmol* 1984;68:293–297.
302. Chylack LT Jr: Mechanisms of senile cataract formation. *Ophthalmology* 1984;91:596–602.
303. Van Heyningen R: Galactose cataract: a review. *Exp Eye Res* 1971;11:415–428.
304. Chylack LT Jr: Classification of human cataracts. *Arch Ophthalmol* 1978;96:888–892.
305. Chylack LT Jr: Classification of human cataractous change by the American Cooperative Cataract Research Group method, in *Human Cataract Formation.* London, Pittman. Ciba Foundation symposium 1984;106:3–24.
306. Kador PF: Overview of the current attempts toward the medical treatment of cataract. *Ophthalmology* 1983;90:352–364.
307. Cobo LM: Aldose reductase and diabetic keratopathy, in *Aldose Reductase and Complications of Diabetes,* Cogan DG, moderator. *Ann Intern Med* 1984;101:82–91.
308. Schultz RO, Van Horn DL, Peters MA, Klewin KA, Schutten WH: Diabetic keratopathy. *Trans Am Ophthalmol Soc* 1981;79:180–199.
309. Hyndiuk RA, Kazarian EL, Schultz RO, Sudman S: Neurotrophic corneal ulcers in diabetes mellitus. *Arch Ophthalmol* 1977;95:2193–2196.
310. Friend J, Thoft RA: The diabetic cornea. *Intl Ophthalmol Clin* 1984;24(4):111–122.
311. Schwartz DE: Corneal sensitivity in diabetes. *Arch Ophthalmol* 1974;91:174–178.
312. Brightbill FS, Myers FL, Bresnick GH: Postvitrectomy keratopathy. *Am J Ophthalmol* 1978;85:651–655.
313. Foulks GN, Thoft RA, Perry HD, Tolentino FI: Factors related to corneal epithelial complications after closed vitrectomy in diabetes. *Arch Ophthalmol* 1979;97:1076–1078.
314. Perry HD, Foulks GN, Thoft RA, Tolentino FI: Corneal complications after closed vitrectomy through the pars plana. *Arch Ophthalmol* 1978;96:1401–1403.
315. Blankenship GW, Machemer R: Pars plana vitrectomy for the management of severe diabetic retinopathy: An analysis of results five years following surgery. *Ophthalmology* 1978;85:553–559.
316. Faulborn J, Conway BP, Machemer R: Surgical complications of pars plana vitreous surgery. *Ophthalmology* 1978;85:116–125.
317. Pfister RR, Schepens CL, Lemp MA, Webster RG: Photocoagulation keratopathy: report of a case. *Arch Ophthalmol* 1971;86:94–96.
318. Kenyon KR, Stark WJ, Stone DL: Corneal endothelial degeneration and fibrous proliferation after pars plana vitrectomy. *Am J Ophthalmol* 1976;81:486–490.
319. Edelhauser HF, Gonnering R, Van Horn DL: Intraocular irrigating solution. A comparative study of BSS plus and lactated Ringer's solution. *Arch Ophthalmol* 1982;96:516–520.
320. Eichenbaum JW, Feldstein M, Podos SM: Extended-wear aphakic soft contact lenses and corneal ulcers. *Br J Ophthalmol* 1982;66:663–666.

321. Kanski JJ: Anterior segment complications of retinal photocoagulation. *Am J Ophthalmol* 1975;79:424–427.
322. Akagi Y, Yajima Y, Kador PF, Kuwabara T, Kinoshita JH: Localization of aldose reductase in the human eye. *Diabetes* 1984;33:562–566.
323. Crepaldi G, Baggio G, Manzato E: Pharmacological approach to the prevention of atherosclerosis, in Schettler FG, Gotto AM, Middlehoff G, Habenicht AJR, Jurutka KR (eds): *Atherosclerosis VI.* New York, Springer-Verlag, 1983, pp 796–804.
324. Jarrett RJ, McCartney P, Keen H: The Bedford survey: Ten year mortality rates in newly diagnosed diabetics, borderline diabetics and normoglycemic controls and risk indices for coronary heart disease in borderline diabetics. *Diabetologia* 1982; 22:79–84.
325. Keen H, Jarrett RJ: Macroangiopathy—its prevalence in asymptomatic diabetes. *Adv Metab Disord* 1975;2(suppl):3–9.
326. Epstein FH: Hyperglycemia. A risk factor in coronary heart disease. *Circulation* 1967;36:609–619.
327. Mainland D: The risk of fallacious conclusions from autopsy data on the incidence of disease with application to heart disease. *Am Heart J* 1953;45:644–654.
328. Liebow IM, Hellerstein HK, Miller M: Atherosclerotic heart disease in diabetes mellitus; clinical study of 383 patients. *Am J Med* 1955;18:438–447.
329. Bryfogle JW, Bradley RF: The vascular complications of diabetes mellitus: A clinical study. *Diabetes* 1957;6:157–159.
330. Anderson RS, Ellington A, Gunter LM: The incidence of arteriosclerotic heart disease in Negro diabetic patients. *Diabetes* 1961;10:114–118.
331. Liebow IM, Newill VA, Oseasohn R: Incidence of ischemic heart disease in a group of diabetic women. *Am J Med Sci* 1964;248:403–407.
332. Klimt CR, Knatterud GL, Meinert CL, Prout TE: A study of the effects of hypoglycemic agents on vascular complications in patients with adult-onset diabetes; Parts I and II. I. Design, methods and baseline results. II. Mortality results. *Diabetes* 1970;19: 747–830.
333. Fein FS, Scheuer J: Heart disease in diabetes, in Ellenberg M, Rifkin H (eds): Diabetes *Mellitus: Theory and Practice,* ed 3. New York, Medical Examination Publishing Co, 1983, pp 851–861.
334. Kannel WB, Dawber TR, Kagan A, Revotski N, Stokes J: III Factors of risk in development of coronary heart disease—six year follow-up experience. *Ann Intern Med* 1961;55:33–50.
335. Epstein FH, Ostrander LD Jr, Johnson BC, et al: Epidemiological studies of cardiovascular disease in a total community—Tecumseh, Michigan. *Ann Intern Med* 1965;62:1170–1187.
336. Blotner H: Coronary disease in diabetes mellitus. *N Engl J Med* 1930;203;709–711.
337. Enklewitz M: Diabetes and coronary thrombosis. *Am Heart J* 1934;9:386–395.
338. Nathanson MH: Coronary disease in 100 autopsied diabetics. *Am J Med Sci* 1932;183:495–502.
339. Root HF, Bland EF, Gordon WH, White PD: Coronary artherosclerosis in diabetes mellitus; post-mortem study. *JAMA* 1939;113:27–30.
340. Lisa JR, Magiday M, Galloway I, Hart JF: Arteriosclersis with diabetes mellitus; study of pathologic findings in 193 diabetic and 2,250 non-diabetic patients. *JAMA* 1942;120:192–195.
341. Sterns S, Schlesinger MJ, Rudy A: Incidence and clinical significance of coronary artery disease in diabetes mellitus. *Arch Intern Med* 1947:80:463–474.
342. Clawson BJ, Bell ET: Incidence of fatal coronary disease in nondiabetic and in diabetic persons. *Arch Pathol* 1949;48:105–106.

343. Goldenberg S, Alex M, Blumental HT: Sequelae of arteriosclerosis of the aorta and coronary arteries; a statistical study in diabetes mellitus. *Diabetes* 1958;7:98–108.
344. Feldman M, Feldman M Jr: Association of coronary occlusion and infarction with diabetes mellitus; necropsy study. *Am J Med Sci* 1954;228:53–56.
345. Goodale F, Daoud AS, Florentin R, Lee KT, Gittelsohn A: Chemico-anatomic studies of arteriosclerosis and thrombosis in diabetics. I. Coronary arterial wall thickness, thrombosis, and myocardial infarcts in autopsied North Americans. *Exp Mol Pathol* 1962;1:353–363.
346. Knowles HC Jr: Long-term juvenile diabetes treated with unmeasured diet. *Trans Assoc Am Phys* 1971:84:95–101.
347. Paz-Guerara AT, Hsu TH, White P: Juvenile diabetes mellitus after forty years. *Diabetes* 1975;24:559–565.
348. Crall FV Jr, Roberts WC: The extramural and intramural coronary arteries in juvenile diabetes mellitus. *Am J Med* 1978;64:221–230.
349. Garcia MJ, McNamara PM, Gordon T, Kannel WB: Morbidity and mortality in diabetics in the Framingham population. Sixteen year follow-up study. *Diabetes* 1974;23:105–111.
350. Gordon T, Castelli WP, Hjortland MC, Kannel WB, Dawber TR: Diabetes, blood lipids, and the role of obesity in coronary heart disease risk for women. The Framingham Eye Study. *Ann Intern Med* 1977;87:393–397.
351. Ostrander LD, Francis T, Hayner NS, Kjelsberg MO, Epstein FH: The relationship of cardio-vascular disease to hyperglycemia. *Ann Intern Med* 1965;62:1188–1198.
352. Epstein FH, Ostrander LD, Johnson BJ, et al: Epidemiological studies of cardiovascular disease in a total community—Tecumseh, Michigan. *Ann Intern Med* 1965; 62:1170–1187.
353. Pell S, D'Alonzo CA: Factors associated with long-term survival of diabetes. *JAMA* 1970;214:1833–1840.
354. Malins J: *Clinical Diabetes Mellitus.* London, Eyre and Spottiswoode, Ltd., 1968.
355. Soler NG, Bennett MA, Pentecost BL, Fitzgerald MG, Malins JM: Myocardial infarction in diabetes. *Q J Med* 1975;44:125–132.
356. Uusitupa O, Siitonen A ARO, Pyorala K: Prevalence of coronary heart disease, left ventricular failure and hypertension in middle-aged newly diagnosed Type 2 (non-insulin-dependent) diabetic subjects. *Diabetologia* 1985;28:22–27.
357. Cooper R, Liu K, Stamler J, et al: Prevalence of diabetes/hyperglycemia and associated cardiovascular risk factors in blacks and whites: Chicago Heart Association detection project in industry. *Am Heart J* 1984;108:827–833.
358. West KM, Ahuja MM, Bennett PH, et al: The role of circulating glucose and triglyceride concentrations and their interactions with other "risk factors" as determinants of arterial disease in nine diabetic population samples taken from the WHO multinational study. *Diabetes Care* 1983;6:361–369.
359. Chait A, Bierman EL, Brunzell JD: Diabetic macroangiopathy, in Alberti KGMM, Krall LP (eds): *The Diabetes Annual/*1. Amsterdam, Elsevier, 1985.
360. Kawate R, Miyanishi M, Yamakido M, Nishimoto Y: Preliminary studies of the prevalence and mortality of diabetes mellitus in Japanese in Japan and on the island of Hawaii. *Adv Metab Dis* 1978;9:201–223.
361. Kannel WB: Diabetes as a risk factor for atherosclerotic cardiovascular disease, in Brodoff BN, Bleicher SJ (eds): *Diabetes Mellitus and Obesity.* Baltimore, Williams & Wilkins, 1982.
362. Kannel WB, McGee DL: Diabetes and cardiovascular disease. The Framingham Eye Study. *JAMA* 1979;241:2035–2038.

363. Robertson WB, Strong JP: Atherosclerosis in persons with hypertension and diabetes mellitus. *Lab Invest* 1968;18:538–551.
364. Hamby RI, Sherman L, Mehta J, Aintablian A: Reappraisal of the role of the diabetic state in coronary artery disease. *Chest* 1976;70(2):251–257.
365. Dortimer AC, Shenoy PN, Shiroff RA, et al: Diffuse coronary artery disease in diabetic patients: fact or fiction? *Circulation* 1978;57:133–136.
366. Leden I, Schersten B, Svensson B: Rheumatic hand syndromes: An early or late manifestation of diabetes mellitus. *Practical Cardiol* 1983;9:209–227.
367. Eaton RP, Sibbitt WL, Harsh A: The effect of an aldose reductase inhibiting agent on limited joint mobility in diabetic patients. *JAMA* 1985;253:1437–1440.
368. Lundbaek K: Stiff hands in long-term diabetes. *Acta Med Scand* 1957;158:447–451.
369. Rosenbloom AL, Frias JL: Diabetes mellitus, short stature and joint stiffness—a new syndrome. *Clin Res* 1974;22:92A.
370. Grgic A, Rosenbloom AL, Weber FT, et al: Joint contracture—common manifestation of childhood diabetes mellitus. *J Pediatr* 1976;88:584–588.
371. Benedetti A, Noacco C, Macor S, Pittaro I: Joint lesions in diabetes. *N Engl J Med* 1975;292:1033–1034.
372. Rosenbloom AL, Silverstein JH, Lezotti DC, Richardson K, McCallum M: Limited joint mobility in childhood diabetes mellitus indicates risk for microvascular disease. *N Engl J Med* 1981;305:191–194.
373. Lawson PM, Maneschi F, Kohner EM: The relationship of hand abnormalities to diabetes and diabetic retinopathy. *Diabetes Care* 1983;6:140–143.
374. Campbell RP, Hawkins SJ, Maddison PJ, Reckless JPD: Limited joint mobility in diabetes mellitus. *Ann Rheum Dis* 1985;44:93–97.
375. Heathcote JG, Cohen H, Noble J: Dupuytren's disease and diabetes mellitus. *Lancet* 1981;1:1420.
376. Beacom R, Kennedy L, Carson D, Campbell SL: Joint contractures in type 1 (insulin dependent) diabetes. *Diabetologia* 1981;21:503.
377. Jung Y, Hohmann TC, Novak J, et al: Diabetic hand syndrome. *Metabolism* 1971;20:1008–1015.
378. Starkman HS, Gleason RE, Rand LI, Miller DE, Soeldner JS: Limited joint mobility (LJM) of the hand in patients with diabetes mellitus: Relation to chronic complications. *Ann Rheum Dis* 1986;45:130–135.
379. Silverstein JH, Fennell R, Donnelly W, et al: Correlates of biopsy-studied nephropathy in young patients with insulin-dependent diabetes mellitus. *J Pediatr* 1985:196–201.
380. Knowles HB: Joint contractures, waxy skin, and control of diabetes. *N Engl J Med* 1981;305 217–219.
381. Slama G, Letanoux M, Thibult N, et al: Quantification of early subclinical limited joint mobility in early diabetes. *Diabetes Care* 1985;8:329–332.
382. Buckingham BA, Uitto J, Sandborg C, et al: Scleroderma-like changes in insulin-dependent diabetes mellitus: Clinical and biochemical studies. *Diabetes Care* 1984; 7:163–169.
383. Hamlin CR, Kohn RP, Luschin JH: Apparent accelerated aging of human collagen in diabetes mellitus. *Diabetes* 1975;24:902.
384. Lieberman LS, Rosenbloom AL, Riley WJ, Silverstein JH: Reduced skin thickness with pump administration of insulin. *N Eng J Med* 1980;303:940–941.

Chapter 2

Hyperglycemia in the Pathogenesis of Diabetic Complications

by Dushan Dvornik, D.Sc.

SYNOPSIS

Since the introduction of insulin and antihyperglycemic agents into clinical medicine and the consequent increase in the survival and longevity of diabetic individuals, the complications of long-term diabetes mellitus have become both more frequent and more apparent. Recent studies of these complications have demonstrated the etiologic role of chronic hyperglycemia in the pathogenesis of specific microvascular and neurologic lesions. Because these conditions have not been susceptible to prevention or treatment by subsequent control of glycemia, attempts have been made to identify new pharmacologic approaches directed at preventing the sequelae of chronic diabetic hyperglycemia. In particular, research efforts have focused on elucidating of possible pathogenetic mechanisms underlying diabetic neuropathy, diabetic nephropathy, diabetic retinopathy and other eye complications, and diabetic vascular disease.

This chapter reviews three mechanisms proposed as explanations for the tissue damage produced by the excess blood glucose of diabetes mellitus:

1. the role of the enzyme aldose reductase in the metabolism of excess glucose via the polyol pathway;
2. non-enzymatic glycation, such as the reaction between glucose and free amino groups of proteins; and
3. intracellular deficiency of myoinositol, a polyol present in most mammalian cells.

Although the measurement of glycated serum proteins, e.g., hemoglobin Alc, offers a clinical advantage in the assessment of glycemia over time, there is not as yet sufficient evidence to determine whether non-enzymatic glycation is related to the changes observed in the known complications of chronic diabetes mellitus.

Myoinositol levels appear to be related to aldose reductase activity, especially in neural tissue. Diabetic nerves in laboratory animals and man have been shown to have elevated levels of glucose, sorbitol, and fructose, and low myoinositol levels. In peripheral neuropathy, where the myoinositol levels are demonstrably low, aldose reductase inhibition can prevent and reverse the deficit.

Observations in laboratory animals have established the critical role of aldose reductase in the pathogenesis of sugar cataract formation. This demonstration inspired the hypothesis that the polyol pathway may also be involved in diabetic complications in other tissues that, like the lens, do not require insulin for glucose uptake and are, therefore, exposed to the glycemia of diabetes mellitus. The hypothesis implies that excess glucose in such tissues is metabolized via the polyol pathway, hence presupposes the presence of aldose reductase in these tissues. The etiologic role of aldose reductase has been confirmed in the pathogenesis of specific diabetic complications in animal models according to the criteria of Kinoshita:[82,142]

the complication and aldose reductase must occur together; the complication must occur in galactosemia as well as in hyperglycemia, and must occur earlier and more severely in galactosemia; the complication must be prevented or delayed by aldose reductase inhibition; and, finally, the effectiveness of aldose reductase inhibition must be confirmed by structurally distinct inhibitors.

According to these criteria, aldose reductase is implicated in the pathogenesis of diabetic neuropathy, diabetic nephropathy, thickening of retinal capillary basement membranes, and keratopathy.

Contents

INTRODUCTION

The association of neuropathy, retinopathy, and nephropathy with diabetes mellitus was recognized even before the discovery of insulin in 1922. With the introduction of insulin into clinical medicine, the survival of young diabetic subjects was prolonged. Development of the sequelae of diabetes thus occurred, and the full extent of the problems of long-term diabetes became apparent. Data from clinical investigations and animal model studies[1–3] acquired over the last 15 years demonstrate that chronic hyperglycemia is a major factor responsible for the development of the specific long-term neurological and microvascular complications of diabetes. Recent clinical trials suggest, however, that in the presence of established neurological and microvascular complications, improved glycemic control as routinely attainable may not suffice to arrest the continuation of the process(es) involved.[4,5] The findings may be interpreted to indicate either that the degree of improved glycemic control was not adequate for detecting the consequences of arrested progression of the process(es) involved or that the lesions were beyond repair, at least for the duration of the treatment. Therefore, treatment appears to be needed earlier or to be more physiological than is currently obtainable. This has led to the concept of a different pharmacological approach to the control of diabetic complications, one aimed at the prevention of the effects of hyperglycemia rather than at complete control of hyperglycemia per se.

Diabetic hyperglycemia occurs because the pathways involved in the metabolism of glucose levels are not set at physiological rates. Based on present knowledge, several different mechanisms have been suggested to explain how tissue damage might be caused by glucose in diabetes. One mechanism is based on the metabolism of excess glucose via the polyol pathway. While this metabolic pathway appears to be virtually dormant under physiological conditions, the hyperglycemia-induced increase in the flux of glucose through the polyol pathway[6–8] results in a correspondingly high rate of sorbitol production and NADPH consumption by aldose reductase, the first enzyme in the polyol pathway. This initiates a series of biochemical changes that result in loss of functional integrity of the cell. The role of the polyol pathway and, in particular, of aldose reductase, is now generally accepted as being critical to the pathogenesis of sugar cataracts.[9–14] Some of the most convincing evidence for implicating aldose reductase in sugar cataract formation emerged from experiments with inhibitors of aldose reductase (AR).[15] An increasing body of evidence also implicates aldose reductase in the pathogenesis of diabetic neuropathy,[15–17] keratopathy, and possibly, diabetic retinopathy[14,18] and nephropathy.[19–21] Again, much of the supporting evidence is being generated with the use of AR inhibitors, both in animal models[22] and in man.

The second mechanism linking glucose to tissue damage in diabetes is based on the capacity of glucose to react chemically with proteins in a process known as "non-enzymatic glycation."* Experimental evidence obtained since the identification of the minor hemoglobin HbA1c as the product of non-enzymatic glycation of hemoglobin[24–26] has made it clear that non-enzymatic glycation can be a common post-translational modification of many proteins. A concept has emerged that excessive non-enzymatic glycation may represent a biochemical link between chronic hyperglycemia and the pathophysiological processes involved in the development of long-term diabetic complications.[27–30]

The third potential mechanism is based mainly on experimental data obtained in laboratory animals that show an intracellular deficiency of myoinositol, a key regulatory factor in neural metabolism and function.[31] According to this hypothesis, disturbed metabolism of myoinositol and its phospholipid derivatives may be the link between hyperglycemia and compromised function of the diabetic nerve leading to impaired axonal transport and decreased conduction velocity characteristic of diabetic neuropathy. These postulates are discussed more extensively in the following sections.

ALDOSE REDUCTASE AND THE PATHOGENESIS OF SUGAR CATARACT

Recent evidence supports the long-standing clinical impression that cataracts are more frequent and occur earlier in diabetic persons than in non-diabetics.[32] The possibility that this is due to diabetes-induced hyperglycemia has stimulated considerable laboratory research on sugar metabolism in the lens, which has resulted in the incrimination of the enzyme aldose reductase in the formation of sugar cataracts.

To provide a background, the pathways of sugar metabolism in the lens that offer insight into the mechanism of sugar cataract formation are reviewed here briefly.

Sugar metabolism in the lens

To fulfill its focusing function, the ocular lens must retain its shape and transparency by virtue of active metabolic processes. In view of its rather undifferentiated structure and its lack of blood supply, the lens was regarded as an inert bag of proteins until 1928, when Kronfeld and Bothman[33] observed that the lens can produce lactic acid in the presence of glucose. Since then, our understanding of the metabolism of the lens has increased very considerably. The current perception of the role of the metabolic processes in the lens is simplified by Kuck's observation that "the lens behaves as a completely transparent robot pump, regulating its own maintenance, growth, and repair with the aid of a power-pack."[34]

*The Joint Commission on Biochemical Nomenclature of the International Union of Biochemistry (IUB) and the International Union of Pure and Applied Chemistry (IUPAC) suggests the term "glycation" rather than "glycosylation" or "glucosylation" for the non-enzymatic reaction between glucose or other sugars, and free amino groups of proteins.[23]

Anatomically, the lens is suspended immediately behind the pupil of the eye by the zonular ligaments anchored to the ciliary muscle (Fig 1). To minimize the scattering of light, there are no blood vessels within the lens. The lens is surrounded by the clear and colorless aqueous and vitreous humors. The main source of nutrients and oxygen required for metabolism is the aqueous humor of the anterior and posterior chambers, which flows slowly past the lens. The nutrient supply is taken up through a one-cell-thick layer of cuboidal epithelial cells.

Since most of the nucleated cells and mitochondria of the lens are localized in its epithelium, most of the transport and accumulation of necessary nutrients and the maintenance of ionic balances[34] are performed by the epithelium. The cells of the lens, like other cells, derive their energy from adenosine triphosphate (ATP), produced by the metabolism of glucose through a series of phosphorylated intermediates constituting two metabolic pathways: glycolysis, or the anaerobic Embden-Meyerhoff pathway, and the oxidative, citric acid pathway, or Krebs cycle. The metabolism in the crystalline lens was recently reviewed by Cheng and Chylack.[35]

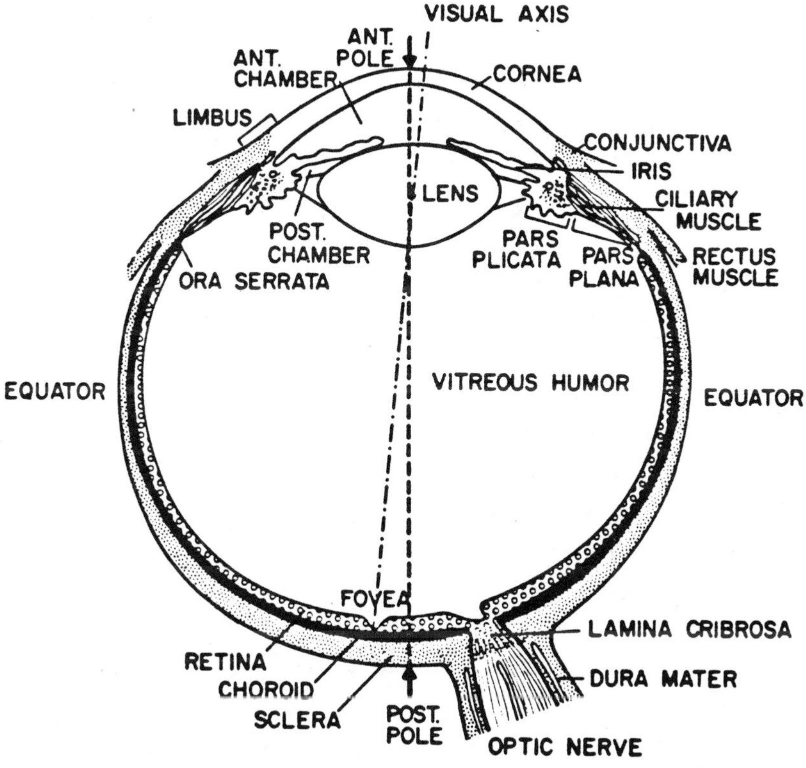

Figure 1. Diagram of the eye. (From The Eye, Academic Press, 1984)

Embden-Meyerhoff pathway of glycolysis

The Embden-Meyerhoff pathway is characterized by the reactions summarized in Fig 2. Occurring under anaerobic conditions in the cytoplasm, the pathway proceeds by way of phosphorylated intermediates and produces only two molecules ATP per molecule glucose. That the lens can derive much of its ATP supply from glycolysis was shown by Kinoshita and associates,[36] who found that the incorporation of amino acids into protein, and the sodium, potassium, and ATP concentrations in the lens were sustained at normal levels in the absence of oxygen, provided that sufficient glucose was present. In the absence of glucose, oxygen enables the bovine lens to derive a substantial amount of energy from its endogenous substrates,[37–39] e.g., from amino acids.[40] About 33% of the ATP in rat lens is derived from oxidative metabolism of glucose,[39,40] thus indicating that mitochondrial oxidation of amino acids via the citric acid cycle can also contribute to the energy produced by the lens.[40] ATP production by anaerobic glycolysis therefore appears adequate to support a variety of metabolic processes, with the exception of tyrosine incorporation into protein.[41] Characteristically, as the calf lens ages, aerobic metabolism assumes relatively greater significance than anaerobic glycolysis in the production of ATP.[39,42]

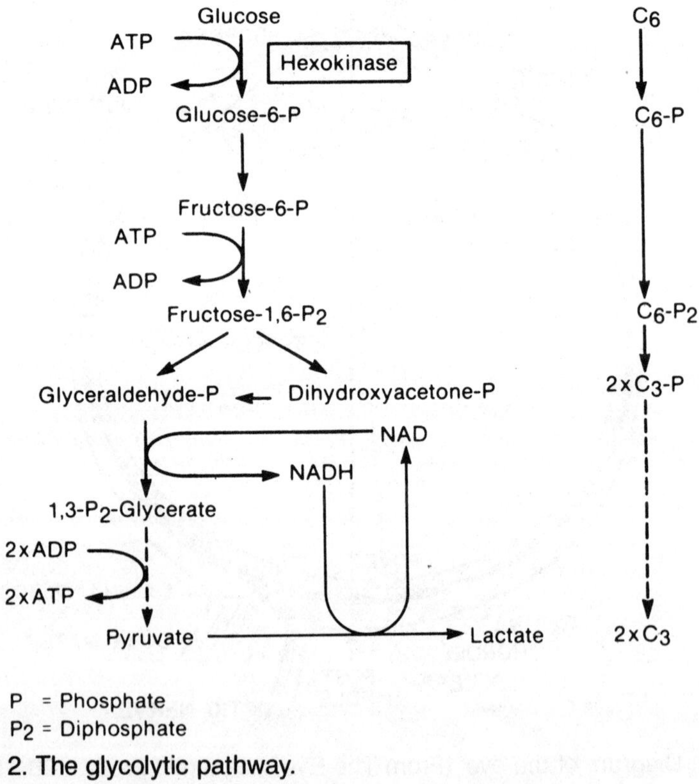

Figure 2. The glycolytic pathway.

Citric acid cycle

The citric acid cycle, occurring in the mitochondria, is the pathway for the oxidation of acetyl-coenzyme A, derived from glucose, fatty acids, and amino acids. From each acetyl-CoA molecule entering the cycle, three molecules of NADH and one of $FADH_2$ are formed. Upon transfer to the respiratory chain located in the inner mitochondrial membrane, the coenzymes generate ATP; from each molecule of acetyl-CoA, 12 molecules of ATP are formed. The events characterizing the citric acid cycle are summarized in Fig 3.

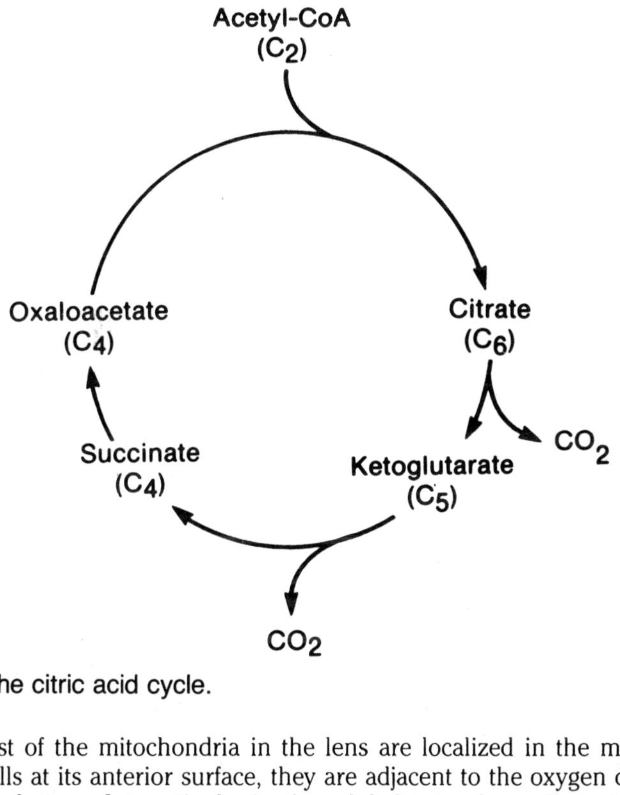

Figure 3. The citric acid cycle.

Since most of the mitochondria in the lens are localized in the monolayer of epithelial cells at its anterior surface, they are adjacent to the oxygen dissolved in the aqueous humor. Interestingly, in the adult bovine lens, the epithelial cells constitute only about 0.1% of the total lens volume, yet they are most likely involved in virtually all metabolic processes involving molecular oxygen.

Hexose monophosphate shunt

In addition to the Embden-Meyerhoff pathway of glycolysis, the lens can also metabolize glucose anaerobically by way of the hexose monophosphate shunt (pentose phosphate shunt, phosphogluconate pathway, or Warburg-Dickens pathway), shown in Fig 4. About 14% of the available glucose is metabolized via the

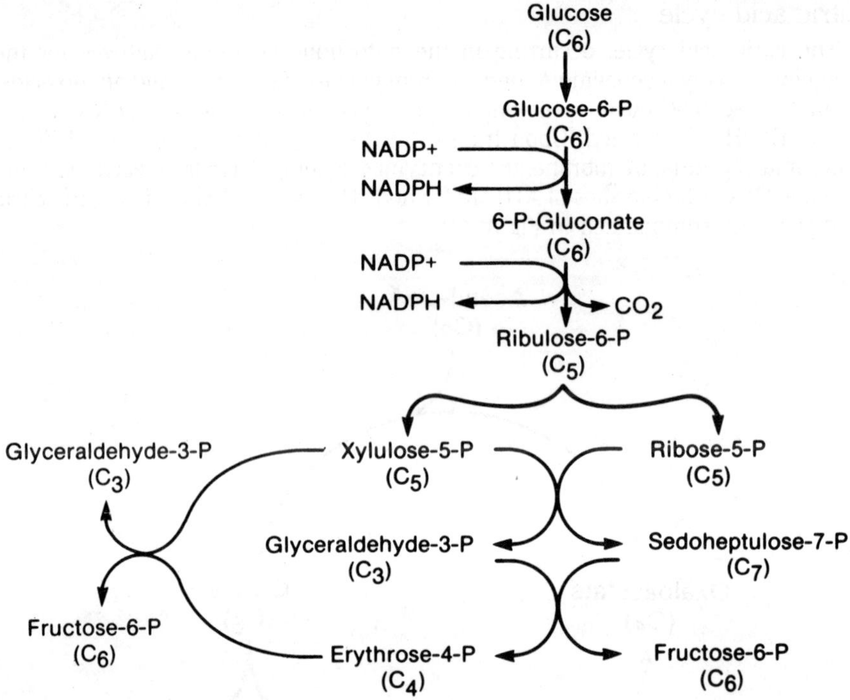

Figure 4. The hexose monophosphate shunt or pentose phosphate pathway.

hexose monophosphate shunt.[43] In the lens, glycolysis serves to generate ATP, while the hexose monophosphate shunt is the principal source of NADPH.[7,44] While in most tissues NADPH is essential for the biosynthesis of fatty acids or steroids, in the lens, NADPH is required by glutathione reductase and aldose reductase.[7,44]

In vitro, the activity of the hexose monophosphate shunt increases linearly in response to increasing glucose concentration in the incubating medium; at 30 to 32 mM glucose, the increase is 6 to 6.5 times that at 5 mM glucose.[36,44] The shunt is also activated by oxidation, albeit to a lower extent than by the polyol pathway.[36,44] The hexose monophosphate shunt is thus activated whenever there is a demand for NADPH. The shunt is, therefore, closely associated with sugar cataractogenesis[35] and detoxification of hydrogen peroxide by glutathione reductase.[45] The competition of glutathione reductase and aldose reductase for NADPH is illustrated in Fig 5.[7]

The initial substrate for the shunt is glucose-6-phosphate, formed by the action of hexokinase; the activity of the hexokinase in the lens thus controls both glycolysis and the hexose monophosphate shunt.

The hexose monophosphate shunt activity in the rat lens diminishes considerably as the animal ages.[46]

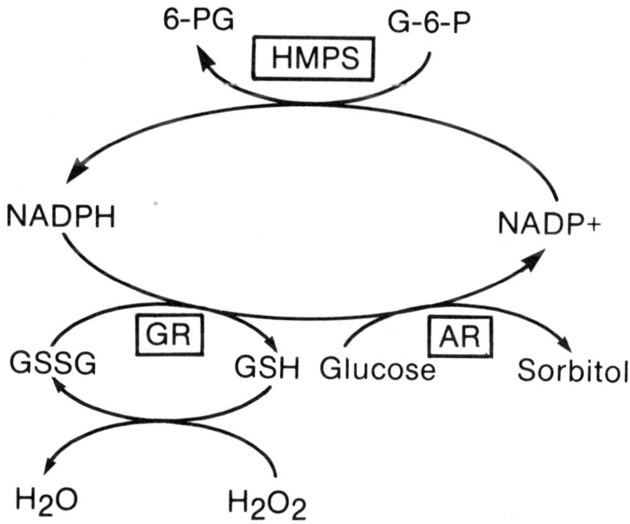

HMPS = Hexose monophosphate shunt
GR = Glutathione reductase
AR = Aldose reductase
G-6-P = Glucose-6-phosphate

6-PG = 3-Keto-6-phosphogluconate
GSH = Glutathione
GSSG = Oxidized glutathione

Figure 5. Schematic representation of the competition of aldose reductase and glutathione reductase for the cofactor NADPH. (From Barnett et al[7])

Control of lens glycolysis

Results obtained with rat, rabbit, and bovine lenses indicate that anaerobic glycolysis is the main source of biological energy required for the maintenance of lenticular function. Under physiological conditions, therefore, glycolysis must occur at a rate that will supply the necessary amounts of ATP without lowering the pH by excessive production of lactic acid, the principal end-product of anaerobic glucose metabolism. As shown by Lou and Kinoshita,[47] the precise control of lens glycolysis seems to reside with two enzymes, the hexokinase and the phosphofructokinase; the activity of the phosphofructokinase is regulated by the availability of ATP, and that of the hexokinase, by the level of its product glucose-6-phosphate. Therefore, when adequate supplies of ATP are available in the lens, excess ATP inhibits the phosphofructokinase, thus increasing the amount of its unused substrate fructose-6-phosphate. Because the equilibrium of the phosphohexose isomerase-catalyzed reaction favors the conversion of fructose-6-phosphate to glucose-6-phosphate, the latter accumulates and, in turn, controls the activity of hexokinase. Recent data suggest that the phosphorylating capacity of the phosphofructokinase decreases with age; in part, this may account for the decrease in glycolytic capacity with increasing age.[48] Other factors involved in the control of glycolysis are cyclic AMP,[49] phosphate ions,[49] and pyruvate kinase.[48]

Lens hexokinase has a high affinity for glucose. Because of the very low concentration of this enzyme, e.g., of 6.1 ± 0.5 mM in rat aqueous humor and of 0.55 mM in rat lens,[47] at physiological glucose levels, lens hexokinase is saturated and raising the glucose concentration in the blood or aqueous humor does not lead to increased glycolytic activity.[49] Therefore, in hyperglycemic states producing sugar concentrations above the binding capacity of the rate-limiting hexokinase, the intracellular sugar level is increased. The metabolic fate of this excess of sugar was not appreciated until Van Heyningen's[50] finding of high polyol levels in rat tissues, namely of sorbitol in alloxan-diabetic rats, of galactitol in galactose-fed rats, and of xylitol in xylose-fed rats. These observations eventually led to the demonstration of the presence of aldose reductase, the first enzyme in the polyol pathway, and its role in the disposition of excess sugar in a number of tissues.

Polyol pathway

The "sorbitol pathway"[36,51,52] or "polyol pathway"[53] involves two enzymatic reactions: in the first, glucose is reduced to sorbitol by the action of aldose reductase (AR)[54] using NADPH, and in the second, sorbitol is oxidized to fructose by the action of polyol dehydrogenase (PDH) using NAD^+:

$$\text{Glucose} + \text{NADPH} + H^+ \xrightarrow{\text{AR}} \text{Sorbitol} + \text{NADP}^+$$

PDH

$$\text{Sorbitol} + \text{NAD}^+ \xrightarrow{\text{PDH}} \text{Fructose} + \text{NADH} + H^+$$

In animal tissues, the polyol pathway was first found by Hers[55] in the seminal vesicles and placenta of sheep and later in the lens of rat and calf[50,56] and in human placenta.[57] Polyol pathway activity in the lens was established by Kinoshita et al[36] by showing that upon incubating intact calf lenses in a medium containing [6-^{14}C] glucose, the specific activities of the isolated glucose, sorbitol, and fructose were virtually identical.

A necessary component of the AR reaction is the coenzyme NADPH. The hydrogen transfer in the human placental aldose reductase catalyzed reaction was shown to be A-side stereospecific,[58] i.e., the pro-4R "A" hydrogen of the dihydronicotinamide ring of NADPH is transferred to the rectus (re) face of the carbonyl group. Aldose reductase is thus an A-type enzyme like liver alcohol dehydrogenase,[59] pig kidney L-hexonate dehydrogenase[60] and sorbitol dehydrogenase.[58]

Crabbe and colleagues have questioned the mechanism through which polyols are formed by aldose reductase and have challenged the NADPH utilization as an index of AR activity, since spontaneous monosaccharide oxidation can generate free radicals that can oxidize NADPH.[61–64] By such a mechanism the hexose would be oxidized to an α-dicarbonyl instead of being reduced to the corresponding polyol.[62] However, Kador et al[65] have conclusively demonstrated that in the presence of NADPH, highly purified rat lens aldose reductase indeed reduced glucose, galactose and xylose to the corresponding polyol sorbitol, galactitol and xylitol. Furthermore, the rates of polyol formation closely mirrored the Km values for the substrates obtained from kinetic measurements that monitored the rate of NADPH disappearance, and no polyol was detected in the absence of aldose reductase.

In the lens, the main source of NADPH is the hexose monophosphate shunt.[66] In the animal lens the hyperglycemia-induced activation of aldose reductase[67] increases the rate of $NADP^+$ production, that in turn, stimulates the hexose monophosphate shunt mechanism.[68] The formation of sorbitol in the lens exposed to high ambient glucose levels is thus favored by low hexokinase, high aldose reductase, and high hexose monophosphate shunt activities[66]; such an environment exists in the epithelium of the lens. The high AR activity and low polyol dehydrogenase activity found in the lenses of rats with alloxan-induced diabetes[69–71] and humans[71] favor lenticular polyol accumulation. In contrast to an earlier report,[67] activation of lens aldose reductase was demonstrated immunohistochemically in galactose-fed rats by using the peroxidase-antiperoxidase method with antibodies produced against purified rat lens aldose reductase.[72] A marked increase in AR activity was also observed in rats fed for five days on a 33% galactose diet.[73] In immunohistochemical studies with antibodies prepared against purified rat lens aldose reductase Akagi et al[74] demonstrated a striking increase in immunoreactive positive staining for aldose reductase in lenses from diabetic rats. The staining appeared beneath the epithelial region where water cleft formation occurred. The intensity of the staining increased with the formation of vacuoles. Similar increases in immunoreactive staining for aldose reductase (with antibodies prepared against purified human placenta aldose reductase) were also observed in the human diabetic lens. In cataractous lenses from diabetic patients, the increased immunoreactive staining for aldose reductase was associated with the presence of vacuoles in both the anterior and posterior superficial cortical layer. Kinetic evaluation of aldose reductase from diabetic lenses revealed no change in the affinity of the enzyme for substrate. These findings suggest that the increased AR activity occurring in diabetic tissues is due to increased amounts of enzyme, rather than to enzyme activation.

The AR activity in rat eye appears to be age-dependent, since a 67% increase was observed in the eyes of 23- to 26-month-old rats as compared with three-month-old animals.[75,76] However, sorbitol dehydrogenase activity in the lens was not age-dependent.[77] According to Williamson et al,[78] the capacity of the lens to accumulate polyols was markedly lower in castrated male rats, either diabetic or non-diabetic, than in intact animals used as control. The results suggest that rat lens AR activity is sex-dependent.

While the physiological role of the polyol pathway in the lens remains unknown, Kuck[52] has suggested that it may serve as a transhydrogenation system in which NADPH is utilized and NADH formed, as shown in Fig 6. Jeffery and Jörnvall[79] regard the polyol pathway as a way to bypass the control points of hexokinase and phosphofructokinase in the glycolytic pathway. Chylack and colleagues,[80,81] on the other hand, have pondered on a cyclical protective role of the polyol pathway, i.e., of counteracting short-lived extracellular, glucose-derived, osmotic stress with the intracellular production of osmotically active sorbitol.

The metabolic flux rate of the polyol pathway in the intact rabbit lens was also measured by [^{13}C]nuclear magnetic resonance spectroscopy.[6] The results demon-

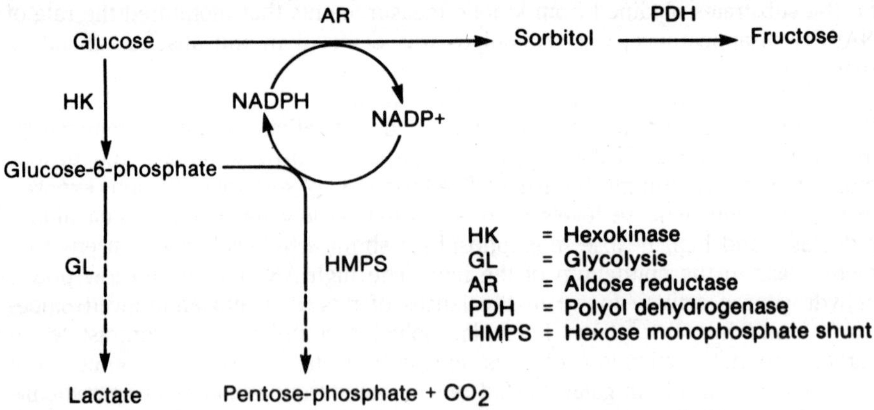

Figure 6. Schematic representation of the interdependence of aldose reductase and the hexose monophosphate shunt.

strated that in the lens exposed to 35.5 mM (640 mg/dL) glucose, the polyol pathway accounted for one-third of the total glucose turnover. The flux of glucose through the polyol pathway thus appears to be more substantial than indicated by polyol accumulation.[82] If this is the case, then a substantial amount of NADPH utilized by aldose reductase may be diverted from reactions in which it is normally used, e.g., by the glutathione reductase.[6–8] According to Lee et al,[83] NADPH levels in the lens decrease and $NADP^+$ levels increase during the first week of cataract formation.

Pathogenesis of sugar cataract

It has been known for quite some time that cataract formation can be induced in rats by feeding them a diet containing xylose[84,85] or galactose,[86–88] and in young diabetic rats, by maintaining blood glucose levels above 12 mM (225 mg/dL).[89] These cataracts are similar in appearance,[90] and in each instance, they develop faster if the condition is severe and if the rats are young.[86,91,92] In fact, adult rats fed on a 35% xylose diet do not develop cataracts[56] and regression of cataracts was observed within 60 days from the time of development of maximal opacity.[85] Since in all cases the blood level of the monosaccharide is elevated,[84] these cataracts are usually referred to as "sugar" cataracts.[50]

The reports that glucose and galactose acted in a synergistic manner [93] and that the two hexoses produce cataracts that are similar in development and appearance suggest that sugar cataracts are produced by a common mechanism.[92]

The formulation of a common cataractogenic mechanism was based on experimental data obtained independently by several groups of investigators.

In 1939, Gifford and Bellows[94] observed a marked increase in the weight and volume of lenses with mature cataract from rats fed on a 50% galactose diet for 27 days. The increase was tentatively attributed to the uptake of water, and the swelling attributed to an increase in osmotic pressure due to "splitting of lens proteins." The occurrence of a great number of vacuoles at various stages of sugar cataract development was regarded by Buschke[95] as strong evidence that osmotic disturbances play an important role in the pathogenesis of sugar cataracts.

In a histopathological study of the sugar (and x-ray) cataracts reported in 1955, Friedenwald and Rytel[96] observed that the earliest morphological change noted in the lens cortex in all types of experimental cataract was the appearance of hydropic lens fibers. Evidence was presented that the accumulation of fluid was intracellular, not extracellular. The hydropic cells ruptured and dissolved in the more advanced stages of cataract development, leading to interfibrillar clefts filled with protein coagulum, which are the common findings in established cataractous lens cortex.

At about the same time, Bounds et al,[97] in an ophthalmoscopic and histologic study of cataracts in alloxan-diabetic rats, described the appearance of vacuoles and swollen fibers under the epithelium or between the epithelium and capsule, their incidence increasing with the progression of cataract development. While the formation and progression of diabetic cataract were related to the severity of diabetes, the authors suggested that defective utilization of glucose may be responsible for the injury to the lens.

In 1957, Dische and colleagues[98] demonstrated that the increase in wet weight of lenses of galactose-fed rats is due almost exclusively to the uptake of water. The authors concluded that the swelling should result in disruption of the physical continuity of the content of lens fibers, thus favoring an increase in protein breakdown.

Of crucial importance was Van Heyningen's[50] finding in 1959 of polyol accumulation in the lenses of rats with sugar cataract induced by alloxan-induced diabetes or by feeding on diets containing either 35% xylose or 35% galactose. Sorbitol accumulated in alloxan-diabetic rats, xylitol in xylose-fed rats, and galactitol (dulcitol) in galactose-fed rats. In addition, Van Heyningen found that dialyzed extracts of rat lens reduced the aldoses glucose, galactose, and xylose in the presence of NADPH, and in turn, oxidized the polyols sorbitol, galactitol, and xylitol in the presence of $NADP^+$. Furthermore, in the presence of NAD^+, the lens extracts oxidized sorbitol and xylitol to the corresponding ketoses fructose and xylulose. The NADPH-dependent reduction of aldoses to polyols was first described by Hers,[54] who used extracts of seminal vesicles and placenta, and named the enzyme "aldose reductase." Van Heyningen's results were the first demonstration that the aldose reductase and polyol dehydrogenase enzyme activities are also present in the lens.

In 1961, Kuck[52] corroborated the presence of the polyol pathway in the lens by showing the formation of fructose in rat lenses incubated in glucose-rich medium. The formation of fructose proceeded via sorbitol as intermediate. In vivo, the amount of fructose formed in the lenses of alloxan-induced diabetic rats increased with the plasma glucose concentration and leveled off at about 12.6 nmol fructose per mg lens. Kuck concluded that "the enhancement of the sorbitol pathway may be a factor in cataract formation."

In 1962, Kinoshita and co-workers[99] integrated the histopathological findings of Friedenwald and Rytel[96] with the biochemical findings of Van Heyningen[50] and Dische et al[98] to postulate that the formation of hydropic lens fibers is due to the osmotic disturbance caused by the intracellular accumulation of polyols produced by the enzyme aldose reductase. The role of aldose reductase in the etiology of diabetic cataracts has been reviewed by Varma.[100]

The postulate of Kinoshita was illustrated by the classical biochemical experiment with lenses from rats fed on a diet of 50% galactose[99] which demonstrated that at every time point, the accumulation of water was proportional to the accumulation of galactitol (Fig 7). The first sign of opacities in the lens, observed after 10 days of access to the galactose-containing diet, was associated with an accumulation of 2.2 μmol of galactitol per lens and an increase in water content of 20% to 35%.[99]

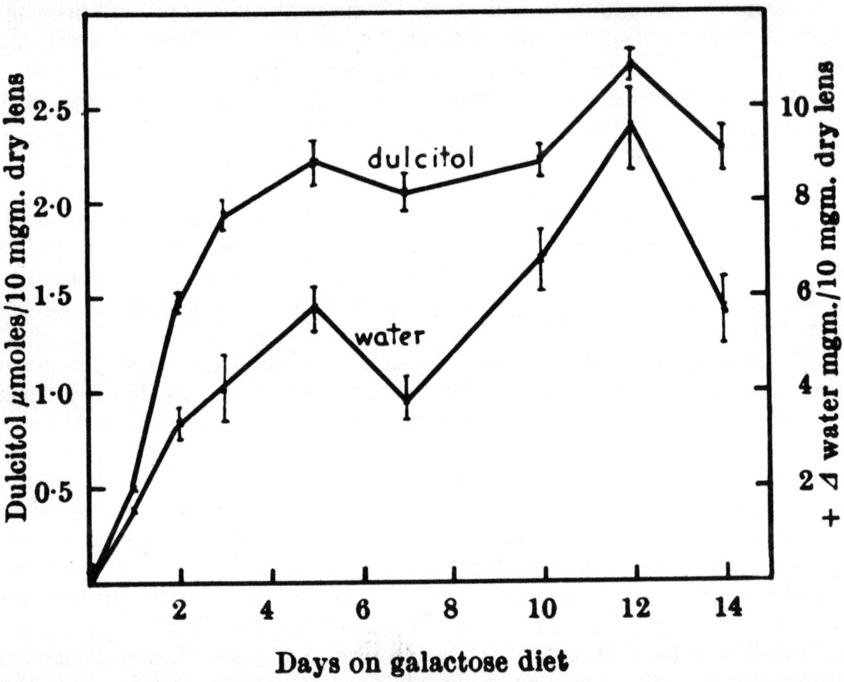

Figure 7. Accumulation of water and dulcitol in the lenses of galactose-fed rats. (From Kinoshita et al[99])

Subsequently, Kuwabara et al[101] used electron microscopy to investigate the morphological changes occurring in the lens of rats fed on a 50% galactose diet for 3, 7, and 10 days. The parallel development of morphological changes and water accumulation in the lens (summarized in Table 1) added strong support to the postulate that the process of sugar cataract formation is initiated by polyol-induced osmotic swelling.[99] In contrast to the finding by light microscopy that fluid accumulation was intracellular,[96] electron microscopy revealed that in addition to cellular swelling, extracellular cysts appear at the early stage.

Kinoshita's "osmotic stress hypothesis" of sugar cataract formation has stimulated numerous studies that have systematically added further support to the

Table 1. Summary of changes detected by electron microscopy in lenses of rats fed on a diet containing 50% galactose.[101]

Days of feeding	Stage	Changes
3	Vacuolar (reversible)	Small vacuoles in equatorial cortex; marked intercellular cyst formation in the superficial cortex of the equatorial and posterior zone; occasional liquefied anterior lens cells.
7	Intermediate vacuolar (partly reversible)	Enlarged intercellular cysts, coalesced into large vacuoles; severely vacuolated epithelial cells; droplets of liquefied lens protein; swollen posterior lens cells.
15	Advanced	Lens is densely opaque; whole corneal portion is liquefied opaque nucleus; markedly irregular anterior epithelium with proliferated cells; posterior lens is liquified and occupied by droplets containing fragmented cell membranes.

hypothesis. Of particular usefulness was the demonstration that many of the early lenticular changes occurring in galactose-fed rats can be duplicated in rabbit lenses incubated in vitro in a high-galactose medium.[102] The lens, being avascular, depends only on the surrounding media for its nutrition. Even though its metabolism is slow, the lens is an ideal tissue for studies in vitro, since the incubation can be carried out under nearly physiological conditions.[103,104] Thus, the fall in lenticular amino acid concentrations in rats fed on a 30% galactose diet[105] was reproduced in vitro and shown to be reversed when the osmotic effect of the accumulating galactitol was counterbalanced by a corresponding increase in the tonicity of the incubating medium.[106] The results demonstrate that the loss of amino acids in the lens exposed to galactose is due to the osmotic swelling produced by the intracellular accumulation of galactitol.

The events occurring in the galactose cataract have been summarized by Kinoshita[107] and are presented in Fig 8. The high systemic galactose concentration results in high galactose concentration in the lens, where it is converted by aldose reductase to galactitol. Because cell membranes are relatively impermeable to polyols,[108] once formed, galactitol accumulates, creating a hypertonic condition. To maintain osmotic equilibrium, water is drawn into the lens fibers. Even at the pre-vacuole stage, before changes in the lens become visible, osmotic swelling has deleterious effects, and the viability of the lens is reduced. The cataractogenic process is reversible only if the galactose load is decreased before membrane damage occurs. The increase in hydration markedly affects membrane permeability, resulting in loss of amino acids, myoinositol and potassium ions, and in a gain of sodium ions. Other secondary changes, such as cessation of protein synthesis and loss of key metabolites, cause opacification of the lens. The same sequence of events applies to sugar cataracts induced by diabetes or xylose feeding; the rate of

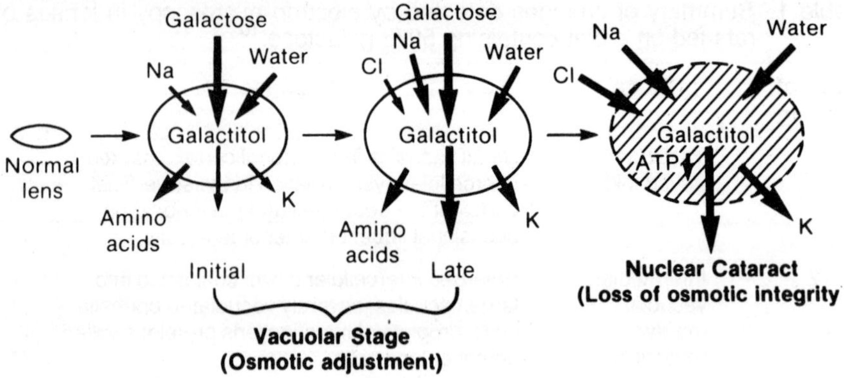

Figure 8. Changes that occur during development of a galactose cataract.[107]

cataract formation reflects the rate of enzymatic conversion of glucose and xylose to the corresponding polyols sorbitol and xylitol.

Supporting evidence for the critical role of aldose reductase in the pathogenesis of sugar cataracts was provided by reports that cataracts are not formed in the absence of aldose reductase in the lens[109,110] and that cataracts develop faster in the presence of higher lenticular aldose reductase activity.[111,112] Thus, no cataracts were detected by Kuck[109] in CFW mice either after 16 days of alloxan-induced diabetes or after access for 73 days to a diet containing 40% galactose. Absence of aldose reductase was also evidenced by the absence of polyols in mouse lens incubated in 1120 mM (20,178 mg/dL) glucose or galactose. Absence of cataracts was also reported by Varma and Kinoshita[110] in mutant strains of mice with congenital diabetes [C57B1/KsJ (db/db) and C57B1/6J (ob/ob)]: in animals with hyperglycemia for five to six months, in spite of a plasma glucose level of 12.5 $\pm$ 0.5 mM (225 $\pm$ 9 mg/dL), the lenses contained only about 1 nmol of sorbitol per mg lens. When mice with hereditary diabetes were given access to a 50% galactose-containing diet for six weeks, no signs of opacity were detected in lenses which contained only about 10 nmol galactitol per mg lens. For comparison, rats fed on a 50% galactose diet accumulate, within four days, lenticular galactitol at a level of 68.8 $\pm$ 2.8 nmol/mg ($\pm$SE)[113] and, within ten days, develop dense nuclear cataract.[114,115]

Similarly, no sorbitol accumulation occurred in the kidney of NSY mice with hereditary hyperglycemia,[116] while in the peripheral nerves of the mutant diabetic mouse strain C57B1/Ks (db/db), the sorbitol and fructose levels remained unchanged despite greatly increased glucose concentrations.[117,118] However, it is pertinent that in the same mouse strain, Robertson and Sima[119] found severely impaired motor nerve conduction velocity (MNCV) that was occurring almost simultaneously with the increase in blood glucose levels. In the early phase, the deficit was reversed by insulin treatment.

Combined, the experimental results demonstrate the absence or very low activity of aldose reductase in the lens, kidney, and peripheral nerves of mice, and there is a striking lack of sugar cataract.

The possibility that cataract formation in mice may be induced by combining feeding on a 50% galactose diet with x-irradiation was investigated by Kodama et al.[120] The unexpected finding of suppressed x-ray cataract development was attributed to the capacity of the accumulated galactose (due to the low levels of aldose reductase) to act as a free radical scavenger.[121]

In contrast to mice, the degu (*Octodon degus*), a rodent native to the Andes, develops nuclear lens opacity within 10 to 12 days of streptozocin-induced diabetes. The rapid rate of cataract development in the degu was associated with a lenticular AR activity three to four times higher than that in rat lens.[111] A similar observation was made in the Mongolian gerbil, another rodent with a lenticular AR activity twice as high as that in rat lens.[112]

For the human lens, analytical data on sorbitol and fructose levels in non-diabetic and diabetic subjects, though variable, demonstrate the presence of both metabolites.[122–126] A deleterious role for the polyol pathway in the human diabetic lens was initially suggested by Pirie and Van Heyningen.[122] The authors cautioned, however, that the lenticular levels of sorbitol and fructose may fluctuate in response to the fluctuating plasma glucose concentration and that the polyol levels in cataracts from diabetic subjects may be minimal, because of the leakiness of the cataractous lens.[127] Accordingly, Varma et al[128] reported a direct correlation between the plasma glucose concentration and the levels of sorbitol and fructose in the lenses of diabetic patients. Strong correlation ($r > 0.8$, $p < 0.005$) between sorbitol and fructose levels in human cataracts and fasting blood glucose as well as hemoglobin A1c levels was also reported.[129] Furthermore, incubation studies by Varma et al[128] and by Chylack et al[130,131] have documented the similarity in response of human and animal lenses to high glucose levels by showing that the adult human lens, clear or cataractous, at an increased load of 35.5 mM (640 mg/dL) glucose, is capable of producing in 24 hours 1 μmol of sorbitol and fructose per lens.

Prompted by reports of lower and deviant AR levels in human lenses[130,132–134] as compared with those found in animal lenses, Jedziniak et al[135] have evaluated the polyol pathway in the human lens at the enzymic level. The results show that the AR activity in the adult human lens is indeed lower than in animal lenses. However, because the enzyme is almost exclusively confined to the epithelium, the AR level present in the juvenile lens epithelium is capable of contributing an osmotic pressure of 380 m0sm* to 570 m0sm sorbitol per epithelium per 24 hours. Such osmolarity was shown to cause cataract formation in intact rabbit lenses.[136]

The accumulation of sorbitol in freshly excised lens from adult diabetic patients[128] was attributed to the age-related decrease in lenticular hexokinase activity found in man by Cheng.[138] The study has also shown that the human lens contains fructose, which can add to the osmotic stress. However, since polyol dehydrogenase was found to be approximately 30 times more active in the fructose to sorbitol direction than in the reverse,[135] it is likely that in the human lens, sorbitol rather than fructose may be an end-point.[139]

The finding of increased AR activity and decreased polyol dehydrogenase activity in human diabetic cataractous lens suggests that the changes brought about

---

*The accumulation of 1 μmol of solute per gram of tissue water is equivalent to 1 m0sm/L in osmotic pressure.[137]

by diabetic conditions favor lenticular polyol accumulation.[71] According to Jedziniak et al,[140] human diabetic cataracts are characterized by a 50% lower level of the isozyme PD-I, which is capable of responding to increased ionic strength. Under such conditions, the diabetic cataract would clear sorbitol less efficiently.

The critical role of aldose reductase in the pathogenesis of sugar cataract formation was supported by the use of inhibitors of aldose reductase, and will be described in Chapter 4.

ROLE OF ALDOSE REDUCTASE IN OTHER DIABETIC COMPLICATIONS

The demonstration of the critical role of aldose reductase in the pathogenesis of sugar cataracts inspired the concept that the polyol pathway may also be involved in the pathogenesis of diabetic complications in other tissues which, like the lens, are exposed to the fluctuating extremes of systemic glycemia caused by diabetes. The concept rests on the premise that excess glucose reaching such tissues is metabolized via the polyol pathway; hence it presupposes the presence of aldose reductase in such tissues.

Experimentally, the presence of aldose reductase in a given tissue can be demonstrated either by isolating and characterizing the enzyme in vitro, by locating it immunohistochemically, or by measuring its products to demonstrate its activity. As shown in Table 2 of Chapter 4, page 229, aldose reductase has been isolated from a variety of mammalian tissues. It was found histochemically in rat brain, spinal cord and sciatic nerve,[141] and immunohistochemically in the eye (lens, cornea, retina, conjunctiva, ciliary processes, optic nerve), the nerve (Schwann cell cytoplasm), the kidney (inner medulla, loop of Henle, collecting tubules, pelvic space epithelium), and the aorta and endothelial lining of muscular arteries (Chapter 4, Table 4, page 231). As discussed in Chapter 4, the activity of aldose reductase in the presence of elevated ambient sugar concentrations was demonstrated by measuring tissue polyol levels in such organs as the lens, sciatic nerve, kidney, retina, and red blood cells. A convenient method to demonstrate the presence of aldose reductase in a given organ is to enhance its activity by exposure to increased sugar levels, and then to elucidate the biochemical, functional, and morphological consequences by the use of AR inhibitors. Inhibition of aldose reductase may well be the best method for establishing the role of the polyol pathway in the pathogenesis of diabetic complications.

To implicate aldose reductase in the pathogenesis of a diabetic complication, based on the experience acquired with AR inhibitors in laboratory animals, Kinoshita[82,142] has formulated five general criteria that should be met in animal models of diabetic complications:

1. aldose reductase should be present;
2. the complication should occur in the galactosemic as well as in the hyperglycemic state;
3. the complication should occur earlier and be more severe in galactosemia than in diabetes;
4. the appearance of the complication should be prevented or delayed by inhibition of aldose reductase;

5. the effectiveness of AR inhibition should be corroborated by structurally distinct inhibitors of aldose reductase.

Based on these criteria, in addition to its critical role in the pathogenesis of sugar cataracts, aldose reductase has been implicated in the pathogenesis of diabetic neuropathy, corneal keratopathy, thickening of retinal capillary basement membranes, and diabetic nephropathy.

Neuropathy

The experimental evidence implicating aldose reductase in the pathogenesis of nerve damage in experimentally-induced diabetes and galactosemia in rats was recently summarized by Greene et al[31] as follows:

> "An array of interacting metabolic abnormalities in diabetic peripheral nerve that are attributable to hyperglycemia may provide a comprehensible basis for metabolically mediated alterations in peripheral nerve function and structure in diabetes. Primary among them is a sequence of defects involving increased polyol pathway activity, reduced MI uptake, reduced tissue myoinositol and impaired sodium-potassium ATPase activity. Although in themselves unlikely to explain the full range of clinical variability of diabetic neuropathy, these metabolic alterations may provide a basis for a conditioning influence of hyperglycemia on the development of diabetic neuropathy. To the extent that they do so, they become logical targets for present and future preventative and therapeutic strategies and are the rationale for much of the current research effort directed at diabetic neuropathy."

It is important to add that inhibition of aldose reductase has been shown by numerous independent groups of investigators to prevent polyol accumulation in the sciatic nerve in either diabetic rats[143–156] or galactosemic rats,[143,157–159] to prevent endoneurial sodium accumulation in galactosemic rats,[160] to prevent the fall of myoinositol in the nerve of diabetic rats[144–146,150,151,154,161] and galactosemic rats,[162] to prevent the impairments of the Na/K-dependent ATPase activity[161] and axonal transport,[144,150,151] as well as to prevent the decrease in nerve conduction velocity in galactosemic[163] and diabetic rats.[145–148,151,153,155,156,164]

Keratopathy

The involvement of aldose reductase in diabetic keratopathy rests on its presence in the corneal and conjunctival epithelium[165] and the corneal endothelium,[168] on the demonstration that a number of structurally distinct inhibitors of aldose reductase have abolished the delayed rate of re-epithelization of denuded corneas in diabetic and galactosemic rats,[167,168] and on the successful treatment of corneal keratopathy in a diabetic patient with an AR inhibitor.[169]

Retinopathy

The presence of aldose reductase in cultured retinal capillary pericytes[170] and retinal microvessels[171] was demonstrated by sorbitol accumulation upon incubation in high-glucose medium. The finding[172] of twice higher rates of protein and collagen synthesis induced by high glucose levels in bovine pericyte cultures suggests that hyperglycemia itself may have an etiological role in the early microvascular basement membrane thickening of diabetic retinopathy. The associated increase in sorbitol content but not the increased collagen synthesis was reduced by 55% upon adding 0.1 mM (23.7 μg/mL) sorbinil to the medium.[173]

The involvement of aldose reductase in the thickening of the basement membranes of retinal capillaries was demonstrated by preventing such thickening from occurring in rats fed on a diet containing 50% galactose and either one of two structurally distinct AR inhibitors, sorbinil, at a dose of 60 mg (253 μmol)/kg/day[174,175] or tolrestat, at a dose of 7 mg (20 μmol)/kg/day.[176]

The presence of aldose reductase in the choroid, retinal pigmented epithelium, and all retinal layers of alloxan-induced diabetic rabbits was indicated by the detection of elevated sorbitol levels associated with a 25% to 30% decrease in myoinositol content and reduced Na/K-dependent ATPase activity.[177]

Nephropathy

Aldose reductase was shown to be present in the inner medulla, Henle's loop, collecting tubules, and glomerular podocytes of the rat kidney[178,179]; in the interstitial cells, Henle's loop, and collecting tubules of the dog kidney,[180] and in human glomeruli.[181] According to Corder et al,[181] the enzymatic activities in human diabetic glomeruli revealed diminished hexokinase, elevated AR activity, and decreased sorbitol dehydrogenase. These changes, coupled with elevated serum glucose levels, suggest that the polyol pathway may be a contributing factor to the pathogenesis of human diabetic glomerulosclerosis via accumulation of intracellular sorbitol.

An interesting preliminary finding was reported by Bagnasco et al,[182,183] who observed that rabbit renal papillary epithelial cells, grown in hypertonic NaCl (300 mM), synthetize large amounts of sorbitol to balance the high extracellular osmotic pressure.[183] This was associated with increased AR activity. Upon return to isotonic medium, cell sorbitol fell due to its rapid efflux and decrease in AR activity.[182] It is pertinent that sorbitol, inositol, betaine, and glycerophosphorylcholine have been identified by Bagnasco et al[184] as the major osmolytes,[185] i.e., intracellular osmotically active organic solutes in renal inner medullae of rats and rabbits during antidiuresis. A six- to eight-fold increase in sorbitol content of the rat renal papillary tip during antidiuresis was reported by Wirthensohn et al.[186] The finding of high sorbitol levels in the renal inner medulla thus coincides with the presence of aldose reductase in rat renal papillae.[179,187,188]

In a preliminary report, Bauman and Farnsworth[189] suggested that sorbitol may be involved in sodium reabsorption.

Vascular permeability

Increased vascular permeability of newly formed vessels by angiogenesis in subcutaneous tissue was demonstrated by Kilzer et al[190] by measuring permeation of [^{125}I]albumin in streptozocin-induced diabetic rats. The increased vascular permeability was associated with a two- to three-fold increase in sorbitol levels and a 17% decrease in myoinositol levels. The involvement of aldose reductase was demonstrated by decreasing albumin permeation by 80% and preventing sorbitol accumulation with the AR inhibitor sorbinil added to the diet at a dose of 25 mg/kg/day.[191] The finding that inhibition of aldose reductase did not affect the solubility of collagen suggests first, that the diabetes-induced increases in collagen cross-linking are independent of the abnormalities in sorbitol/myoinositol metabolism and second, that the diabetes-induced vascular permeability changes are independent of collagen cross-linking changes. Since the changes in tissue levels of sorbitol and myoinositol[191] as well as the increase in vascular permeability were prevented by castration, Williamson et al[192] postulated that aldose reductase is sex steroid-dependent. Relevantly, administration of testosterone to castrated bulls produced in the seminal vesicles a five-fold increase in the activities of aldose reductase and sorbitol dehydrogenase.[193]

Subsequently, Chang et al[194] demonstrated that feeding rats for three weeks on diets containing 10% to 50% galactose increased [^{125}I]albumin permeation of the aorta and the vessels of the eye, kidney, sciatic nerve, and new granulation tissue analogous to that observed in diabetic rats. However, collagen solubility in the galactosemic rats was increased, in contrast to the decreased solubility observed in diabetic rats[191]; the observations virtually exclude the possibility that the differences in collagen solubility are linked to non-enzymatic glycation.[194]

The glucose uptake by the endothelial cells of large vessels is insulin-independent; the presence of aldose reductase was shown by the accumulation of glucose and sorbitol in human endothelial cells incubated in a medium containing 20 mM (360 mg/dL) glucose.[195] The intracellular accumulation of glucose and sorbitol may have osmotic consequences and account for the disturbed proliferation and other ill-effects of high glucose on vascular endothelium.

ALDOSE REDUCTASE AND HUMAN MUSCULAR DYSTROPHY

The postulate that the polyol pathway may play a key role in human muscular dystrophy was formulated by Ellis et al[196–198] on evidence that can be summarized as follows. Despite a six-fold increase in glucose content, caused by a selective leakiness of the dystrophic muscle membrane to glucose,[198] rather than following the normal glycolytic pathway, glucose in dystrophic muscle is converted to fructose via the polyol pathway. The sorbitol content in the dystrophic muscle rises six-fold, and that of fructose, three-fold as compared to normal muscle; moreover, there is a 13-fold increase in the activity of aldose reductase and a more variable 3.5-fold increase in polyol dehydrogenase activity.[197] Also, upon incubation of the dystrophic muscle with [^{14}C]glucose in the presence of the AR inhibitor tetramethyleneglutaric acid (TMG),[199] the metabolism of glucose was inhibited by 84%.[197] Relevantly, in the dystrophic muscle, the activity of the hexose monophosphate shunt is enhanced, thus providing the NADPH needed to sustain the increased activity of aldose reductase.

The shift of glucose metabolism in the dystrophic nerve from the glycolytic pathway to the polyol pathway is attributed to a dysfunction of the rate-limiting hexokinase. The dysfunction is caused by genetic alteration in the kinetic properties of the hexokinase isoenzyme II, which is characteristically abundant in skeletal muscle.[200] The net effect of the abnormal glucose metabolism in the dystrophic muscle is that one half the usual production of metabolic energy in terms of ATP is lost.

According to Ellis,[198] "an altered specificity of a hexokinase component may lead to a build-up of glucose within the muscle fiber from fetal life on, from which adaptation to less-efficient pathways brings about a downward spiral of energy metabolism which has the chronic effects associated with dystrophy." Of interest is the parallelism between the non-physiological intracellular abundance of glucose, its metabolic disposition by aldose reductase, and the ensuing complications occurring in chronic diabetes and in muscular dystrophy. In both situations, the abnormal disposition of glucose can be controlled by inhibiting the rate limiting aldose reductase.

The possible role of increased AR activity in muscular dystrophy in chicken was considered by Davidson and Murphy,[201] who have tentatively attributed the reported restoration of righting ability by treatment with diphenylhydantoin (phenytoin)[202,203] to inhibition of aldose reductase. In fact, aldose reductase was isolated from chicken breast muscle, and more AR activity was found in the breast muscle of the dystrophic birds than in controls.[204] The isolated enzyme was inhibited in vitro by the AR inhibitors alrestatin and sorbinil.[204,205] However, phenytoin possesses very weak intrinsic AR inhibitory activity, causing 31% inhibition at 1×10^{-3}M.[204] As expected, in vivo, in rats fed for four days on a diet containing 20% galactose, phenytoin had no effect on galactitol accumulation in the diaphragm, sciatic nerve, and lens upon addition to the diet at a dose of 145 mg/kg/day.[206]

OTHER POTENTIAL MECHANISMS

Non-enzymatic glycation of proteins

Over 90% of the protein present in the red blood cells (RBC) of human subjects is hemoglobin A.[207] Among the minor components of hemoglobin, the most abundant is hemoglobin A1c, which comprises 4% to 7% of the total hemoglobin.[208–210] Hemoglobin A1c is an aldimine, or a Schiff-base, i.e., a condensation product between a hexose and the amino group of the N-terminal valine residue in the β-chain of hemoglobin.[24,25]

Interest in hemoglobin A1c was aroused by the finding that its levels in diabetic patients were about twice as high as in non-diabetics.[211–213] Hemoglobin A1c is formed by the reaction between glucose and hemoglobin A, as originally proposed by Dixon[214] and corroborated and amplified by Bunn et al,[215] who demonstrated that the condensation between D-glucose and valine is followed by an Amadori rearrangement of the aldimine to a ketoamine. Subsequently, Bunn et al[26] postulated that the reaction is non-enzymatic, that hemoglobin A1c is formed slowly during the 120-day life-span of the erythrocyte, and that the levels of hemoglobin A1c should reflect the adequacy of glucose control in diabetics during that time period. Flückiger and Winterhalter[216] confirmed that the glycation of hemoglobin is non-enzymatic.

The usefulness of hemoglobin A1c as a clinical measurement was underscored by the following findings: first, in diabetic patients, the hemoglobin A1c levels and area under the curve of the glucose tolerance test are linearly correlated[217]; second, the hemoglobin A1c levels reflect the degree of carbohydrate control[218]; and third, after normalization of blood sugar, the hemoglobin A1c levels decrease at the rate proportional to the appearance of newly formed erythrocytes.[218] The measurement of hemoglobin A1c thus provides an objective, retrospective index of the control of hyperglycemia.[218–228]

In addition to its utility as a clinical measurement, the non-enzymatic formation of hemoglobin A1c has provided a conceptual basis for the pathogenesis of complications of long-term diabetes: if a protein such as hemoglobin can undergo glycation,[216] then other functional or structural proteins may also be modified by reacting with glucose available in abundance in diabetes.[217,218] Non-enzymatic glycation has been known for some time in food science as an intermediate step of the Maillard-reaction[229]: food proteins that are stored or heated in the presence of reducing sugars eventually become insoluble and have yellow and fluorescent products attached to them. In fact, the reaction of glucose (naturally present in foodstuffs) with amino groups of proteins accounts for the golden brown color commonly observed during cooking.[230] The interest in the possibility that such reaction(s) could also occur in diabetes was enhanced by the observation that in vitro the ketoamine can undergo, albeit very slowly, a series of further chemical reactions. However, as pointed out by Candiano et al,[231] most of the published results on foodstuffs and on model browning reactions have been obtained under non-physiological conditions and cannot be applied readily to biological systems. Yet, the authors have shown that under simulated physiological conditions, lysine can react with 2-amino-2-deoxyglucose, a hexose present at a fairly high concentration in the blood.[231]

The process of non-enzymatic glycation starts with the reaction between the open-chain aldehyde form of glucose and a free amino group on a protein (Fig 9). The rate and extent of reaction between an amine and a sugar carbonyl depends on the basicity (pK) of the amine and on the steric factors affecting its accessibility.[232] Since it involves a nucleophilic attack by a non-protonated amino group, the reaction is a function of the pK of the amine, hence is pH-dependent. Aldimine formation may become rate-limiting at pH values higher than the pK of the amine. Except for very weakly basic amines, aldimine formation may be rate-limiting under physiological conditions.[232,233] Practically, non-enzymatic glycation occurs primarily at intra-chain lysine residues.[29] Steric factors may affect glycation by controlling both the accessibility of the free amino group(s) to the sugar and the rearrangement of the aldimine to the ketoamine.[233,234] Once formed, the ketoamine is immediately stabilized by cyclic hemiacetal formation. By analogy to D-fructose, it is expected that about 75% of the cyclic hemiacetal would be in the β-pyranose form and about 21% in the β-furanose form.[232,235] High-resolution NMR spectra of the mutarotated N-(1-deoxy-D-fructos-1-yl)-L-amino acids in D_20 indicated 64% of β-pyranose, 15% of α-furanose, 15% of β-pyranose, and of 6% of α-pyranose forms.[193]

Under physiological conditions, glucose in solution exists mainly as the stable cyclic hemiacetal in pyranose form, in equilibrium with the open aldehyde form

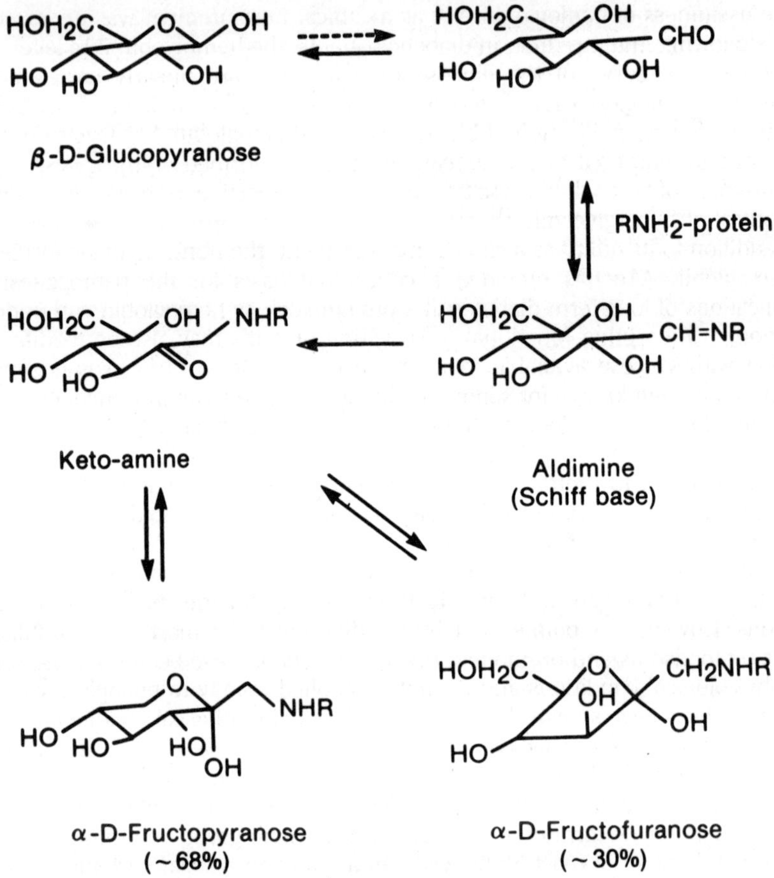

Figure 9. Reaction of glucose with proteins.

present at only 0.02%.[236] As shown by Bunn and Higgins,[237] various monosaccharides react with hemoglobin, with the rate of condensation dependent on the extent to which a monosaccharide exists in the open chain aldehyde structure. Of all the monosaccharides tested,[238,239] glucose has the most stable ring structure; hence it cannot readily react with a protein.[237] Supporting evidence was obtained in vitro with human albumin[240] and in vivo in rats fed on a high galactose diet.[241–243] Because of the lower stability of galactose in hemiacetal form,[236] in vitro, the extent of glycation of human albumin with galactose was three times greater than with glucose. Non-enzymatic glycation of lens crystallin in galactose-fed rats was at least twice as high as in normal rats and higher than in alloxan-[241] or streptozocin-induced diabetic rats.[242] Galactosemia in rats also resulted in elevated hemoglobin A1c levels.[243,244]

The relatively high stability of glucose in hemiacetal form thus allows high concentrations of glucose and proteins to coexist in various tissues, with a minimal risk of covalent bond formation.[237] However, based on the 4% to 7% content of glycated hemoglobin in non-diabetic subjects, it seems unlikely that aldimine formation in vivo involves only glucose in open aldehyde form.[29]

As discussed by Brownlee et al,[28] the aldimine is a relatively labile condensation product,[245] the rate of formation of which is approximately equal to its rate of dissociation. Over a period of weeks, however, the aldimine rearranges to the more stable ketoamine at a rate corresponding to approximately 1.6% of the rate of aldimine formation. The existence of two forms of glycated hemoglobin that are chromatographically indistinguishable was shown by Goldstein et al[246]: the chemically labile aldimine, which is acutely responsive to changes in blood glucose, and the stable ketoamine, representing 80% to 90% of the total hemoglobin A_{1c}, which does not appear to be altered by short-term changes in the blood-glucose level.

Although ketoamine formation is reversible,[247] the ketoamine accumulates until equilibrium is attained. Steady state ketoamine levels are dependent on the rates of glycated protein formation and elimination and on the protein life-span. The lower hemoglobin A_1 content in normal rats, about 1.5% as compared with about 4% in normal humans, probably reflects the 53- as opposed to the 120-day life-span of rat versus human RBC.[243]

Non-enzymatic glycation represents a relatively general post-translational modification of proteins, especially of proteins with slow turnover. Most proteins can therefore undergo glycation even at physiological sugar levels, the rate of glycation being increased in diabetic hyperglycemia. In proteins with a slow rate of turnover, the ketoamine may slowly undergo a series of other chemical reactions, such as dehydration, rearrangement and cleavage, resulting in vitro in highly cross-linked, insoluble, pigmented and fluorescent carbohydrate-protein polymers. Such reactions also occur during the aging of stored foods and are referred to as the "Maillard reaction,"[229] or "non-enzymatic browning."[248] The question arises whether the presence of glycated proteins and/or of potential final products of their additional structural modifications can affect normal cellular function, and if so, whether accumulation of such products can play a role in the development of some of the long-term complications of diabetes, and in aging.[249] Non-enzymatic glycation and the browning reactions were discussed in 1981 at a symposium organized by the Kroc Foundation, the proceedings of which were published in 1982.[250] Non-enzymatic glycation was reviewed recently by Kennedy and Baynes,[27] Brownlee et al,[28] Peterson and Formby[29] Wieland et al,[251] Vlassara et al,[30] and a monograph was written by Cohen.[252]

Currently available information on the subject will be considered in the following sections.

Red blood cell proteins

Glycation of hemoglobin occurs at ε-chain valine residues and ε-amino groups of lysine residues. Since the terminal valine plays a part in the binding site for 2,3-diphosphoglycerate, the physiological regulator of hemoglobin's affinity for oxygen, glycation of hemoglobin might contribute to pathology through an effect on oxygen affinity.[253] In vitro, the glycated hemoglobin A1c exhibits altered oxygen saturation curves and/or decreased sensitivity to the allosteric effects of organic phosphate.[254] In vivo, however, the higher affinity of hemoglobin for oxygen occurring in diabetic patients does not seem to depend on the degree of glycation.[255] Furthermore, the oxygen saturation curves of whole blood from normal and diabetic populations are essentially identical.[210,256] It is therefore unlikely that glycation of hemoglobin has any pathological effects.[27,257]

The proteins of the erythrocyte membrane are also subject to increased glycation in diabetes.[258–260] However, there is no evidence at present linking glycation with such abnormalities of the erythrocyte known to occur in diabetes as changes in deformability,[261] doublet formation,[262] and microviscosity.[263] Glycation of the integral membrane protein, which mediates glucose transport in RBC, has no effect on transport function under physiological conditions.[264] Based on results obtained in a study of the microrheologic characterization of deformability in the diabetic erythrocyte and of the dependence of deformability on cell age, Williamson et al[265] have concluded that none of the more substantive differences in membrane and hemoglobin glycation, cell volume, and lipid phosphorus content between diabetic and control cells significantly affects the viscoelastic properties of diabetic erythrocytes. In particular, glycation of its constituents appeared to be of no consequence to the rheologic erythrocyte behavior. Pertinently insulin infusion seems to improve erythrocyte deformability within hours.[266] Lowered erythrocyte membrane fluidity observed in IDDM patients was attributed by Watala et al[267] to non-enzymatic glycation of membrane protein.

Plasma proteins

Albumin

Human albumin is a single-chain polypeptide comprising about 60% of the plasma proteins. Because of its capacity to bind a great variety of ligands, albumin is considered a multifunctional plasma transport protein. Although larger than hemoglobin, albumin reacts with glucose with greater specificity.[233,234]

Non-enzymatic glycation of albumin[234,268,269] and of other plasma proteins[270] seems to provide an alternate index of control of glycemia during the preceding one to two weeks.[225,235,271–275] About 10% of albumin in normal human serum was reported to be glycated.[234] While fresh albumin from normal human subjects is glycated to the level of about 0.25 mol glucose per albumin,[276] the level is about three times higher in diabetic patients.[272,276]

Lysine residue 525 of human serum albumin[234] was reported to be the first lysine to be glycated.[277] Subsequent results suggested that, in addition to the lysine residues 525 and 199, other lysine residues must be modified in diabetic patients.[278] Based on a total of 59 lysines per human serum albumin molecule, Candiano et al[231] concluded that about 35% of the lysine residues on the surface of albumin are glycated. Approximately 33% of the overall glycation occurs at lysine 525[279] as well as at lysine sites 199, 281 and 439. The site specificity of glycation was attributed to localized catalysis of the Amadori rearrangement by positively charged basic amino acid residues.[279]

Glycation of albumin was shown to induce a conformational change accompanied by a considerably reduced affinity for α-parinaric acid, a C_{18}-chain fatty acid containing four conjugated double bonds and expected to bind to the strongest binding site for fatty acids.[280] The finding is compatible with an earlier observation that fatty acid-free albumin was more susceptible to reacting with glucose.[269] These results suggest a link between the sites of fatty acid binding and non-enzymatic glycation of albumin. However, glycation with up to 3 mol glucose per mol human serum albumin did not affect the binding of up to 2 mol palmitate.[281] The authors concluded that, even though glycation may induce a conformational change, the capacity of glycated albumin to bind and deliver a physiologically useful fatty acid remains unaffected.[281]

According to Ghiggeri et al,[282] the conformational status of albumin rather than its electrical charge appears to determine its handling by the kidney. The conclusion is based on the observation that the increase in the urinary excretion rate of albumin in diabetic patients correlated with an increase in free SH groups, which, in turn, correlated with the degree of glycation.[278] The authors imply that the hyperfiltration of albumin occurring in diabetic patients may be due to a glycation-induced conformational change of albumin.

A four-fold increase in glycated albumin levels was found in streptozocin-diabetic rats.[277] A similar observation was made in diabetic dogs.[283] In alloxan-induced diabetic dogs glycation of albumin increased its catabolic rate by 33% and decreased its half-life of elimination to 125 $\pm$ 6 hr as compared to 179.5 $\pm$ 5 hr calculated for non-diabetic dogs.[284]

A number of drugs usually taken by diabetic subjects had no effect on the non-enzymatic glycation of albumin in vitro[274]; however, aspirin was shown to decrease the extent of glycation of bovine serum albumin.[285,286] It has been suggested that, by proceeding faster, aspirin-induced acetylation of human serum albumin could decrease the extent of its glycation.[287]

Glycation was reported to alter the binding of bilirubin to albumin[288] and to decrease the binding of some acidic drugs.[269,289,290] The free fraction of phenytoin was found to be linearly related to the amount of glycated albumin thus indicating that, in IDDM patients, glycation reduces the extent of phenytoin binding.[291] However, in subjects with diabetes, we have observed no difference in the binding of tolrestat, an aldose reductase inhibitor, containing a free carboxylic acid function.[206]

Lipoproteins

Since no unique pathogenic factor has yet been implicated as the link between diabetes and the accelerated atherosclerosis affecting patients with diabetes, there is great interest in whether diabetes alters the interactions between the cellular elements of the vessel wall and the most atherogenic, low density lipoproteins (LDL). Among other factors, non-enzymatic glycation of LDL was investigated by Schleicher et al[292] and Witztum et al[293] and subsequently, by Lorenzi et al.[294] According to the latter, exposure of cultured human endothelial cells to 20 mM (360 mg/dL) glucose for up to 12 days affected neither the relationship between the degree of confluency of the monolayer and the extent of LDL degradation, nor the dose-dependent LDL uptake and degradation. However, seven-day pre-incubation of human LDL with 80 mM (1441 mg/dL) glucose decreased its uptake and degradation, particularly when the ketoamine was reduced. The authors concluded that the reactive ε-amino groups of lysine involved (together with arginine) in the recognition of human LDL by fibroblast receptors[295] are also important for the interaction of LDL with the receptors on the human endothelial cells.

According to Steinbrecher and Witztum,[296] incubation of human LDL for five to nine days with varying glucose concentrations resulted in great variability in degree of glycation, maximally 6% glycation being attained even with 200 mM (3600 mg/dL) glucose. However, the clearance by guinea pigs of intravenously injected LDL with 2% to 5% of lysines glycated was decreased from 5% to 25%. Since in some diabetics up to 5% of the lysine residues of isolated LDL can be glycated,[293] the authors suggested that glycation might also decrease the rate of LDL catabolism in human diabetics, thus causing an increase in plasma LDL levels.

Witztum et al[297] reported that in some diabetic patients the clearance of the glucitolyl-lysine adducts of LDL, i.e., the cyano-borohydride reduction products of the ketoamine adducts of LDL, was increased. It is pertinent that glucitolyl-lysine differs chemically from fructosyl-lysine, the glycated molecular species that appears to predominate in vivo.[257,298] Although an enzyme capable of generating reduced glucitolyl-lysine adducts in vivo is not known to exist, the authors have interpreted the rapid clearance as immune-mediated. Since borohydride reduction may alter protein structure, it is not surprising that the altered protein was treated as foreign.[29] According to Etchells et al,[299] glucitolyl-lysine adducts of LDL can be specifically bound to human adipocyte plasma membranes.

In contradistinction, Schleicher et al[300] found no effect of glycation on the metabolism of human LDL by human fibroblasts after three days of incubation with up to 1100 mM (19,818 mg/dL) glucose. By concluding that it is the chemical nature of a modification rather than the number of lysine residues that is recognized by the high-affinity receptor, the authors dismissed the usefulness of borohydride reduction of glycated LDL as a tool for studying the possible effect of hyperglycemia on LDL catabolism. Interestingly, Curtiss and Witztum,[301] by using mouse monoclonal antibodies to glucitolyl-lysine,[298] demonstrated in hyperglycemic diabetic subjects the presence of immunoreactive glucitolyl-lysine in plasma apolipoproteins A, B, C and E. The physiological significance of this observation remains to be determined.

Electrophoretic mobility of LDL was used by Sampietro et al[302] as index of LDL glycation. LDL electrophoretic mobility was increased in 36% of well-controlled and in 63% of poorly-controlled IDDM patients.

The results obtained with glycated LDL are still inconclusive, possibly due to the relatively low degree of 2% to 5% glycation usually present,[27] though higher values were reported by Jack et al,[303] i.e., 4.6 ± 1.0% in non-diabetic subjects and 9.4 ± 3.5% in diabetic patients. Internalization and degradation of glycated LDL does not differ from that of native LDL unless the modification exceeds 12 glucose molecules per mol apolipoprotein B. Since in diabetic patients only 0.6 to 2.0 mol lysine-bound glucose per mol apolipoprotein B was found as compared to 0.2 to 0.6 mol in normal subjects, this effect may not have relevance to diabetes.[304] The rate of catabolism of highly glycated, high-density lipoprotein was, however, accelerated. As pointed out by Kennedy and Baynes,[27] it is theoretically possible that in diabetic subjects even a slight increase in lipoprotein glycation may affect the rate of metabolism, thus inducing a gradual development of vascular disease.

Increased LDL glycation was also found in a group of relatively well-controlled IDDM patients. LDL glycation was more closely correlated with mean plasma glucose and plasma protein glycation than with hemoglobin $A1_c$.[305]

The potential relevance of non-enzymatic glycation to atherosclerosis was reviewed by Cerami et al.[306] Of interest is the finding by Barrett-Connor et al[309] of a statistically significant correlation between glycated hemoglobin with total and LDL cholesterol in non-diabetic subjects of both sexes.

Immunoglobulins

Incubation of purified human and rabbit immunoglobulin G (IgG) with glucose results in glycation concomitant with a marked decrease in complement-fixing capacity.[308] This decrease was observed at glycation levels comparable to those found in diabetic patients. The degree of glycation, expressed in mmol 5-hydroxymethylfurfural per mol IgG, ranged from 42 to 77 in normal, and from 59 to 310 in diabetic sera.[308]

Approximately 15 times more IgG and over 4 times more IgM was reported to be trapped by peripheral nerve myelin isolated from human diabetic subjects as compared with non-diabetics. This excessive high-affinity trapping was tenatively attributed to non-enzymatic glycation of the immunoglobulins.[309]

Other proteins

Ney et al[310] have demonstrated that human transferrin, α_2-macroglobulin, and fibrinogen undergo non-enzymatic glycation upon incubation with 20 mM (360 mg/dL) glucose for seven days. However, no difference in the function was detected between the glycated and non-glycated proteins. Thus, the rate and extent of iron binding were identical for both glycated and non-glycated transferrin; the clearance of methylamine-treated α_2-macroglobulin was identical for the glycated and non-glycated sample, and glycated fibrinogen had the same clotting time as control fibrogen. The discrepancy between the results obtained with glycated fibrinogen and those reported earlier[311] was attributed to the high glucose concentration [500 mM (9008 mg/dL)] and the 23-day incubation period used by Brownlee et al[311] compared with the three- to four-day half-life of fibrinogen. When fibrinogen was glycated in vitro to a glucose content of greater than 20 mol per mol fibrinogen, its clottability was inhibited by more than 90%.[312]

Lutjens et al[313] isolated glycated fibrinogen from human plasma: in non-diabetic subjects, 0.95 $\pm$ 0.17 mol glucose was bound per mol fibrinogen, and in IDDM patients, 1.33 $\pm$ 0.21 mol ($p<0.001$). Lysine was suggested as the site of glycation.

Sampietro et al[314] demonstrated non-enzymatic glycation of human platelet membrane proteins both in vitro and in vivo. Platelet proteins from poorly controlled patients with IDDM showed about four times higher glycation than platelet proteins from non-diabetics, thus exceeding the glycation of plasma proteins.

Glycated antithrombin III was found in the plasma of diabetic subjects,[315] and non-enzymatic glycation of human antithrombin III was reported to reduce its activity in vitro.[314,316,317] According to a recent report,[318] by improving the degree of metabolic control, the reduced antithrombin III acitivity in diabetic subjects was increased and correlated inversely with protein glycation. In contrast to antithrombin III, the slightly impaired activity of the α_1-proteinase inhibitor in diabetic patients is not due to glycation.[319]

Repeated injections of glycated plasma proteins into normal mice resulted in glomerular basement membrane thickening;[320] a similar preferential binding of glycated proteins to renal basement membranes was not detected in rats.[321] Therefore, a link between glycation of plasma proteins and their deposition along basement membranes is still tentative.[27]

The excretion of glycated proteins in the urine of diabetic subjects was reported to depend on the degree of renal damage, judged by the degree of proteinuria; while the excretion of glycated proteins was facilitated in diabetic patients with normal urinary protein levels, it was decreased in patients in proportion to the increase in proteinuria.[322,323] The preferential urinary excretion of glycated albumin was shown to decrease with age in normal subjects while in IDDM patients the decrease correlated with microproteinuria.[324]

While non-enzymatic glycation of alkaline phosphatase was detected in vitro,[325] no evidence was found for the occurrence of the ketoamine form of glycated alkaline phosphatase in vivo.[326]

In vitro, ribonuclease A underwent glycation at lysine sites 7, 37, 41 and 98. The associated decrease in enzymatic activity was attributed to modification of lysine 41 in the active site.[327]

Non-enzymatic glycation of extracellular granuloma tissue proteins was detected in STZ-diabetic rats with carrageenan-induced granuloma.[328] Coupled with the unexpected increase in free amino groups in diabetic granuloma, attributed to increased proteolytic activity, glycation could contribute to impairment of wound healing during diabetes.

Lens proteins

The crystallin of the human lens has a much longer life-span than other proteins in the body. It is synthesized in the epithelial cells, which then divide and transform into elongated fiber cells. Approximately 90% of the soluble protein within the fiber cells is crystallin. Since the lens never stops growing, i.e., adding layer upon layer of fiber cells around its core, the cells at the nucleus are believed to be as old as the lens itself, and a portion of the protein in the core of the lens may be as old as the individual. As it ages, human lens crystallin undergoes various post-translational modifications,[329–331] including non-enzymatic glycation.[241,242,332–340]

Non-enzymatic glycation of lens proteins was first demonstrated by Stevens et al[341] with bovine lens crystallin, which, upon incubation with [^{14}C)-labeled glucose (or glucose-6-phosphate), led with time to incorporation of radioactivity into acid-precipitable proteins. A similar increase was found upon incubation of rat lens crystallin. The concomitant opacification of the lens and its protection by reducing agents led to the hypothesis that glycation offers another possible mechanism for cataract formation by increasing the susceptibility of crystallin sulfhydryl groups to oxidation, thus inducing formation of disulphide-linked aggregates.[241,341] Results obtained in vitro with calf α-crystallin suggested that non-enzymatic glycation may facilitate such oxidation by unfolding the protein, thus exposing the sulfhydryl groups.[342]

This hypothesis was examined by several groups of investigators. Glycation of human lens crystallin was established by Garlick et al,[338] who demonstrated that the amount of crystallin monomers containing glycated lysine increases from 1.3% in an infant to 4.2% at 100 years of age. The extent of crystallin glycation in diabetic lenses was about twice as high as in normal lenses, ranging from 2.3% to 3.0% of crystallin monomers. However, the glycated lysine content of diabetic lens crystallin samples did not increase with age. Additionally, in contrast to the small extent of glycation (1% to 3% of total lysine residues) of either normal or non-diabetic cataractous human lenses reported by Pande et al,[332] markedly higher levels of glycated proteins were found in cataractous lenses from diabetic subjects.[336] Ansari et al,[333] however, found no correlation between glycation and sulfhydryl oxidation of protein fractions obtained either from normal, senile, or diabetic cataractous lenses.

That glycation of lens cortical proteins, but not of nuclear proteins, is significantly higher in the diabetic as compared with the non-diabetic patients with senile cataract was reported by Lee et al[339] and confirmed by Liang et al.[340] The finding implies that, in adulthood, the lens nucleus may not be exposed to as much metabolic variation as the cortex.[339]

Compared to albumin and hemoglobin, the rate of glycation of human lens crystallin is exceedingly slow. Thus, in contrast to human albumin, which with a 19-day half-life is 7% to 12% glycated[234,235] and hemoglobin, which with a life-span of 120 days, is about 7.5% glycated,[343] human lens crystallin contains only 2.7% glycated lysine[338] despite its very much longer residence time in the body. The difference is attributed to the six times lower glucose concentration in the lens as compared with that in plasma or erythrocytes, to the low degree of conformational flexibility imposed by the tightness of packing, and to the lower lysine content of the crystallins as compared with that of hemoglobin and albumin.[338]

Liang et al[340] have found that in human diabetic lens, about 80 years of age, the extent of glycation in α-crystallin was approximately two to four times that observed in β- or γ-crystallin. The authors concluded that the extent of glycation depends on the accessibility of the lysine residues which, in turn, is determined by the conformational flexibility of the protein.

Chiou et al[242] showed that glycation of lens protein was not involved in the initiation of sugar cataract formation in rats fed on a 50% galactose diet when cataract development was prevented by treatment with the AR inhibitor sorbinil[143] The fact that the same amount of glycated lysine was found in both galactosemic rats with cataracts and in galactosemic rats treated with an AR inhibitor and having no cataracts, excludes the possibility that glycation of lens proteins plays a role in the initiation of sugar cataract.[27,335]

Glycation was also found to occur in the human lens capsule and was significantly greater in subjects with diabetes.[337] The lens epithelial basement membrane is formed very early during the embryonal development and remains intact as lens capsule throughout life. It is unknown whether glycation of lens capsule can be considered a degenerative process playing a role in cataractogenesis.

Neural proteins

Increased glycation was found in the peripheral nerves of 3-month alloxan-induced diabetic rats and of 60-month experimentally diabetic dogs.[344] Subsequently, a five-fold increase in glycation was noted in myelin isolated from the peripheral nerves of 3-month alloxan-induced diabetic rats, and a four-fold increase was detected in myelin isolated from whole brain.[345] Glycation was also found in peripheral nervous tissue[346] obtained post mortem from diabetic and non-diabetic subjects.

Renal proteins

Fibronectin is a major component of the glomerular basement membrane and mesangium and serves as an adhesion protein, primarily for cells of mesodermal origin as well as for other cell types, e.g., for epithelial cells. In diabetes, fibronectin is increased, both in the mesangial matrix and in the capillary walls.[347] According to Tarsio et al,[348] glycation of fibronectin is increased 2.3-fold in dogs with alloxan-induced diabetes as compared with age-matched controls. In vitro, time-dependent non-enzymatic glycation of human plasma fibronectin was shown upon incubation in 500 mM (9008 mg/dL) glucose. Glycation occurred only on lysine residues.

A 25% increase in 5-hydroxymethylfurfural (derived from glycated proteins subjected to acid hydrolysis) was reported to occur in the renal glomeruli of 8-week streptozocin-induced diabetic rats. No difference from matched controls was detected after two weeks of experimental diabetes.[349]

Uitto et al[350] have reported that glycation of glomerular basement membrane isolated from human kidneys was about twice as high in patients with diabetes than in non-diabetic subjects. However, there were no differences in the relative content of hydroxylysine-0-glycosides in glomerular basement membrane collagen between diabetic and control samples. In addition, the amino acid composition of glomerular basement membrane collagen isolated from diabetic and control kidneys was similar; in particular, no marked differences were detected in the degree of hydroxylation of the lysyl or prolyl residues. The enzymatic hydroxylation and glycation of the glomerular basement membrane collagen is thus unaltered in diabetes. The authors speculated that glycation could stabilize the intermolecular cross-links of collagen, thus possibly increasing resistance to proteolysis, and by decreasing solubility, prolonging the turnover of basement membrane collagen. However, in bovine retinal capillary cultures incubated in glucose-rich medium, the increase in non-enzymatic glycation was accompanied by increased solubility.[351]

Similarly, Trueb et al[352] have found 1.7 times higher degree of glycation of Type IV collagen in kidneys of patients with long-term diabetes as compared with kidney collagen from sex- and age-matched controls. The 1 to 2 residues of hexose per triple helical molecule were regarded as insufficient to affect the function and turnover of Type IV collagen, unless they were bound to a crucial site on the collagen molecule. Non-enzymatic glycation of collagen was therefore considered by the authors as a consequence of the metabolic disturbances rather than as a cause of the late complications of diabetes.

A 34% to 40% increase in glycation of renal tubular basement membrane was found in genetic diabetic mice as compared with non-diabetic controls.[353]

Collagen

Collagen, the major extracellular component of connective tissue, represents a family of glycoproteins that contain galactosyl and glucosyl-galactosyl residues attached to hydroxylysine.[354] Attachment occurs through an 0-glycosidic linkage, which is catalyzed by the collagen galactosyl transferase and collagen glucosyl transferase. Collagens are likely to be good substrates for non-enzymatic glycation, first, because they are rich in lysine and hydroxylysine, and second, because collagens are characterized by an unusually slow rate of turnover, estimated to correspond to a half-life of about 2.5 years.[355]

Because collagens are continuously exposed to glucose in the vascular and extravascular fluids, glycation may be expected to occur. Accordingly, glycation of aortic[356] and glomerular[357] basement membrane collagens was found in normal rats and was increased upon induction of diabetes with streptozocin. Glycation of collagens from human diaphragmatic tendon[358] and skin[359] was found to increase both with age and with the presence of diabetes. Samples from young diabetic patients gave values in the range of those of older non-diabetics.[360] However, according to Vogt et al,[346] who have measured the level of glycation in a variety of tissues obtained post mortem from diabetic and non-diabetic subjects, the levels of bound glucose in tendon, aorta, coronary artery, peripheral nerve, lung parenchyma, and glomerular basement membrane were, on the average, at least twice as high in diabetic as compared with non-diabetic subjects.

That collagen from normal non-diabetic subjects becomes less soluble and less susceptible to enzymatic digestion with advancing age[359,361] was attributed to the gradual formation and increasing stabilization of cross-links between and within collagen molecules.[362] In diabetic subjects a marked premature increase in collagen resistance to pepsin and collagenase digestion was observed.[359,363] However, results obtained with human skin collagen in vitro suggest that increased ketoamine formation by glycation has no effect on collagen resistance to digestion by collagenase.[364]

Kohn et al[365] reported that incubation of rat-tail tendon fibers with glucose, glucose-6-phosphate, or ribose resulted in a prolonged breaking time, similar to that occurring with aging. The authors attributed the age-like changes in collagen to the cross-linking associated with non-enzymatic glycation. Glycation of collagen followed by cross-linking was shown to alter normal stability of collagen fibers from rat tail tendons.[366]

Kent et al[369] described a readily controlled model, using rabbit forelimb tendons, for the study of the chemistry of the changes induced in collagen by non-enzymatic glycation, such as increases in hydrometric tension, increased amounts of polymeric collagen and decreased solubility.

Based upon examination of physicochemical parameters in vitro, Guitton et al[368] reported that non-enzymatic glycation of acid-soluble collagen (extracted from rat tail tendon) introduced no structural modification detectable by circular dichroism with up to 5% substituted lysine or hydroxylysine residues per molecule. The authors concluded that the addition of glucose did not interfere with the molecular structure of collagen and that the additional hydrophilic functions are not sufficient to disturb the hydrogen bonding involved in triple helical stability. However, close packing of fibers is expected to be less effective when collagen is glycated.

Based on a 2.7 times higher level of glycated collagen isolated from sheep carotid arteries as compared with that from the jugular veins, Davis and Stehbens[369] concluded that blood glucose concentration may not be the only factor controlling non-enzymatic glycation of vascular collagen. Interestingly, the level of glycation of arterial collagen was higher than that of the collagen from venous tissue damaged by surgical arteriovenous shunt. The finding does not support the view that the link between increased systemic sugar levels and vascular complications of diabetes is mediated by the degree of non-enzymatic glycation.

Preliminary experiments reported by Le Pape et al[370] suggest that, in diabetes, human placentae contain both collagenous and non-collagenous materials with increased platelet-aggregating potency. Both materials had higher levels of ketoamine linked glucose.

Hamlin et al[363] reported an apparently accelerated "aging" of tendon collagen obtained from insulin-dependent diabetic as compared with non-diabetic subjects. The observation was attributed to alteration of the properties of diabetic collagen in ways that simulate accelerated aging. In accordance with this "aging" phenomenon, the absorbance and fluorescence of solubilized dura collagen samples from insulin-dependent diabetic patients were reported to correspond to the amounts of pigment found in samples from much older subjects.[371] The formation of such pigments was attributed to "browning" reactions of the non-enzymatically glycated proteins.

The collagen-linked fluorescence (excitation at 360 nm and emission at 454 nm) found by Monnier et al in 41 IDDM patients[372] and thought to be derived from glycated collagen by the "browning" reactions, was shown to be associated with the severity of diabetic complications, particularly with retinopathy.[373] It is pertinent that in the same group of diabetic patients no correlation was found between the mean level of reduced Amadori products, i.e., ϵ-glucitolyl-lysine, and age, diabetes duration, or severity of retinopathy, nephropathy, arterial stiffness, and joint stiffness.[374] It is therefore likely that, per se, Amadori adducts, i.e., ketoamines, are not involved in the pathogenesis of diabetic complications. Evidence supporting this view is the finding that, along with reversal of the Amadori rearrangement, Amadori adducts undergo oxidative cleavage between C-2 and C-3 of the fructosyl-chain to give ϵ-carboxymethyl-lysine and erythronic acid.[375] ϵ-Carboxymethyl-lysine was detected in hydrolysis of lens protein from a patient with NIDDM as well as in hydrolysates of tendon collagen. The finding suggests that oxidative cleavage may have a role in limiting the consequences of protein glycation in the body.

To explain the resistance of some diabetic patients to retinopathy, Monnier et al[376] have postulated the existence of mechanism(s) that either prevent excessive "browning" of collagen, or are efficient in removing the modified collagen.

In absence of a specific test for non-enzymatic "browning" products, other mechanisms of collagen-linked fluorescence formation must be taken into consideration.[373] In fact, Jones et al[377,378] have found similar fluorescence properties in serum IgG and albumin of diabetic patients and have attributed such protein-linked fluorescence to more immediate free-radical-induced oxidation rather than to long-term cumulative glycemia.[379] The formation of fluorescent monomeric and aggregated IgG in vivo was also found in fresh rheumatoid sera and synovial fluid by Lunec et al.[380] The authors believe that fluorescence formation (excitation at 360 nm, emission at 454 nm) specifically characterizes free-radical-induced damage to any protein. The extent of the fluorescent "damage" would then seem to be related to the periodicity of and content of aromatic amino acids within the protein.

Buckingham et al[381] detected increased glycation of collagen in the skin of children with poorly controlled insulin-dependent diabetes who had joint contractures. No comparison was made with diabetic patients free of joint limitation. However, when Lyons and Kennedy[382] directly compared the extent of skin collagen glycation in IDDM patients with and without limited joint mobility, no significant difference was detected. This finding does not support the concept that non-enzymatic glycation, at least as reflected by the ketoamine link, is central to the development of limited joint mobility.[382]

Keratin

Keratin, a hard and insoluble fibrous protein (scleroprotein), is the principal constituent of epidermis. The stratum corneum, the superficial horny layer of human epidermis acting as principal defensive barrier, consists of several layers of dead epithelial cells completely filled with keratin. Keratin proteins in the hair[383] and stratum corneum[384,385] were shown to undergo non-enzymatic glycation. The degree of keratin glycation in the stratum corneum of the sole of diabetic subjects was related to diabetic control.[385] It was hypothesized that alterations in non-enzymatic glycation of keratin might be associated with changes in the physical properties in the superficial layers of the skin.[385] The levels of furosine, the acid-hydrolysis product of fructose-lysine derived from hair, were found to be significantly higher in diabetic patients than in healthy subjects, and correlated with hemoglobin A_1 levels.[386] Approximately 2.6 times higher furosine levels were found in the nails of patients with NIDDM as compared with non-diabetic controls.[389] The furosine levels were significantly higher in patients with background ($p<0.05$) and proliferative retinopathy ($p<0.01$) than in those without retinopathy.

Quantitation of non-enzymatic glycation

Measurement of non-enzymatically glycated proteins has been critically reviewed by Duncan and Heiss,[224] and comprehensive reviews of the available methods for glycated hemoglobin measurements have been prepared by Goldstein et al.[388,389]

In all currently available procedures, only the ketoamine adducts are determined.[27,28] Among the several methods proposed to measure the ketoamine adducts,[335] the most widely used is the thiobarbituric acid procedure[343] originally developed by Flückiger and Winterhalter[216] for the quantitation of hemoglobin glycation: the 1-deoxyfructosyl-protein adduct is hydrolyzed to 5-hydroxymethylfurfuraldehyde, which forms an adduct with thiobarbituric acid that is measured colorimetrically. Very careful standardization is essential to obtain reproducible results.[390] Other methods for the determination of ketoamine adducts are based on the fluorimetric quantitation of formaldehyde formed by periodate oxidation[391]; on the analysis of furosine formed upon vigorous acid hydrolysis[276]; on the ability of ketoamines to act as reducing agents in alkaline solution[392–398] ("fructosamine test"), and on the reaction with phenylhydrazine.[399] Among these tests, the determination of serum fructosamine is used by many investigators because of its simplicity, reproducibility, and good correlation with hemoglobin A1c levels.[400–403]

An affinity chromatography system is now widely used[303,404–409] to separate the ketoamines, which are characterized by the presence of vicinal diols and hence react with *m*-aminophenyl boronic acid.[410] Separation is also achieved by anion exchange chromatography with boronate buffers.[233] A fully automated, high performance liquid chromatography method for hemoglobin A1c determination was introduced for use in the multicenter Diabetes Control and Complications Trial.[411] According to Shah et al,[412] glycated hemoglobin measured by the thiobarbituric acid procedure more accurately represents the ketoamine linked sugar, is less subject to handling artifacts, and more accurately reflects the blood glucose values during the preceding four weeks.

Greater sensitivity and accuracy is provided by radiochemical methods based on the reduction of the ketoamine adduct with tritiated borohydride, followed by hydrolysis and chromatography.[343,413] Usually, only data from identically treated normal and diabetic or galactosemic samples were compared[241,242]; however, with appropriate standards and controls, the method can be used for absolute quantitation of glycation.[27]

A specific method for the quantitative determination of plasma glucitol-lysine, the stable, chemically reduced glucose/lysine adduct, has been described by Schmid et al.[414]

While several methods are available to measure the initial condensation products of glucose and a protein,* direct quantitative detection of the accumulated chemically defined end-products of subsequent reactions is at present not possible.[28] Development of such procedures will be essential for evaluating the relevance of these compounds to the complications of long-term diabetes.[27] According to Candiano et al,[416] the browning products react with a diazonium salt and produce a chromophore with maximal absorbance at 490 nm. Diazonium salts may, therefore, be useful to detect "late" products of glycation.

*According to Trueb et al,[415] the test most frequently used, i.e., incubation of isolated proteins with radioactively labeled glucose, can lead to erroneous results, due to the presence of radioactive impurities which bind covalently to proteins.

Recapitulation

Non-enzymatic glycation, the chemical reaction between a sugar and an accessible free amino group on a protein, is a common post-translational event. The extent to which glycation occurs in vivo depends on the levels of systemically available sugar, the number of accessible free amino groups, and on the time during which a protein is exposed to the sugar levels which, in turn, is influenced by the biological half-life, or turnover, of the protein. While glycation occurs very slowly, particularly with glucose, the ketoamine(s), the relatively stable products of glycation of most proteins, can be detected in normal healthy subjects. Since some of them are distinctly increased in the presence of excessive glucose levels, as in diabetes, their measurement provides a convenient test for the assessment of glucose control achieved over the lifetime of the glycated protein examined. The measurement of glycated serum protein or the glycated hemoglobin test provide information about the degree of intermediate (two to three weeks) and long-term (six to eight weeks) glucose control that is not otherwise obtainable in the usual clinical setting.[417,418] By providing improved means of assessing cumulative hyperglycemia, the non-enzymatically glycated protein markers afford significant advantages over the classical measures of hyperglycemia.[29]

Since the accessible amino groups of any protein can potentially interact with a sugar, and since glycated protein can undergo additional chemical reactions, there has been much speculation concerning the potential effect of non-enzymatic glycation on the function of a given protein and its involvement in the development of chronic diabetic complications, especially in tissues not requiring insulin for glucose uptake.[419] Currently available evidence is not sufficient to establish a link between non-enzymatic glycation and either functional or morphological alterations associated with chronic diabetes in man. Thus, though attractive, the hypothesis that non-enzymatic glycation of proteins produces important functional consequences still needs testing.

Myoinositol metabolism

Originally, interest in myoinositol was stimulated by the report that it may be an essential dietary factor for the growth of the mouse.[420] Of the nine possible stereoisomers of hexahydroxycyclohexane, myoinositol greatly predominates in biological systems and is thus the isomer of primary metabolic and functional interest.[421]

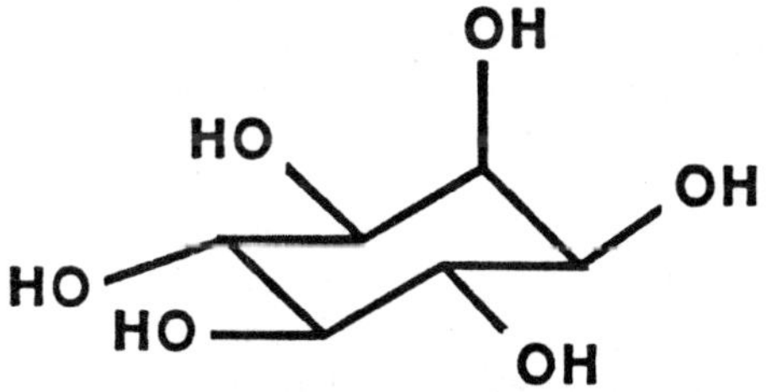

Myoinositol

In animal tissues, myoinositol (inositol) exists mainly in its free form and as part of the polar headgroup of three myoinositol-containing phosphatides: phosphatidylinositol [1,3-sn-phosphatidyl)-D-myoinositol], phosphatidylinositol-4-phosphate or diphosphoinositide, and phosphatidylinositol-4,5-biphosphate or triphosphoinositide. They are highly active metabolically. Most of the polyphoinositides are in the plasma membranes.[421]

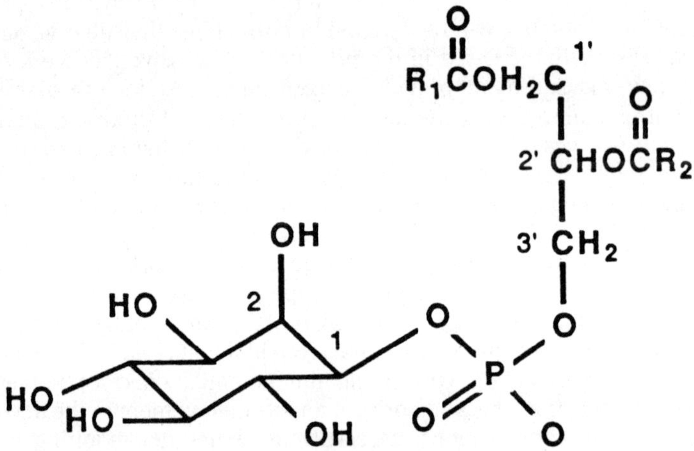

Phosphatidylinositol

The predominant phosphatidylinositol species isolated from almost all mammalian tissues is the 1-stearoyl-2-arachidonoyl derivative.[422]

In many tissues, the turnover of myoinositol containing phospholipids is increased by hormones and neurotransmitters.[423–425] The interaction of these agonists with their receptors is believed to activate phospholipase C, which catalyzes the hydrolysis of phosphatidylinositol and/or its phosphates. Hydrolysis of phosphatidylinositol diphosphate produces diacylglycerol and inositol triphosphate. There is now compelling evidence that both cleavage products are second messengers:[426] inositol-1,3,5-triphosphate, for the release of calcium from the endoplasmic reticulum[427] and diacylglycerol, for the activation of a Ca/phospholipid-dependent protein kinase, also known as "protein kinase C."[428,429] It seems likely, therefore, that activation of protein kinase C results from the synergistic actions of increases in the intracellular concentrations of both Ca^{++} and diacylglycerol. It is likely that protein kinase C is involved in many functions in the nervous system.[429]

The metabolism and function of myoinositol and inositol phospholipids was recently reviewed by Holub,[430] and the role of inositol triphosphate and diacylglycerol in intracellular signaling, by Berridge.[431]

Although myoinositol is an essential growth factor for most mammalian cells in tissue culture,[432] myoinositol deficiency states have not been observed in man. Actually, as shown by Clements and Diethelm,[433] the normal human kidney synthesizes daily about 4 g of myoinositol as compared with a usual dietary myoinositol intake of about 1 g per day.[434] Since the average daily myoinositol turnover of 9.8 g is considerably greater than the sum of myoinositol ingested with the diet and that produced by the kidney, in man, as in the rat,[435] extra-renal tissues contribute substantially to the endogenous formation of myoinositol.

Most mammalian tissues maintian free myoinositol concentrations that are much higher than those in plasma.[436] In the rat, for example, the mean tissue/plasma gradients are as high as 30, 84, and 106 for the sciatic nerve,[437,438] pituitary and thyroid glands,[436] respectively. The existence of this very considerable concentration gradient of free myoinositol between the tissues and plasma implies a considerable permeability barrier to intracellular free myoinositol in the cell wall.[436] The high concentration of myoinositol in tissue cells can be contrasted with glucose, for which a concentration gradient between tissues and plasma has not been found. Since the transport of myoinositol from the plasma into the tissues can occur against a large concentration gradient, at least part of the tissue myoinositol is of dietary origin.[436]

While it is clear that tissue myoinositol is regulated, the physiological role of the high myoinositol levels normally maintained in most tissues has eluded clarification. In view of the low affinity [Km, 1.5 mM[439]; 2.5 mM[440]] of the cytidine-diphosphate diacylglycerol:inositol transferase for myoinositol, it has been suggested that a high concentration gradient may facilitate the incorporation of myoinositol into membrane phospholipids[434] and that the normally high myoinositol levels serve to permit rapid turnover of phosphatidylinositol, thus functioning in metabolic regulation[433,441] through changes in Na/K-ATPase activity.[442]

Lens

The levels of myoinositol found by Van Heyningen[443] in the mammalian ocular lens, ranging from 2.6 nmol/mg in the rat to 25.7 nmol/mg in the sheep and human, were higher than in any other tissue. Myoinositol is also the largest free polyol component of human lens tissue, ranging (in nmol/mg lyophilized lens) from 11 to 104 in non-cataractous lenses, from 16.5 to 126 in uncomplicated senile cataractous lenses, and from 38.5 to 159 in senile cataractous lenses from diabetic patients.[126]

A marked fall in rabbit lens myoinositol occurred when cataracts were produced by x-rays. A similar decrease in lens myoinositol levels was also found in senile human cataract (19.2 nmol/mg) when compared with normal human lens (32.9 nmol/mg).[444] The inverse relationship between lens myoinositol and glucose levels in senile human cataracts was originally observed by Van Heyningen and Pirie.[122]

As shown by Wada and Tsumita[445] in Fisher 344 rats, lenticular myoinositol levels increased rapidly during the first seven months of age and reached a plateau level of 148 nmol/lens. With the appearance of senile cataract at 32 months of age, the myoinositol fell to 21 nmol/lens and corresponded to the intensity of turbidity.

An active transport and slow efflux of myoinositol and the presence of a myoinositol specific transport mechanism in the lens was shown by Cotlier[446,447] and by Varma et al.[448]

The loss of myoinositol from the cataractous lens of galactosemic rats, first reported by Stewart et al,[449] was accompanied by very high galactitol levels; conversely, rats fed on a 40% galactose diet and then changed to galactose-free diet, showed in the lens a decrease in galactitol and an increase in myoinositol levels. The finding was corroborated in rats made diabetic with alloxan or fed 40% galactose in the diet.[450] In 50- to 60-day-old rats with streptozocin-induced diabetes, the fall in lens myoinositol levels occurred between 7 and 15 days after the induction of diabetes.[451]

In vitro, by using the incubation technique of Kinoshita et al,[106] Broekhuyse[450] demonstrated that, like the lenticular amino acid uptake mechanism, the cation pump-coupled mechanism of lenticular myoinositol uptake was also inhibited by the osmotic swelling caused by the hyperglycemia-induced polyol accumulation. The reduced myoinositol uptake was accompanied by increased myoinositol efflux from lenses incubated in high galactose medium, thus leading to low lenticular myoinositol levels. The finding was confirmed and amplified by Kinoshita et al,[452] who demonstrated that such depletion of myoinositol was prevented by the AR inhibitor tetramethyleneglutaric acid.[453] In contrast, addition to the medium of 10 mM myoinositol had no effect on the uptake of myoinositol or on the depressed Na/K-ATPase activity.[454]

In vivo, the involvement of aldose reductase in the process of lens myoinositol depletion was shown by inhibiting aldose reductase in streptozocin-induced diabetic rats. Upon twice daily administration of sorbinil at a dose of 20 mg/kg/day for 14 days, the loss of free myoinositol was decreased to 58% of control.[455] The depletion of myoinositol in the lens of 2-week streptozocin-induced diabetic rats (from 2.31 to 0.41 nmol/mg) was shown to be associated with an increase in lenticular sorbitol levels (from 0.39 to 38.26 nmol/mg) and a 50% reduction in Na/K-pump activity.[456] The changes were prevented by administration of sorbinil.

A protective effect of 2% myoinositol in the diet on cataract development in streptozocin-induced diabetic rats was reported by Bucci et al.[457]

Retina

In spite of very pronounced increases in retinal glucose, sorbitol, and fructose concentrations, no change in retinal myoinositol levels was detected by Hutton et al[451] in rats with streptozocin-induced diabetes of 20-days' duration. However, in rabbits with alloxan-induced diabetes, MacGregor et al[177,458] noted a 25% to 30% decrease of myoinositol content in microscopically defined retinal layers.

Nerve

Comprehensive reviews on the role of hyperglycemia-induced defectiveness of neural myoinositol metabolism have been provided by Clements,[459,460] Greene,[461] Greene and Lattimer,[462] Winegrad,[442] and Greene et al.[463]

Animal data

As part of their pioneering work on the polyol pathway in the nerves of diabetic and galactosemic rats,[464–466] Stewart et al[467] reported that the sciatic nerve myoinositol levels were decreased by 22% in alloxan-induced diabetic rats, and by

72% in rats ingesting 40% galactose with the diet. Subsequently, Stewart et al[449] found that in the sciatic nerve, as in the lens, the decrease in myoinositol content was associated with increased levels of galactitol and water, and hence was possibly due to the osmotic effect of galactitol accumulation rather than to direct inhibition of myoinositol uptake or synthesis. The authors postulated that hypertonicity and the resulting edema may damage cell membranes thus affecting the active uptake and retention of myoinositol, or allowing a faster leakage of myoinositol from the cells. However, the role of osmotic hypertonicity in the deficient myoinositol metabolism in rats with acute experimental diabetes[468,469] is controversial,[442,460–462,470] unless the accumulation of sorbitol is anatomically highly localized.[462,471] Of importance is the demonstration of Nishimura and Kinoshita[469] that the known 30 mM (540 mg/dL) hexose-induced interference with myoinositol uptake by an intact sciatic nerve preparation[472] is readily compensated by increasing the tonicity of the incubating medium to 350 m0sm. The findings in the sciatic nerve are thus similar to those in the lens.[106]

Major interest in nerve myoinositol was stirred in 1975 by the finding of Greene et al[437] that acute streptozocin-induced diabetes in rats impaired their capacity to maintain normal myoinositol concentrations in peripheral nerve, thus creating a myoinositol deficit, which, in turn, was related to a decrease in motor nerve conduction velocity (MNCV). A 31% decrease in nerve myoinositol levels occurred, despite similar plasma myoinositol concentrations in normal and diabetic rats of about 200 μM (3.6 mg/dL). The impaired MNCV in rats with acute experimental diabetes was modified or prevented by supplementing the diet with 1% myoinositol,* without affecting the nerve sorbitol and fructose levels. The decreases in nerve myoinositol levels and MNCV in diabetic rats were also prevented by insulin treatment.

The findings were confirmed and expanded by Palmano et al[438] who showed that the depletion of myoinositol in the sciatic nerve of mildly diabetic rats was progressive. Jeffreys et al,[476] however, were unable to reproduce the results of Greene et al[437] in diabetic rats fed on diets containing either 1% or 35% myoinositol. The lack of response was ascribed by Clements et al[477] to the fact that the rats were old (weighing 410–510 g) and less hyperglycemic (310 mg/dL) than those used by Greene et al (547 mg/dL).[437] To exclude the possible influence of continued growth on nerve conduction velocity, Thomas et al[478] used old rats (weighing 490–660 g) made diabetic with streptozocin (mean blood glucose, 446

*However, feeding normal rats on a diet containing 3% myoinositol and raising plasma myoinositol concentration to 499 μM (9.1 mg/dL) was associated with impaired sciatic MNCV.[437] A similar adverse effect of elevated plasma myoinositol levels on peripheral nervous function had been reported by Clements et al[473] in normal rats fed 35% myoinositol with the diet for one week: a striking decrease in sciatic MNCV developed which improved upon withdrawal of myoinositol. These and additional experiments in the rat supported the possibility that elevated plasma myoinositol levels may contribute to the pathogenesis of uremic polyneuropathy in subjects with chronic renal failure.[474] In a relevant study, Reznek et al[475] have found that, in uremic patients, the elevations in plasma myoinositol levels were related to a decrease in sural nerve conduction velocity, but a relationship with clinically evident neuropathy was not established.

mg/dL) and, again, detected no effect of the 1% myoinositol supplement on tibial MNCV.

These discrepancies were addressed by Greene et al,[479] who investigated the time-dependent effects of experimental diabetes and dietary myoinositol supplementation on MNCV in two different populations of large myelinated motor nerve fibers in the rat hind limb. These fiber populations were differentially affected by growth, by streptozocin-induced diabetes, and by supplementation of 1% myoinositol in the diet. The diabetes-induced nerve conduction impairment was, however, ameliorated by myoinositol in both fiber populations, albeit with different time courses. The authors have attributed the reported discrepancies[476,478] in part, at least, to physiologic or metabolic differences existing among different populations of large nerve fibers.

The postulate of Greene et al[437] that lowered neural myoinositol levels rather than elevated neural sorbitol levels account for the reduced MNCV in diabetic rats appeared to be supported by a report[117] that genetically diabetic mice have impaired MNCV and decreased neural myoinositol levels but unchanged sorbitol levels. However, the reported decrease was associated with a large mismatch of variances of the group means[118]; moreover, nerves of mice with either short-term genetic or streptozocin-induced diabetes were found to exhibit unchanged myoinositol levels, normal MNCV, and no sorbitol accumulation, consonant with low levels or absence of aldose reductase in the nerve.*[118] Evidence supporting the primary role of myoinositol depletion rather than sorbitol accumulation in the initiation of diabetic neuropathy was obtained by Greene et al[480] by showing that the paranodal fiber swelling of peripheral nerves in BB rats and the associated MNCV slowing was reversed by oral myoinositol administration without affecting nerve sorbitol levels.

The significantly lower specific activity of the enzymes involved in the synthesis of phosphatidylinositol and its 4,5-biphosphate found in nerves of diabetic rats suggests that altered metabolism of inositol lipids may also contribute to the decrease in nerve conduction velocity.[481] The decreased rate of myoinositol incorporation into nerve phosphatidylinositol was also attributed to a depression of myoinositol transport due to lack of insulin.[482,483]

In 1982, Simmons et al[441,484] postulated the existence of small, discrete pools of phosphatidylinositol, with rapid turnover, which serve in the nerve as mechanisms of metabolic regulation. A link between the rapid turnover of phosphoinositides and neural activity was originally suggested by Kai and Hawthorne.[485] High neural myoinositol levels were believed necessary to ascertain prompt resynthesis of phosphatidylinositol, which is markedly affected by relatively small decreases in myoinositol. The authors concluded that approximately 25% of the resting energy

*However, Robertson and Sima[119] found severely impaired MNCV in the mutant diabetic mouse of the C57BL/ks (db/db) strain. The decrease in MNCV developed promptly during the early phase of the diabetic syndrome and occurred almost simultaneously with the elevation of blood glucose levels. The temporal discrepancy between the occurrence of functional and morphometric deficits was regarded as a strong indication that the neuropathy was primarily metabolic in origin. The conclusion was supported by the positive effect of insulin treatment on MNCV during the early phase of diabetes, but not during the late phase. Unfortunately, neural myoinositol levels were not measured in the study.

utilization in normal peripheral nerve axons and Schwann cells, including a component of Na/K-dependent ATPase activity, was regulated through phosphatidylinositol turnover. A greatly diminished rate of ATP hydrolysis catalyzed by the membrane-bound Na/K-dependent ATPase in myoinositol-deficient cells was demonstrated earlier by Charalampous.[486] Simmons et al[484] concluded that hyperglycemia could affect the metabolism and composition of peripheral nerve by impairing the maintenance of adequately high myoinositol levels in the nerve, thus deranging the phosphatidylinositol turnover. Indeed, incorporation of [^{3}H]myoinositol into phosphatidylinositol in nerves of streptozocin-induced diabetic rats was decreased by 32% after 20 weeks of diabetes;[487] incorporation of [^{32}P]orthophosphate into phosphatidyl-4,5-biphosphate and polyphosphoinositides was, however, increased.[488] The observations indicate that hyperglycemia results in abnormal nerve polyphosphoinositide metabolism.

Based on the published results listed in Table 2, the magnitude of neural myoinositol depletion in rats with short-term experimentally-induced diabetes corresponds to a median decrease of 22% as compared with non-diabetic rats. Considerably greater loss of myoinositol was found in the sciatic nerves of rats fed on diets containing 40% to 50% galactose (Table 3).

Energy utilization in peripheral nerves, as in the brain, depends on a exogenous glucose supply, which is not insulin-dependent.[497] Nevertheless, in streptozocin-induced diabetic rats, energy and substrate utilization is decreased by about 26% to 31%, despite an increase in tissue glucose and fructose concentrations.[498] The about 50% fall in the Na/K-dependent, ouabain-sensitive ATPase activity in sciatic nerves of streptozocin-induced diabetic rats, first reported by Das et al,[499] was later shown to be selectively prevented by 1% myoinositol supplementation.[490] Subsequently, it was demonstrated that the decrease in energy and substrate utilization by the diabetic nerve can be equated with the decrease in Na/K-dependent ATPase activity.[500] By integrating the above findings, Greene et al[31,500] have proposed the existence in the nerve of a self-reinforcing cycle between the myoinositol-dependent activity of the Na/K-dependent ATPase and the sodium-dependent uptake of myoinositol.

Confirming his earlier speculation,[501] Greene et al[502] have shown that, in the BB rat, direct correlations exist between the myoinositol-related Na/K-dependent ATPase defect and both hyperglycemia and the reversible component of nerve conduction slowing. The evidence was obtained by measuring the effects of rigorous insulin replacement on myoinositol content, peripheral nerve conduction velocity, and on Na/K-dependent ATPase activity. Supporting evidence was provided by the 46% decrease in Na/K-dependent ATPase activity found in the dorsal root ganglia of rats with streptozocin-induced diabetes.[503]

A further explanation of the decrease in Na/K-dependent ATPase activity in diabetes was provided by Greene and Lattimer[504] by showing that the activity can be normalized by activating protein kinase C activity.

The Na/K-dependent ATPase is believed to be localized primarily in the nodal and paranodal regions of large myelinated nerve fibers.[505] The reduced axonal Na/K-dependent ATPase activity in the spontaneously diabetic BB rat is, therefore, postulated to lead to increased axonal sodium concentration, followed by subthreshold membrane potential and conduction block that decreases MNCV and

Table 2. Sorbitol and myoinositol levels in sciatic nerves of rats with short-term experimentally induced diabetes.

Strain (body wt)	Diabetes induced by (mg/kg)	Duration of diabetes	Group	nmol/mg ± SE Sorbitol	nmol/mg ± SE Myoinositol	Ref. No.
Holtzman (200 g)	Alloxan (120, i.p.)	4 months	ND	0.15 ± 0.01	2.74 ± 0.33	467
			D	3.46 ± 0.53	2.15 ± 0.15	
Wistar albino (200 g)	STZ (75–85, i.p.)	3 days to 3 months	ND	0.23 ± 0.03	2.18 ± 0.10	489
			D	1.69 ± 0.19	2.00 ± 0.20	
Wistar (250–350 g)	STZ (35, i.p.)		ND	0.14 ± 0.09	3.10 ± 0.34	438
		2 weeks	D	0.57 ± 0.44**	2.66 ± 0.97*	
		13 weeks	D	0.89 ± 0.53**	2.44 ± 0.48**	
Wistar[a] (410–510 g)	STZ (60, i.p.)	4 weeks	ND	0.08 ± 0.05	2.37 ± 0.64	476
			D	0.54 ± 0.19***	1.97 ± 0.68	
Wistar (225 g)	STZ (60, i.v.)	14 weeks	ND	—	2.76 ± 0.06	479
			D	—	2.27 ± 0.17*	
Wistar (180–200 g)	STZ (60, i.v.)	4 weeks	ND	—	2.98 ± 0.20	490
			D	—	2.21 ± 0.08**	
Wistar (270–320 g)	STZ (50, i.p.)	2 weeks	ND	0.13 ± 0.01	3.40 ± 0.18	147
			D	1.47 ± 0.20***	2.51 ± 0.10**	
		10 weeks	ND	0.25 ± 0.01	3.63 ± 0.15	
			D	2.38 ± 0.17***	2.40 ± 0.18***	
Wistar (290–310 g)	STZ (50, i.p.)	3 weeks	ND	0.08 ± 0.01	2.30 ± 0.10	146, 151
			D	1.56 ± 0.22	1.47 ± 0.10***	
		42 days	ND	0.05 ± 0.01	2.33 ± 0.15	
			D	1.48 ± 0.14	1.73 ± 0.17**	

Wistar (270–320 g)	STZ (35, i.p.)	15 weeks	ND	0.24 ± 0.02	3.92 ± 0.07	145
			D	2.90 ± 0.22***	2.98 ± 0.11***	
Wistar (180–200 g)	STZ (60, i.p.)	2 weeks	ND	0.24 ± 0.01	2.86 ± 0.17	491
			D	0.78 ± 0.07***	2.12 ± 0.11**	
Wistar (180–200 g)	STZ (60, i.p.)	4 weeks	ND	—	2.79 ± 0.11	492
			D	—	2.26 ± 0.11**	
Wistar (350–360 g)	STZ (60, i.p.)	20 days	ND	0.17 ± 0.05	3.54 ± 0.22	150
			D	2.03 ± 0.28	2.66 ± 0.18**	
Wistar (310–330 g)	STZ (50, i.p.)	29 days	ND	0.01 ± 0.00	3.31 ± 0.15	493
			D	2.19 ± 0.13	2.65 ± 0.16**	
Wistar inbred (178 ± 25 g)	STZ (70, i.p.)	2 weeks	ND	0.22 ± 0.07	5.01 ± 0.39	494
			D	1.58 ± 0.67**	3.93 ± 0.67**	
Sprague Dawley (109–113 g)	STZ (55, i.v.)	4 weeks	ND	0.21 ± 0.14	3.35 ± 0.22	495
			D	1.06 ± 0.12***	2.42 ± 0.09***	

STZ = Streptozocin; ND = Non-diabetic; D = Diabetic.
[a]Diet containing 0.023% myoinositol.
*$p<0.05$; **$p<0.01$; ***$p<0.001$.

Table 3. Galactitol and myoinositol levels in sciatic nerves of galactose-fed rats.

Strain (body wt)	Galactose in diet	Duration of galactosemia	Group	nmol/mg ± SE		Ref. No.
				Galactitol	Myoinositol	
Holtzman (200 g)	40%	5 weeks	C G	0.15 ± 0.01 17.4 ± 1.50	4.06 ± 0.26 1.03 ± 0.09	467
		5 months	C G	0.22 ± 0.02 19.30 ± 0.70	4.50 ± 0.29 1.27 ± 0.20	
Holtzman (150–200 g)	40%	2 months	C G	0.24 ± 0.02 20.2 ± 1.20	4.33 ± 0.35 1.16 ± 0.05	449
Wistar inbred (178 ± 25 g)	50%	2 weeks	C G	— —	6.01 ± 0.40 4.84 ± 0.52*	494
Sprague Dawley (45–60 g)	50%	9 days	C G	— 25.0 ± 3.0	5.50 ± 0.70 3.20 ± 0.30**	496

C = Control rats; G = Galactose-fed rats.
*$p<0.01$; **$p<0.001$.

the evoked action potentials.[506,507] The increased intra-axonal sodium levels in the first four weeks of diabetes were accompanied by marked paranodal swelling of large myelinated axons and were prevented by two weeks of insulin replacement[508] or oral myoinositol treatment.[480] However, the tibial MNCV slowing produced by 12 weeks of insulin deficiency was only partially corrected by six weeks of insulin replacement.[507] The poorly reversible impairment of nerve conduction in the chronically diabetic BB rat was attributed by Sima et al[507] to poorly reversible structural damage characterized by loss of paranodal axo-glial junctional complexes. These junctions are thought to limit lateral migration of axolemmal Na/K-dependent ATPase away from the nodes of Ranvier.

That the described metabolic abnormalities and impaired function in the diabetic rat nerve are, in fact, linked with the increased flux of glucose through the polyol pathway was demonstrated by inhibiting aldose reductase. The experimental evidence was obtained by several groups of investigators by using structurally distinct AR inhibitors, i.e., sorbinil, ICI-105,552, statil, and tolrestat. The results indicate that inhibition of aldose reductase in the nerve of diabetic rats prevented the decreases in myoinositol levels[144–147,151,491–495,509] (Chapter 4, Tables 40 and 41 page 267), in Na/K-dependent ATPase activity[492,510] (Chapter 4, Table 42, page 271), in sodium-dependent amino acid uptake,[511] in axonal transport[146,151,165,493] (Chapter 4, Table 40, page 267), and in nerve conduction velocity,[144–147,151] respectively (Chapter 4, Tables 38, 39, and 41, pages 265, 266 and 267). Sorbinil treatment of diabetic rats also reversed myoinositol depletion and decreased nerve conduction velocity.[145]

The relationship between hyperglycemia, the polyol pathway, myoinositol, Na/K-dependent ATPase, and nerve conduction in diabetes as postulated by Greene et al[31] fails, however, to explain[460,468] the observation that in vivo myoinositol is readily taken up by the nerve of diabetic rats administered either myoinositol[437] or an AR inhibitor.[144–147,150,151,491–495,509] The competitive inhibition by glucose of the sodium-dependent neural myoinositol uptake demonstrable in vitro[472] is thus readily overcome in vivo, despite high systemic glucose levels, either by inhibiting aldose reductase or by elevating systemic myoinositol levels. Since the AR inhibitors used do not affect either systemic intracellular glucose levels in vivo (Chapter 4, Tables 24, 32 and 33, pages 252, 260, 261), competitive inhibition of myoinositol uptake by glucose may not play a role in vivo. It thus appears that in the diabetic nerve excess glucose spills into the polyol pathway; that sorbitol and fructose accumulate, and by affecting the integrity of cell membranes, impair the tissue's capacity to maintain the supply of myoinositol needed to control the performance of the membrane-bound Na/K-dependent ATPase which, in turn, modulates the activity of diverse metabolic and biological processes in the nerve (Fig 10). By inhibiting aldose reductase, the conversion of glucose to sorbitol is arrested and, in concert with the rate of elimination of the intracellularly accumulated sorbitol and fructose, the functional integrity of the cell membranes and its constituents is restored. The mechanism by which hyperglycemia induces decreased Na/K-ATPase activity and functional alterations in peripheral nerve, as well as in the kidney, and retina has been recently modified[442,512] to include adenosine in local energy control. Regarding the replenishment of nerve

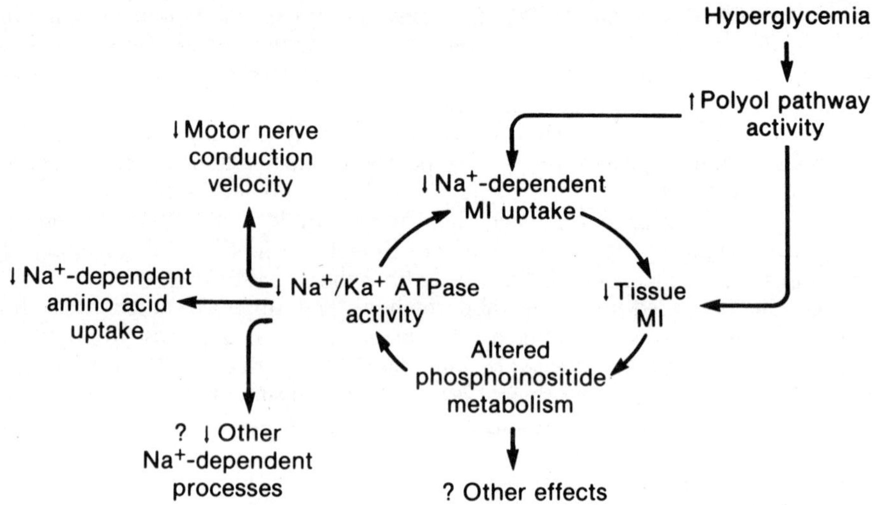

Figure 10. Relationship between hyperglycemia, polyol pathway, myoinositol, Na/K-dependent ATPase, and nerve conduction velocity in diabetes. (Modified scheme of Greene et al[31])

myoinositol content in diabetic rats by myoinositol administration in the absence of a functioning myoinositol uptake mechanism, it is likely that uptake occurs due to the greatly increased concentration gradient between systemic and intracellular myoinositol levels[513] separated by a "leaky" membrane with compromised functional integrity.

In a six-month study in rats with streptozocin-induced diabetes, Cameron et al[514] have investigated the time-course of changes in MNCV, myoinositol levels and morphology in the peripheral nerves. The pattern of axon growth in the larger myelinated fibers closely paralleled the trend shown in the conduction velocity data: both axon area and conduction velocity remained at onset levels. While there was neural myoinositol depletion after three months, none was evident after six months. We have confirmed[515] these observations in rats with streptozocin-induced diabetes of six months' duration and fed on either normal diet or on a diet supplemented with 68% sucrose to exacerbate the hyperglycemia.[155,516,517] Despite greatly increased levels of sorbitol and fructose, no significant differences in neural myoinositol content were found between any of the non-diabetic and diabetic rats (Table 4). The results suggest[514] that the myoinositol deficit is transient, lasting only until the metabolic derangement reaches steady state. The argument is supported by results from other long-term studies in rats (Table 4) with 4,[467] >8,[518] or 14 months[437] of experimental diabetes in which neural myoinositol was found to be within the normal range. Pertinently, in chronic diabetic rats, after 14 months of persistent hyperglycemia (478 $\pm$ 15 mg/dL), sciatic MNCV was normal compared with age-matched controls.[519] While it is established that neural

Table 4. Glucose, sorbitol, fructose and myoinositol levels in the sciatic nerve of rats with long-term experimentally induced diabetes.

Duration of diabetes	nmol/mg ± SE					Ref. No.
	Group	Glucose	Sorbitol	Fructose	Myoinositol	
4 months	ND	2.26 ± 0.11	0.15 ± 0.01	0.39 ± 0.68	2.74 ± 0.33	467
	D[a]	13.50 ± 0.94	3.46 ± 0.53	4.88 ± 0.67	2.15 ± 0.15	
6 months	ND	—	0.39 ± 0.06	1.71 ± 0.24	4.55 ± 0.47	514
	D[b]	—	4.21 ± 0.35	9.18 ± 0.92	3.99 ± 0.47	
6 months	ND	1.58 ± 0.10	0.04 ± 0.02	0.51 ± 0.04	3.17 ± 0.28	
	D[c]	14.81 ± 1.95	1.48 ± 0.25	8.36 ± 1.48	2.88 ± 0.41	206
	ND + sucr.[d]	1.99 ± 0.11	0.09 ± 0.01	0.83 ± 0.08	2.82 ± 0.27	
	D + sucr.	43.63 ± 3.72	3.76 ± 0.43	9.63 ± 0.80	2.09 ± 0.18	
>8 months	ND	1.65 ± 0.08	0.15 ± 0.02	0.79 ± 0.72	2.08 ± 0.10	518
	D[e]	9.45 ± 2.55	1.30 ± 0.19	6.51 ± 1.15	2.05 ± 0.22	

[a]Induced with alloxan (120 mg/kg, i.p.).
[b]Induced in male Sprague Dawley rats, b.w. 554 to 588 g, with streptozocin (45 mg/kg, i.p.).
[c]Induced in female Wistar rats, b.w. about 200 g, with streptozocin (35 mg/kg, i.v.).
[d]68% sucrose admixed to the diet.
[e]Induced in male Wistar rats, b.w. 200 g, with streptozocin.

myoinositol depletion contributes to neurological disturbances in experimental diabetes of short duration,[144–147,151,479,493] the recent findings[514,515] suggest that, in long-term diabetes, alterations in nerve myoinositol may not be necessary for the functional deficit. This is also supported by the finding of normal myoinositol levels in spontaneously diabetic db/db or streptozocin-treated mice.[118] However, it is possible that the recovery of neural myoinositol levels does not fully restore the more specific smaller phosphatidylinositol pools,[520] whose rapid turnover has been postulated to play a part in the control of Na/K-ATPase activity.[441,442,512]

In contrast to the reports that myoinositol depletion is not detectable in long-term diabetic rats,[437,467,514,515,518] we have found a 60% decrease in myoinositol content of the sciatic nerves of rats fed for 178 days on a 50% galactose diet[162] (Chapter 4, Table 37, page 264). In view of the very considerable difference between the neural sorbitol levels in six-month diabetic rats fed on a 68% sucrose diet (3.8 $\pm$ 0.4 nmol/mg) ($\pm$SE)[515] and neural galactitol levels in rats fed for six months on a 50% galactose diet (30.0 $\pm$ 4.0 nmol/mg) ($\pm$ SE),[162] it is possible that the persisting neural myoinositol deficiency in long-term galactosemic rats is due to the much higher polyol levels.

Human data

The observation[437] that ingestion of myoinositol can improve MNCV in diabetic rats in spite of persisting hyperglycemia has been followed by the desire to test its relevance to diabetic polyneuropathy in man.[521] Such studies were initiated by Clements and Reynertson,[434] who have compared the metabolism of myoinositol in diabetic and non-diabetic subjects. While dietary intake and fecal excretion of myoinositol were similar in both groups, urinary myoinositol excretion in diabetic patients was ten times higher. In diabetic patients ingesting 3 g of myoinositol, despite the expected increase in urinary myoinositol excretion,[473,522–528] plasma myoinositol concentrations were significantly higher [about 140 μM (2.6 mg/dL) versus about 90 μM (1.6 mg/dL) in non-diabetic subjects]. Both the impaired oral myoinositol tolerance and the abnormal urinary myoinositol excretion were corrected by insulin treatment. The finding suggested that hyperglycemia may condition an impairment of intracellular myoinositol transport and that chronic oral myoinositol administration could be used to elevate the plasma myoinositol concentrations in human diabetics.

The first study on the effect of myoinositol administration on peripheral nerve function was carried out by Gregersen et al[529,530] in 59 diabetic patients given 1 g of myoinositol three times daily for 24 weeks. A double-blind, parallel study design was used. The results indicated that vibratory perception threshold on pulpa of the great toes was the same in placebo- and myoinositol-treated patients and that the differences in peroneal MNCV found during the tests (repeated every four weeks) were not significant. The authors mentioned, however, that measurements of sensory nerve conduction velocities might have disclosed alterations which they were unable to see with the technique used.

A statistically significant increase in the median and sural sensory nerve conduction velocity was indeed observed by Clements et al[477] in 20 patients with symptomatic distal symmetrical diabetic polyneuropathy given 1.3 $\pm$ 0.3 g myoinositol per day for 16 weeks. Interestingly, in control subjects, daily administration of 1.6 $\pm$ 0.3 g of myoinositol resulted in a slight, but significant fall in median sensory nerve conduction velocity ($p<0.05$).

In a double-blind, placebo-controlled crossover trial with seven diabetic patients, 0.5 g of myoinositol given twice-daily for two weeks failed to improve the nerve conduction velocities in the median, sural, and popliteal nerves, but increased the amplitude of the evoked action potentials by an average of 76%, 160%, and 40%, respectively.[531]

In a comprehensive study, Dyck et al[532] measured the sorbitol, fructose, and myoinositol content of biopsied sural nerves from 20 diabetic patients with neuropathy of varying severity and compared these with values in the nerves obtained from 15 healthy volunteers. Neuropathy was detected and graded by a scored evaluation of neurological symptoms and signs, by computer-assisted sensory examination, by measurements of nerve conduction velocity and needle electromyography, and by pathological and morphometric evaluation of the sural nerve. The increased contents of sorbitol and fructose in the nerve were related to the patients' median fasting blood sugar levels for the preceding six months ($p<0.001$). The variability of sorbitol and fructose levels in diabetic nerves was greater than in non-diabetic nerves. However, more than one third of the diabetic nerves had sorbitol and fructose values above the highest levels of controls. No relationship was evident between the elevated sorbitol or fructose levels and the presence or severity of neuropathy. Actually, the highest levels were found in untreated diabetic patients without neuropathy. The results demonstrated that the polyol pathway in the nerve of diabetic patients is activated, thus resulting in elevated sorbitol and fructose levels. However, no myoinositol deficiency was detected in any diabetic nerve; in fact, the myoinositol levels were more consistently elevated in the diabetic than in non-diabetic nerves.

The effect of myoinositol in chronic insulin-treated diabetic patients with distal symmetrical, primarily sensory polyneuropathy was investigated by Greene et al.[533] All subjects had sensory deficits in their legs, and all but two had sensory deficits in their arms. Their neuropathy was classified as mild to moderate in severity. Myoinositol or placebo was given in divided doses totaling 2 g to 3 g per day. A single-blind design was used. After six months of treatment, clinical improvement had occurred in four of 13 patients (31%), in legs and arms, as judged by improvement both in symptoms and in the extent of deficits in pin-prick and temperature perception. However, abnormalities in sensory modalities mediated by large myelinated fibers (detectable by nerve conduction velocity measurements) were generally unaltered. In spite of small increases in peroneal and ulnar MNCV, clinical improvement was not accompanied by evidence of a consistent pattern of improvement in the non-uniform distribution of abnormal electrophysiological tests recorded at the outset. The authors concluded, however, that the finding of some degree of clinical improvement over a six-month period raised the possibility that a significant portion of diabetic patients with painful distal symmetrical, primarily sensory polyneuropathy may have the potential to improve.

In 1983 Gregersen et al[534] conducted a double-blind, placebo-controlled study on the effect of 6 g of myoinositol per day in 28 young diabetic subjects with subclinical diabetic neuropathy. After two months' treatment, measurements of vibratory perception threshold, of motor and sensory conduction velocity, and of the amplitude of nerve potential did not disclose any effect of the administered myoinositol. Furthermore, there was no lack of myoinositol in diabetic blood or muscle tissue. The plasma myoinositol concentration in diabetic patients was normal or high, even though the myoinositol excretion in urine was greater than in non-diabetic subjects. Additionally, the myoinositol content in the muscle tissue of diabetic patients was not affected by myoinositol administration.

An observation supporting the view that human diabetic nerves are deficient in myoinositol was provided by Mayhew et al,[535] who have found approximately 40% lower levels of free and lipid myoinositol in post mortem sciatic nerves from 23 diabetic patients as compared with those from 15 non-diabetic subjects. As shown below, the levels of glucose, sorbitol, and fructose were greatly increased in the nerves of diabetic patients. The significance of these values has been questioned, however, because of the relatively large inter-patient variation of the reported myoinositol values.[536]

Variable	**Content in sciatic nerve (nmol/mg ± SD)**	
	Normal subjects	**Diabetic patients**
Myoinositol,		
free	3.33 ± 2.07	1.91 ± 1.34*
lipid	1.11 ± 0.60	0.71 ± 0.38*
Glucose	0.46 ± 0.29	1.61 ± 1.26**
Sorbitol	0.09 ± 0.10	0.39 ± 0.49*
Fructose	0.08 ± 0.13	1.24 ± 1.88*

*$p<0.03$; **$p<0.003$

In contrast, no difference in nerve myoinositol concentrations between diabetic and non-diabetic subjects was detected by Hale et al,[537] who have measured glucose, sorbitol, fructose and myoinositol concentrations in proximal nerve biopsies taken above (sciatic) and below knee (common peroneal) amputations performed for either neuropathic sepsis or peripheral vascular disease in non-diabetic and diabetic patients. As expected, glucose, sorbitol, and fructose levels were higher in diabetic subjects.

From the preceding discussion it is clear that the available clinical data on the effect of orally administered myoinositol on diabetic neuropathy are inconclusive.[459,538] However, in view of the relationship of aldose reductase (AR) activity and myoinositol levels in peripheral nerves of experimentally diabetic animals, it is reasonable to conclude that myoinositol depletion in diabetic nerve is readily prevented by inhibiting aldose reductase.

Kidney

Beyer-Mears et al[19] reported a 52% decrease in glomerular myoinositol content in rats with streptozocin-induced diabetes of nine weeks' duration (5.46 ± 1.32

nmol/mg protein, ± SE) as compared with non-diabetic rats (11.37 ± 1.56 nmol/mg protein). The decrease was prevented by administration of the AR inhibitor sorbinil at a daily oral dose of 20 mg/kg.

That the glomeruli contain a sodium-dependent transport system for myoinositol, similar to that in peripheral nerve, was demonstrated by Ulbrecht et al[539]; in isolated renal glomeruli, the myoinositol uptake was significantly reduced ($p<0.05$) in the presence of 20 mM (360 mg/dL) glucose. While the glucose-induced decrease in myoinositol uptake was not affected by sorbinil, either in vitro or in vivo, addition to the incubation medium of 15 mM (270 mg/dL) sorbitol decreased the myoinositol uptake by 12% ($p<0.05$).[540]

Measurement of Na/K-dependent ATPase activity in membranes prepared from the glomeruli indicated a 32% decrease in rats with streptozocin-induced diabetes of 11 to 18 days' duration. The decrease was prevented by administration of the AR inhibitor sorbinil.[20,21,541] It is of interest that, in the glomeruli of acutely diabetic rats, Cohen et al[542] were unable to detect changes in phosphatidylinositol hence questioned the hypothesis that the reduction in Na/K-dependent ATPase activity in diabetes arises from diminished endogenous phosphatidylinositol as a result of decreased intracellular myoinositol levels.

According to Goldfarb et al,[543] the increase in glomerular filtration rate occurring in rats with streptozocin-induced diabetes of seven to ten days' duration is significantly reduced by supplementing the diet with 1% myoinositol or by inhibiting aldose reductase with sorbinil injected intraperitoneally at a dose 25 mg/kg/day for eight days. The observations suggest that hyperglycemia, inducing cellular myoinositol depletion via increased aldose reductase activity, may contribute to the pathogenesis of glomerular hyperfiltration in diabetes of short duration.

Red blood cells

A correlation between plasma and red blood cell myoinositol concentrations was found by Servo et al[544] in both normal subjects and in severely uremic patients. Since myoinositol, like other polyols, passes slowly from the intra- to the extracellular space, after dialysis, the myoinositol level in the red blood cells exceeded that in plasma, thus creating an osmotic gradient. A correlation between plasma and red blood cell myoinositol levels was also found in diabetic patients, the height of the levels depending on the degree of glomerular filtration rate.[545] In spite of the increased urinary myoinositol excretion in diabetic patients,[434,545] the myoinositol levels in plasma and red blood cells are normal, or above normal.[545] The correlation between plasma and red blood cell myoinositol levels was corroborated by Gregersen et al[534] in normal subjects and diabetic patients taking 2 g of myoinositol three times daily for two months. The presence of higher plasma and red blood cell myoinositol levels in the diabetic patients was confirmed by Malone et al.[546]

The more recent interest in red blood cell myoinositol content was prompted by two lines of observations. First, that in diabetic rats erythrocyte sorbitol concentrations parallel the sorbitol content of both peripheral nerve and lens over a wide range of hyperglycemia[547]; second, that the increase in sorbitol content was due to the hyperglycemia-induced activation of aldose reductase since it was prevented by an AR inhibitor, sorbinil.[547] Combined, the observations suggested that in diabetic patients the AR activity in red blood cell could be used as a model for its activity in less accessible tissues.[547–549] The approach promised to be particularly useful for monitoring the activity of AR inhibitors in human subjects. Indeed, the elevated red blood cell sorbitol content in diabetic patients was shown to be normalized by treatment with several structually distinct inhibitors of aldose reductase. (For more detailed information see Chapter 4, Tables 50, 51, and 52, on pages 296 and 297). However, the expectation that, as in the peripheral nerve, the increase in tissue sorbitol levels would be associated with myoinositol depletion was not confirmed in the red blood cells. Several investigators were unable to find an association between sorbitol and myoinositol levels in the erythrocytes of normal or diabetic subjects.[546,550–553] In fact, in 65 diabetic patients, no correlation was found between red blood cell sorbitol levels and neural sensory tests.[554]

A dissimilarity between the red blood cell and the peripheral nerve was also found by Dasmahapatra et al[555]: while decreased in the nerve of diabetic rats, the Na/K-dependent ATPase in the erythrocytes was increased.

Aorta

Incubation of rabbit thoracic aortic smooth muscle in a glucose-rich medium resulted in increased polyol pathway activity, increased water content, and decreased myoinositol content. The decrease in myoinositol was inversely related to the glucose concentration in the medium.[556] Addition of ibuprofen, considered to be an AR inhibitor, to the incubation medium containing 50 mM (901 mg/dL) glucose resulted in higher tissular myoinositol levels.

Conceptus

In studies on the dysmorphogenic effects of high glucose in the cultured rat conceptus (including embryo, visceral yolk sac, and ectoplacental cone), Hod et al[557] (Table 5) have found in the intact conceptus a four- to six-fold increase in

Table 5. Effects of AR inhibitors on sorbitol and myoinositol levels in rat conceptuses cultured in high glucose medium. (From Hod et al[557])

Glucose in the medium (nM)	AR inhibitor (× 10^{-5}M)	ng/intact conceptus ± SE: Sorbitol	ng/intact conceptus ± SE: Myoinositol
6.7 (control)	—	144 ± 32	481 ± 31
16.7	—	565 ± 28	327 ± 21
16.7	Sorbinil (1)	233 ± 89	320 ± 28
16.7	Statil (2.5)	336 ± 56	323 ± 14
66.6	—	880 ± 114	122 ± 11
66.6	Sorbinil (1)	275 ± 102	150 ± 15
66.6	Statil (2.5)	391 ± 102	161 ± 11

Significance brackets (as printed): Sorbitol — 144 vs 565 ***; 565 vs 233 **; 565 vs 336 **; 144 vs 880 ***; 880 vs 275 **; 880 vs 391 *. Myoinositol — 481 vs 327 **; 481 vs 122 ***.

*$p<0.05$; **$p<0.01$; ***$p<0.001$

sorbitol levels and a 32% to 75% decrease in myoinositol levels. While the addition to the culture medium of two structurally distinct AR inhibitors, sorbinil (1×10^{-5}M) and statil (2.5×10^{-5}M), significantly attenuated the rise in sorbitol levels, the myoinositol depletion was not affected by either AR inhibitor.

References

1. Pirart J: Diabetes mellitus and its degenerative complications: Prospective study of 4000 patients observed between 1947 and 1973. *Diabetes Care* 1978;1:168–188, 252–263.
2. Brownlee M, Cerami A: The biochemistry of the complications of diabetes mellitus. *Ann Rev Biochem* 1981;50:385–432.
3. Ludworth AG, Bodansky HJ, West KM: Genetic and metabolic factors in relationship to the prevalence and severity of diabetic complications, in Keens H, Jarret J (eds): *Complications of Diabetes,* ed 2. London, E Arnold Ltd, 1982, pp 1–10.
4. Kohner EM: Recent advances in diabetic retinopathy, in Alberti KGMM, Krall LP (eds): *The Diabetes Annual 1.* Amsterdam, New York, Oxford, Elsevier Science Publishers, 1985, pp 257–287.
5. Viberti GC, Bilous RW, Mackintosh D, Bending JJ, Keen H: Long term correction of hyperglycemia and progression of renal failure in insulin-dependent diabetes. *Br Med J* 1983;286:598–602.
6. Gonzalez RG, Barnett P, Aguayo J, Chen HM, Chylack LT Jr: Direct measurement of polyol pathway activity in the ocular lens. *Diabetes* 1984;33:196–199.
7. Barnett PA, Gonzalez RG, Chylack LT Jr, Cheng HM: The effect of oxidation on sorbitol pathway kinetics. *Diabetes* 1986;35:426–432.
8. Cheng HM, Gonzalez RG: The effect of high glucose and oxidative stress on lens metabolism, aldose reductase, and senile cataractogenesis. *Metabolism* 1986;35 (suppl 1):10–14.
9. Kinoshita JH: Mechanisms initiating cataract formation. *Invest Ophthalmol* 1974; 13:713–724.
10. Kinoshita JH, Kador P, Datiles M: Aldose reductase in diabetic cataracts. *JAMA* 1981;246:257–261.
11. Varma DS, Richards RD: Etiology of cataracts in diabetes. *Int Ophthalmol Clin* 1984;24:93–110.
12. Kupfer C: Bowman Lecture. The conquest of cataract: A global challenge. *Trans Ophthalmol Soc UK* 1984;104: 1–10.
13. Kador PF, Kinoshita JH: Diabetic and galactosemic cataracts, in *Human cataract formation.* Ciba Foundation Symposium 106. London, Pitman, 1984, pp 110–131.
14. Kinoshita JH: Aldose reductase in the diabetic eye. XLIII Edward Jackson memorial lecture. *Am J Ophthalmol* 1986;102:685–692.
15. Ward JD: Diabetic neuropathy, in Alberti KGMM, Krall LP (eds): *The Diabetes Annual 1.* Amsterdam, New York, Oxford, Elsevier Science Publishers, 1985, pp 288–308.
16. Dvornik D: Chronic complications of diabetes. *Ann Rep Med Chem* 1978;13:159–166.
17. Lipinski CA, Hutson NJ: Aldose reductase inhibitors as a new approach to the treatment of diabetic complications. *Ann Rep Med Chem* 1984;19:169–177.
18. Kinoshita JH, Kador P, Robison WG, et al: Aldose reductase and complications of diabetes. *Ann Intern Med* 1984;101:82–91.

19. Beyer-Mears A, Ku L, Cohen MP: Glomerular polyol accumulation in diabetes and its prevention by oral sorbinil. *Diabetes* 1984;33:604–607.
20. Cohen MP, Dasmahapatra A: Reduced glomerular Na/K ATPase in diabetes and its prevention by oral sorbinil. *Clin Res* 1984;32:796A.
21. Cohen MP, Dasmahapatra A: Glomerular Na/K ATPase activity is reduced in diabetes and restored by sorbinil or insulin treatment. *Clin Res* 1985;33:583A.
22. Kador PF, Kinoshita JH, Sharpless NE: Aldose reductase inhibitors: A potential new class of agents for the pharmacological control of certain diabetic complications. *J Med Chem* 1985;28:841–849.
23. Nomenclature Committee of IUB (NC-IUB), IUB-IUPAC Joint Commission on Biochemical Nomenclature (JCBN). Newsletter 1984, International Union of Biochemistry (IUB), International Union of Pure and Applied Chemistry (IUPAC). *Hoppe-Seyler's Z Physiol Chem* 1984;365:I–V.
24. Holmquist WR, Schroeder WA: A new terminal blocking group involving a Schiff base in hemoglobin Alc. *Biochemistry* 1966;5:2489–2503.
25. Bookchin RM, Gallop PM: Structure of hemoglobin Alc; nature of the N-terminal -chain blocking group. *Biochem Biophys Res Comm* 1968;32:86–93.
26. Bunn HF, Haney DN, Kamin S, Gabbay KH, Gallop PM: The biosynthesis of human hemoglobin Alc: Slow glycosylation of hemoglobin in vivo. *J Clin Invest* 1976;57: 1652–1659.
27. Kennedy L, Baynes JW: Non-enzymatic glycosylation and the chronic complications of diabetes: An overview. *Diabetolotogia* 1984;26:93–98.
28. Brownlee M, Vlassara M, Cerami A: Nonenzymatic glycosylation and the pathogenesis of diabetic complications. *Ann Intern Med* 1984;101:527–537.
29. Peterson CM, Formby B: Glycosylated proteins, in Alberti KGMM, Krall LP (eds): *The Diabetes Annual 1.* Amsterdam, New York, Oxford, Elsevier Science Publishers, 1985, pp 178–197.
30. Vlassara H, Brownlee M, Cerami A: Nonenzymatic glycosylation: Role in the pathogenesis of diabetic complications. *Clin Chem* 1986;32:B37–B41.
31. Greene DA, Lattimer S, Ulbrecht J, Carroll P: Glucose-induced alterations in nerve metabolism: Current perspective on the pathogenesis of diabetic neuropathy and future direction for research and therapy. *Diabetes Care* 1985;8:290–299.
32. Leske MC, Sperduto RD: The epidemiology of senile cataracts: A Review. *Am J Epidemiol* 1983;118:152–165.
33. Kronfeld P, Bothman L: Zur Frage de Linsenatmung. *Z Augenheilkunde* 1928;65:41–62.
34. Kuck JFR Jr: Metabolism of the lens, in Graymore CN (ed): *Biochemistry of the Eye.* Academic Press, 1970, p 262.
35. Cheng HM, Chylack LT Jr: Lens metabolism, in Maisel H (ed): *The Ocular Lens.* New York, Basel, M Dekker Inc, 1985, pp 223–264.
36. Kinoshita JH, Futterman S, Satoh K, Merola LO: Factors affecting the formation of sugar alcohols in ocular lens. *Biochim Biophys Acta* 1963;74:340–350.
37. Kinoshita JH, Kern HL, Merola LO: Factors affecting the cation transport of calf lens. *Biochim Biophys Acta* 1961;47:458–486.
38. Sippel TO: The relationship of rat lens respiration to oxygen concentration and pH. *Invest Ophthalmol* 1962;1:385–389.
39. Trayhurn P, Van Heyningen R: The role of respiration in the energy metabolism of the bovine lens. *Biochem J* 1972;129:507–509.
40. Trayhurn P, Van Heyningen R: The metabolism of amino acids in the bovine lens. Their oxidation as source of energy. *Biochem J,* 1973;136:67–75.

41. Van Heyningen R, Linklater J: The metabolism of bovine lens in air and nitrogen. *Exp Eye Res* 1975;20:393–396.
42. Trayhurn P, Van Heyningen R: Anaerobic metabolism in the bovine lens. *Exp Eye Res* 1971;12:315–327.
43. Kinoshita JH, Wachtl C: A study of the C-14 glucose metabolism of the rabbit lens. *J Biol Chem* 1958;233: 5–7.
44. Cheng HM, Fagerholm P, Chylack LT Jr: Response of the lens to oxidative-osmotic stress. *Exp Eye Res* 1983;37:11–21.
45. Giblin FJ, McCready JP, Reddy VN: The role of glutathione metabolism in the detoxification of H 0 in rabbit lens. *Invest Ophthalmol Vis Sci* 1982;22:330–335.
46. Lerman S: Carbohydrate metabolism in the rat lens as related to the age of the animal. *Arch Ophthalmol* 1961;65:181–183.
47. Lou MF, Kinoshita JH: Control of lens glycolysis. *Biochim Biophys Acta* 1967; 141:545–559.
48. Chylack LT Jr, Cheng HM: Sugar metabolism in the crystalline lens. *Surv Ophthalmol* 1978;23:26–34.
49. Levari R, Wertheimer E, Kornblueth W: Interrelation between the various pathways of glucose metabolism in the rat lens. *Exp Eye Res* 1964;3:99–104.
50. Van Heyningen R: Formation of polyols by the lens of the rat with "sugar" cataract. *Nature* 1959;184:194–195.
51. Van Heyningen R: The lens: Metabolism and cataract, in Davson H (ed): *The Eye, Vol 1*, ed 2. New York, London, Academic Press, 1969, p 389.
52. Kuck J: The formation of fructose in the ocular lens. *Arch Ophthalmol* 1961; 65:840–846.
53. Kinoshita JH, Varma SD, Fukui HN: Aldose reductase in diabetes. *Jap J Ophthalmol* 1976;20:399–410.
54. Hers HG: L'Aldose-reductase. *Biochim Biophys Acta* 1960;37:120–126.
55. Hers HG: Le mécanisme de la formation du fructose séminal et du fructose foetal. *Biochim Biophys Acta* 1960;37:127–138.
56. Van Heyningen R: Metabolism of xylose by the lens. 2. Rat lens in vivo and in vitro. *Biochem J* 1959;73:197–207.
57. Ritter P, Leuthardt F: Die Bildung von Fructose und Sorbit aus Glukose in der menschlichen Placenta. *Helv Physiol Acta* 1963;21:212–215.
58. Feldman HB, Szczepanik PA, Havre P, et al: Stereo-specificity of the hydrogen transfer catalyzed by human placental aldose reductase. *Biochim Biophys Acta* 1977; 480:14–20.
59. Popjak G: Stereospecificity of enzymic reactions, in Boyer PD (ed): *The Enzymes, Vol 1*, ed 3. New York, London, Academic Press, 1970, pp 134–157.
60. Flynn TG, Shires J, Walton DJ: Properties of nicotin-amide adenine dinuclotide phosphate-dependent aldehyde reductase from pig kidney. *J Biol Chem* 1975;250:2933–2940.
61. Crabbe MJC, in Nugent J, Whelan J (eds): *Human cataract formation.* Ciba Foundation Symposium 106. London, Pitman Publishing Ltd, 1984, pp 123–127.
62. Wolff SP, Crabbe MJC, Thornalley PJ: The autoxidation of glyceraldehyde and other simple monosaccharides. *Experientia* 1984;40:244–246.
63. Wolff SP, Crabbe MJC: Low apparent aldose reductase activity produced by monosaccharide autoxidation. *Biochem J* 1985;226:625–630.
64. Crabbe MJC, Petchey M, Wolff SP: Monosaccharide-induced NADPH oxidation (aldose reductase activity) and the uptake of sorbinil and myoinositol in incubated rat lenses. *Lens Res* 1986;3:69–91.

65. Kador PF, Kinoshita JH, Brittain DR, et al: Purified rat lens aldose reductase. Polyol production in vitro and its inhibition by aldose reductase inhibitors. *Biochem J* 1986;240:233–237.
66. Kinoshita JH: Pathways of glucose metabolism in the lens. *Invest Ophthalmol* 1965;4:619–628.
67. Varma SD, Kinoshita JH: Sorbitol pathway in diabetic and galactosemic rat lens. *Biochim Biophys Acta* 1974; 338:632–640.
68. Gonzalez AM, Sochor M, Hothersall JS, McLean P: Effect of aldose reductase inhibitor (sorbinil) on integration of polyol pathway, pentose phosphate pathway, and glycolytic route in diabetic rat lens. *Diabetes* 1986; 35:1200–1205.
69. Collins JG, Corder CN: Aldose reductase and sorbitol dehydrogenase distribution in substructures of normal and diabetic rat lens. *Invest Ophthalmol Vis Sci* 1977; 16:242–243.
70. Efimov AS, Obrosova IG, Veliki NN: The sorbitol pathway of glucose metabolism in streptozotocin diabetes of varying duration and gravity. *Probl Endokrinol* 1984; 30:71–76.
71. Ahmad SS, Tsou KC, Ahmad SI, Ataur Rahman M: Studies on cataractogenesis in humans and in rats with alloxan-induced diabetes. II. Histochemical evaluation of lenticular enzymes. *Ophthalmic Res* 1985;17:12–20.
72. Akagi Y, Kador PF, Shiono T, Kinoshita JH: Aldose reductase distribution and activation in diabetic and galactosemic rat lens. *Invest Ophthalmol Vis Sci* 1984; 25(suppl):136.
73. Libondi T, Menzione M, Iuliano G, et al: Changes of some biochemical parameters of the lens in galactose-treated weaned rats with and without vitamin E therapy. *Ophthalmic Res* 1985;17: 42–48.
74. Akagi Y, Kador PF, Kinoshita JH: Immunohistochemical localization for aldose reductase in diabetic lenses. *Invest Ophthalmol Vis Sci* 1987;28:163–167.
75. Cao Danh H, Strolin-Benedetti M, Mousset A, Pasquier-Bechet P: Age-related changes in the activities of the amine metabolizing enzymes of rat eye. *J Pharm Pharmacol* 1985;37:357–361.
76. Cao Danh H, Strolin-Benedetti M, Boucher T: Age-related changes in aldose reductase activity in rat lens, in Biggio G (ed): *Symposia in neuroscience 3. Modulation of central and peripheral transmitter function.* New York, Springer-Verlag, 1986; pp 273–276.
77. Cao Danh H, Strolin-Benedetti M, Dostert P: Age-related changes in sorbitol dehydrogenase activity in rat brain, liver, kidney and eye. *J Pharm Pharmacol* 1985;37:910–912.
78. Williamson JR, Chang K, Jeffery JR, et al: Sex steroid modulation of diabetes-induced increases in lens polyol content. *Invest Ophthalmol Vis Sci* 1986;27(suppl):136.
79. Jeffery J, Jornvall H: Enzyme relationships in a sorbitol pathway that bypasses glycolysis and pentose phosphates in glucose metabolism. *Proc Natl Acad Sci* 1983;80:901–905.
80. Cheng HM, Gonzalez RG, Barnett PA Aguayo JB, Wolfe J, et al: Sorbitol/fructose metabolism in the lens. *Exp Eye Res* 1985;40:223–229.
81. Chylack LT Jr, Tung W, Harding R: Sorbitol production in the lens: a means of counteracting glucose-derived osmotic stress. *Ophthalmic Res* 1986;18:313–320.
82. Kador PF, Robison WG, Kinoshita JH: The pharmacology of aldose reductase inhibitors. *Ann Rev Pharmacol Toxicol* 1985;25:691–714.
83. Lee SM, Sehade SZ, Doughty CC: Aldose reductase, NADPH and NADP in normal, galactose-fed and diabetic rat lens. *Biochim Biophys Acta* 1985;841:247–253.
84. Darby WJ, Day PL: Xylose as a cataractogenic agent. *Proc Soc Exp Biol Med* 1939;41:507–508.

85. Booth AM, Wilson RH, Deeds F: Effects of prolonged ingestion of xylose in rats. *J Nutr* 1953;49:347–355.
86. Mitchell HS, Dodge WM: Cataract in rats fed on high lactose rations. *J Nutr* 1935;9:37–49.
87. Yudkin AM, Arnold CH: Cataract formation in rats fed on a diet containing galactose. *Proc Soc Exp Biol Med* 1935;32:836–837.
88. Day PL: Blood sugar in rats rendered cataractous by dietary procedures. *J Nutr* 1936;12:395–404.
89. Patterson JW: Course of diabetes and development of cataracts after injecting dehydroascorbic acid and related substances. *Am J Physiol* 1951;165:61–65.
90. Sterling RE, Day PL: Blood sugar levels and cataract in alloxan-treated galactose-fed and xylose-fed weanling rats. *Proc Soc Exp Biol Med* 1951;78:431–433.
91. Sasaki T: Untersuchungen der Linse, des Blutes und des Kammerwassers von Ratten bei Galaktosverfütterung. I. Klinische Beobachtungen bei der Galaktosekatarakt. *Graefe's Arch Ophthalmol* 1938;138:351–364.
92. Patterson JW: Cataractogenic sugars. *Arch Biochem Biophys* 1955;58:24–30.
93. Patterson JW: Cataracts caused by carbohydrates. *Am J Ophthalmol* 1953; 36:143–149.
94. Gifford SR, Bellows J: Histologic changes in the lens produced by galactose. *Arch Ophthalmol* 1939;21:346–358.
95. Buschke W: Classification of experimental cataracts in the rat: Recent observations on cataract associated with tryptophen deficiency and with other experimental conditions. *Arch Ophthalmol* 1943;30:735–750.
96. Friedenwald JS, Rytel D: Contribution to the histopathology of cataract. *Arch Ophthalmol* 1955;53:825–831.
97. Bounds GW Jr, Janes RG, Leinfelder PJ: Cataracts induced by alloxan diabetes in rats and rabbits. *Arch Ophthalmol* 1955;54:564–572.
98. Dische Z, Zelmenis G, Youlus J: Studies on protein and protein synthesis. *Am J Ophthalmol* 1957;44:332–341.
99. Kinoshita JH, Merola LO, Satoh K, Dikmak E: Osmotic changes caused by the accumulation of dulcitol in the lenses of rats fed with galactose. *Nature* 1962;194: 1085–1087.
100. Varma SD: Aldose reductase and the etiology of diabetic cataracts. *Curr Topics Eye Res* 1980;3:91–155.
101. Kuwabara T, Kinoshita JH, Cogan DG: Electron microscopic study of galactose-induced cataract. *Invest Ophthalmol* 1969;8:133–149.
102. Kinoshita JH, Merola LO, Dikmak E: The accumulation of dulcitol and water in rabbit lens incubated with galactose. *Biochim Biophys Acta* 1962;62:176–178.
103. Kinsey VE, Wachtl C, Kuck JFR Jr, Reddy DVN: Current research on the culture of lenses. *Acta Conc Ophthalmol* 1958;18:865–872.
104. Levari R, Kornblueth W, Wertheimer E: The effect of insulin on the uptake of monosaccharides by the rat lens. *J Endocrinol* 1961;22:361–369.
105. Reddy DVN: Amino acid transport in the lens in relation to sugar cataracts. *Invest Ophthalmol* 1965;4:700–708.
106. Kinoshita JH, Merola LO, Hayman S: Osmotic effects on the amino acid-concentrating mechanism in the rabbit lens. *J Biol Chem* 1965;240:310–315.
107. Kinoshita JH: Cataracts in galactosemia. *Invest Ophthalmol* 1965;4:786–799.
108. Lefevre PG, Davies RI: Active transport into the human erythrocyte: Evidence from comparative kinetics and competition among monosaccharides. *J Gen Physiol* 1951; 34:515–524.

109. Kuck JFR: Response of the mouse lens to high concentrations of glucose or galactose. *Ophthalmol Res* 1970;1:166–174.
110. Varma SD, Kinoshita JH: The absence of cataracts in mice with congenital hyperglycemia. *Exp Eye Res* 1974; 19:577–582.
111. Varma SD, Mizuno A, Kinoshita JH: Diabetic cataracts and flavonoids. *Science* 1977;195:205–206.
112. El-Aguizy HK, Richards RD, Varma SD: Sugar cataracts in Mongolian gerbil (Meriones unguiculatus). *Exp Eye Res* 1983;36:839–844.
113. Simard-Duquesne N, Greselin E, Gonzalez R, Dvornik D: Prevention of cataract development in severely galactosemic rats by the aldose reductase inhibitor, tolrestat. *Proc Soc Exp Biol Med,* 1985;178:599–605.
114. Beyer-Mears A, Cruz E, Nicolas-Alexandre J: Sorbinil effect on sugar cataract progression and recovery. An initial study. *Invest Ophthalmol Vis Sci* 1982;21:154.
115. Hu T, Datiles M, Kinoshita JH: Reversal of galactose cataract with sorbinil in rats. *Invest Ophthalmol Vis Sci* 1983;24:640–644.
116. Ono H, Shibata M: Sorbitol in the kidney of NSY mice with congenital hyperglycemia. *J Japan Diab Soc* 1982;25:243–245.
117. Gillon KRW, Hawthorne JN: Metabolism of inositol and inositol lipids in peripheral nerve of diabetic and control animals, in Serratric G, Desnuelle C, Pellissier JF, et al (eds): *Neuromuscular diseases.* New York, Raven Press, 1984; pp 225–230.
118. Whiteley SJ, Tomlinson DR: Motor nerve conduction velocity and nerve polyols in mice with short-term genetic or streptozotocin-induced diabetes. *Exp Neurol* 1985;89:314–321.
119. Robertson DM, Sima AAF: Diabetic neuropathy in the mutant mouse [C57BL/ks(db/db)]. A morphometric study. *Diabetes* 1980;29:60–67.
120. Kodama T, Reddy VN, Giblin F, Kinoshita JH, Harding C: Scanning electron microscopy of X-ray-induced cataract in mice on normal and galactose diet. *Ophthalmol Res* 1983;15:324–333.
121. Litchfield WJ, Wells WW: Effect of galactose on free radical reactions of polymorphonuclear leucocytes. *Arch Biochem Biophys* 1978;188:26–30.
122. Pirie A, Van Heyningen R: The effect of diabetes on the content of sorbitol, glucose, fructose and inositol in the human lens. *Exp Eye Res* 1964;3:124–131.
123. Pirie A: Epidemiological and biochemical studies of cataract and disease. *Invest Ophthalmol* 1965;4:629–637.
124. Kuck JFR: Carbohydrates of the lens in normal and precataractous states. *Invest Ophthalmol* 1965;4:638–642.
125. Heaf DJ, Galton DJ: Sorbitol and other polyols in the lens, adipose tissue and urine in diabetes mellitus. *Clin Chim Acta* 1975;63:41–47.
126. Pfaffenberger, CD, Szafranek J, Horning EC: Gas chromatographic study of free polyols and aldoses in cataractous human lens tissue. *J Chromatogr* 1976; 126:535–545.
127. Kinoshita JH, Merola LO, Dikmak E: Osmotic changes in experimental galactose cataracts. *Exp Eye Res* 1962;1:405–410.
128. Varma SD, Schocket SS, Richards RD: Implications of aldose reductase in cataracts in human diabetes. *Invest Ophthalmol Vis Sci* 1979;18:237–241.
129. Lerner BC, Varma SD, Richards RD: Polyol pathway metabolites in human cataracts. Correlation of circulating glycosylated hemoglobin content and fasting blood glucose levels. *Arch Ophthalmol* 1984;102:917–920.
130. Chylack LT Jr, Henriques HF, Tung WH: Inhibition of sorbitol production in human lenses by an aldose reductase inhibitor. *Docum Ophthalmol Proc Series* 1979; 18:65–75.

131. Chylack LT Jr, Henriques HF, Cheng HM, Tung WH: Efficacy of alrestatin, an aldose reductase inhibitor, in human diabetic and nondiabetic lenses. *Ophthalmology* 1979;86:1579–1585.
132. Pottinger PK: A study of three enzymes acting on glucose in the lens of different species. *Biochem J* 1967;104:663–670.
133. Friedburg, D: Enzyme activity patterns and some intermediates in human senile cataract. *Ophthalmol Res* 1972;3:224–232.
134. Friedburg D: Enzyme activity patterns in clear human lenses and in different types of human senile cataract, in *The Human Lens — in relation to cataract.* Ciba Symposium 19. New York, Elsevier Excerpta Medica, 1973, pp 117–128.
135. Jedziniak JA, Chylack LT Jr, Cheng HM, et al: The sorbitol pathway in the human lens: Aldose reductase and polyol dehydrogenase. *Invest Ophthalmol Vis Sci* 1981;20:314–326.
136. Chylack LT Jr, Kinoshita JH: A biochemical evaluation of a cataract induced in high-glucose medium. *Invest Ophthalmol* 1969;8:401–412.
137. Gabbay KH: The sorbitol pathway and the complications of diabetes. *N Engl J Med* 1973;288:831–836.
138. Cheng HM: Thiol oxidation in the lens. *Invest Ophthalmol Vis Sci* 1979;18(suppl):99.
139. Wolfe JK, Gillis MK, Chylack LT Jr: Glucose metabolism in calf lens. *Exp Eye Res* 1985;40:629–641.
140. Jedziniak J, Arredondo LM, Meys M: Polyol dehydrogenase the human lens. *Invest Ophthalmol Vis Sci* 1986;27(suppl):137.
141. Orosz SE, Townsend SF, Tornheim PA, Brownscheidle CM: Localization of aldose reductase and sorbitol dehydrogenase in the nervous system of normal and diabetic rats. *Acta Diabet Lat* 1981;18:373–381.
142. Kinoshita JH: Concept of aldose reductase and diabetic cataracts, in Cogan DG (moderator): Aldose reductase and complications of diabetes. *Ann Intern Med* 1984;101:82–91.
143. Peterson MJ, Sarges R, Aldinger CE, MacDonald MP: CP-45,634: A novel aldose reductase inhibitor that inhibits polyol pathway activity in diabetic and galactosemic rats. *Metabolism* 1979;28(suppl 1):456–461.
144. Mayer JH, Tomlinson DR: The influence of aldose reductase inhibition and nerve myo-inositol on axonal transport and nerve conduction velocity in rats with experimental diabetes. *J Physiol* 1983;340:25P–26P.
145. Gillon KRW, Hawthorne JN: Sorbitol, inositol and nerve conduction in diabetes. *Life Sci* 1983;32:1943–1947.
146. Mayer JH, Tomlinson DR: Prevention of defects of axonal transport and nerve conduction velocity by oral administration of myo-inositol for an aldose reductase inhibitor in streptozotocin-diabetic rats. *Diabetologia* 1983;25:433–438.
147. Gillon KRW, Hawthorne JN, Tomlinson DR: Myo-inositol and sorbitol metabolism in relation to peripheral nerve function in experimental diabetes in the rat: The effect of aldose reductase inhibition. *Diabetologia* 1983;25:365–371.
148. Kikkawa R, Hatanaka I, Yasuda H, et al: Effect of a new aldose reductase inhibitor, (E)-3-carboxymethyl-5-[(2E)-methyl-3-phenyl-propenyli-dene]rhodanine (ONO-2235) on peripheral nerve disorders in streptozotocin-diabetic rats. *Diabetologia* 1983; 24:290–292.
149. Asano T, Mochio S, Kuwata T, et al: Effect of aldose reductase inhibitor (ONO-2235) on somatic and autonomic nervous dysfunction in streptozotocin-induced diabetic rats. *J Japan Diab Soc* 1983;26:1105–1111.
150. Fretten P, Tomlinson DR, Townsend J: Prevention of axonal transport defects, in vagus and sciatic nerves of diabetic rats, by aldose reductase inhibition. *Br J Pharmacol* 1984;82:265P.

151. Tomlinson DR, Moriarty RJ, Mayer JH: Prevention and reversal of defective axonal transport and motor nerve conduction velocity in rats with experimental diabetes by treatment with the aldose reductase inhibitor sorbinil. *Diabetes* 1984;33:470–476.
152. Malone JI, Leavengood H, Peterson MJ, O'Brien MM, Page MG: Red blood sorbitol as an indicator of polyol pathway activity. Inhibition by sorbinil in insulin-dependent diabetic subjects. *Diabetes* 1984;33:45–59.
153. Kikkawa R, Hatanaka I, Yasuda H, Kobayashi N, Shigeta Y: Prevention of peripheral nerve dysfunction by an aldose reductase inhibitor in streptozotocin-diabetic rats. *Metabolism* 1984;33:212–213.
154. Mayer HJ, Tomlinson DR, McLean GW: Slow orthograde axonal transport of radiolabelled protein in sciatic motoneurons of rats with short-term experimental diabetes: Effects of treatment with an aldose reductase inhibitor or myo-inositol. *J Neurochem* 1984;43:1265–1270.
155. Hotta N, Kakuta H, Fukasawa H, et al: Effects of a fructose-rich diet and the aldose reductase inhibitor, ONO-2235, on the development of diabetic neuropathy in streptozotocin-treated rats. *Diabetologia* 1985;28:176–180.
156. Stribling D, Mirrless DJ, Harrison HE, Earl DCN: Properties of ICI 128,436, a novel aldose reductase inhibitor, and its effects on diabetic complications in the rat. *Metabolism* 1985;34:336–344.
157. Dvornik D, Simard-Duquesne N, Kraml M, et al: Polyol accumulation in galactosemic and diabetic rats: Control by an aldose reductase inhibitor. *Science* 1973; 182:1146–1148.
158. Hu T, Merola LO, Kuwabara T, Kinoshita JH: Prevention and reversal of galactose cataract in rats with topical sorbinil. *Invest Ophthalmol Vis Sci* 1984;25:603–605.
159. Simard-Duquesne N, Greselin E, Dubuc J, Dvornik D: The effect of a new aldose reductase inhibitor (tolrestat) in galactosemic and diabetic rats. *Metabolism* 1985; 34:885–892.
160. Mizisin AP, Powell HC, Myers RR: Edema and increased endoneurial sodium in galactose neuropathy. *J Neurol Sci* 1986;74:35–43.
161. Greene DA, Lattimer SA: Relationship of polyol (sorbitol) pathway inhibition to a myo-inositol-mediated defect in sodium-potassium ATPase activity. *Diabetes* 1984;33:712–716.
162. Dvornik D, Millen J, Kemper C: Prevention by tolrestat of the biochemical and morphological changes in galactose-fed rats. *Diabetes* 1986;35(suppl 1):215A.
163. Gabbay KM: Role of sorbitol pathway in neuropathy, in Camerini-Davalos RA, Cole HS (eds): *Vascular and Neurological Changes in Early Diabetes.* New York, Academic Press, 1973, pp 417–424.
164. Yue DK, Hanwell MA, Satchell PM, Turtle JR: The effect of aldose reductase inhibition on nerve conduction velocity in diabetic rats. *Diabetes* 1982;31:789–794.
165. Akagi Y, Kador PF, Kuwabara T, Kinoshita JH: Aldose reductase localization in human retinal mural cells. *Invest Ophthalmol Vis Sci* 1983;24:1516–1519.
166. Schultz RO, Matsuda M, Yee RW, Edelhauser HF, Schultz KJ: Corneal endothelial changes in Type I and Type II diabetes mellitus. *Am J Ophthalmol* 1984;98:401–410.
167. Kinoshita JH, Fukushi S, Kador P, Merola LO: Aldose reductase in diabetic complications of the eye. *Metabolism* 1979;28(suppl 1):462–469.
168. Datiles MB, Kador PF, Fukui HN, Hu TS, Kinoshita JH: Corneal re-epithelization in galactosemic rats. *Invest Ophthalmol Vis Sci* 1983;24:567–569.
169. Cobo LM: Aldose reductase and diabetic keratopathy, pp 87–89, in Cogan DG (moderator): Aldose reductase and complications of diabetes. *Ann Intern Med* 1984;101: 82–91.
170. Buzney SM, Frank RN, Varma SD, Tanashima T, Gabbay KH: Aldose reductase in retinal mural cells. *Invest Ophthalmol Vis Sci* 1977;16:392–396.

171. Kennedy A, Frank RN, Varma SD: Aldose reductase activity in retinal and cerebral microvessels and cultured vascular cells. *Invest Ophthalmol Vis Sci* 1983; 24:1250–1258.
172. Li W, Shen S, Khatami M, Rockey JH: Stimulation of retinal capillary pericyte protein and collagen synthesis in culture by high-glucose concentration. *Diabetes* 1984; 33:785–789.
173. Li W, Khatami M, Rockey JH: The effects of glucose and an aldose reductase inhibitor on the sorbitol content and collagen synthesis of bovine retinal capillary pericytes in culture. *Exp Eye Res* 1985;40:439–444.
174. Robison WG, Kador PF, Kinoshita JH: Retinal capillaries: Basement membrane thickening by galactosemia prevented with aldose reductase inhibitor. *Science* 1983;221:1177–1179.
175. Frank RN, Kern RJ, Kennedy A, Frank KW: Galactose-induced retinal capillary basement membrane thickening: Prevention by sorbinil. *Invest Ophthalmol Vis Sci* 1983;24:1519–1529.
176. Unpublished results from the Ayerst Research Laboratories.
177. MacGregor LC, Matschinsky F: Correlation of biochemical and electrophysiological abnormalities in retinas of experimentally diabetic animals. *Diabetes* 1985;34 (suppl 1):13A.
178. Ludvigson MA, Sorenson RL: Immunohistochemical localization of aldose reductase. I. Enzyme purification and antibody preparation. Localization in peripheral nerve, artery and testis. *Diabetes* 1980;29:438–449.
179. Ludvigson MA, Sorenson RL: Immunohistochemical localization of aldose reductase. II. Rat eye and kidney. *Diabetes* 1980;29:450–459.
180. Kern TS, Engerman RL: Immunohistochemical distribution of aldose reductase. *Histochem J* 1982;14:507–515.
181. Corder CN, Braughler JM, Culp PA: Quantitative histochemistry of the sorbitol pathway in glomeruli and small arteries of human diabetic kidney. *Folia Histochem Cytochem* 1979;17:137–146.
182. Bagnasco S, Bedford J, Balaban R, Uchida S, Burg M: High levels of sorbitol and aldose reductase are induced in renal papillary epithelial cells by hypertonic (high NaC1) medium. *Fed Proc* 1986;45:1839.
183. Bagnasco S, Uchida S, Balaban R, Burg M: Renal papillary cells cultured in hypertonic medium synthesize large amounts of intracellular sorbitol. *Kidney Int* 1986;29:412.
184. Bagnasco S, Balaban R, Fales HM, Yang YM, Burg M: Predominant osmotically active organic solutes in rat and rabbit renal medullas. *J Biol Chem* 1986;261:5872–5877.
185. Yancey PH, Clark ME, Hand SC, Bowlus RD, Somero GN: Living with water stress: evolution of osmolyte systems. *Science* 1982;217:1214–1222.
186. Wirthensohn G, Beck F, Guder WG: Glycerophosphoryl-choline and sorbitol in osmoregulation of rat renal papilla. *J Clin Chem Clin Biochem* 1986;24:679.
187. Gabbay KH, O'Sullivan JB: The sorbitol pathway in diabetes and galactosemia: Enzyme and substrate localization and changes in kidney. *Diabetes* 1968;17:300.
188. Corder CN, Collins JG, Brannan TS, Sharma J: Aldose reductase and sorbitol dehydrogenase distribution in rat kidney. *J Histochem Cytochem* 1977;25:1–8.
189. Bauman JW Jr, Farnsworth PN: Effect of aldose reductase inhibition on natriuresis and proteinuria in diabetic rats. *Kidney Int* 1986;29:391.
190. Kilzer P, Chang K, Marvel J, et al. Albumin permeation on new vessels is increased in diabetic rats. *Diabetes* 1985;34:333–336.
191. Williamson JR, Chang K, Rowold E, et al: Sorbinil prevents diabetes-induced increases in vascular permeability but does not alter collagen cross-linking. *Diabetes* 1985;34:703–705.

192. Williamson JR, Chang K, Rowold E, et al: Diabetes-induced increases in vascular permeability are prevented by castration and by sorbinil. *Diabetes* 1985;34(suppl 1):108A.
193. Roper H, Roper S, Heyns, K: NMR Spectroscopy of N-(1-deoxy-D-fructose-1-yl)-L-amino acids ("fructose-amino acids"). *Carbohydr Res* 1983;116:183–195.
194. Chang K, Tomlinson M, Jeffery JR, et al: Galactose ingestion increases vascular permeability and collagen solubility in normal male rats. *J Clin Invest* 1987;79:367–373.
195. Lorenzi S, Lane M: Polyol and glucose accumulation by human endothelial cells cultured in high glucose are not prevented by sorbinil. *Clin Res* 1985;33:63A.
196. Ellis DA, Strickland JM: Differences in the metabolism of glucose between normal and dystrophic human muscle. *Biochem J* 1972:130:17P–18P.
197. Ellis DA, Strickland JM, Eccleston JF: The direct interconversion of glucose and fructose in human skeletal muscle with special reference to childhood muscular dystrophy. *Clin Sci* 1973;44:321–334.
198. Ellis DA: Intermediary metabolism of muscle in Duchenne muscular dystrophy. *Br Med Bull* 1980;36:165–171.
199. Kinoshita JH, Dvornik D, Kraml M, Gabbay KH: The effect of aldose reductase inhibitor on the galactose-exposed rabbit lens. *Biochem Biophys Acta* 1968;158:472–475.
200. Strickland JM, Ellis DA: Isoenzymes of hexokinase in human muscular dystrophy. *Nature* 1975;253:464–466.
201. Davidson WS, Murphy DG: Aldehyde reductases and their involvement in muscular dystrophy, in Flynn TG, Weiner H (eds): *Enzymology of carbonyl metabolism 2: Aldehyde dehydrogenase, aldo-keto reductase, and alcohol dehydrogenase.* New York, AR Liss Inc, 1985, pp 251–263.
202. Cosmos E, Butler J: Animal models of muscle diseases. III. Compilation of therapeutic trials for hereditary muscular dystrophy. *Muscle & Nerve* 1980;3:427–435 and references cited.
203. Hudecki MS, Pollina CM, Heffner RR, Bhargava AK: Enhanced functional ability in drug-treated dystrophic chickens: Trial results with indomethacin, diphenylhydantoin, and prednisolone. *Exp Neurol* 1981;73:173–185.
204. Murphy DG, Williamson WS: Chicken muscle aldose reductase: Purification, properties and relationship to other chicken aldo/keto reductases. *Int J Biochem* 1986;18:215–221.
205. Murphy DG, Davidson WS: Inhibition studies on chicken muscle aldose reductase. *Biochem Pharmacol* 1985;34:2961–2965.
206. Unpublished results from the Ayerst Research Laboratories.
207. Allen DW, Schroeder WA, Balog J: Observation on the chromatographic heterogeneity of normal adult and fetal human hemoglobin: A study of the effects of crystallization and chromatography on the heterogeneity and isoleucine content. *J Am Chem Soc* 1958;80:1628–1634.
208. Clegg MD, Schroeder WA: A chromatographic study of the minor components of normal adult human hemoglobin including a comparison of hemoglobin from normal and phenylketonuric individuals. *J Am Chem Soc* 1959;81:6065–6069.
209. Schnek AG, Schroeder WA: The relation between the minor components of whole normal adult hemoglobin as isolated by chromatography and starch block electrophoresis. *J Am Chem Soc* 1961;83:1472–1478.
210. Ditzel J, Andersen H, Peters ND: Oxygen affinity of hemoglobin and red blood cell 2,3-diphosphoglycerate in childhood diabetes. *Acta Pediatr Scand* 1975;64: 355–361.
211. Rahbar S, Blumenfeld O, Ranney HM: Studies of an unusual hemoglobin in patients with diabetes mellitus. *Biochem Biophys Res Comm* 1969;36:838–843.

212. Paulsen EP: Hemoglobin Alc in childhood diabetes. *Metabolism* 1973;22:269–272.
213. Trivelli LA, Ranney HM, Lai HT: Hemoglobin components in patients with diabetes mellitus. *N Engl J Med* 1981;284:353–357.
214. Dixon HBF: A reaction of glucose with peptides. *Biochem J* 1972;129:203–208.
215. Bunn HF, Haney DN, Gabbay KH, Gallop PM: Further identification of the nature and linkage of the carbohydrate in hemoglobin Alc. *Biochem Biophys Res Comm* 1975;67:103–109.
216. Flückiger R, Winterhalter KH: In vitro synthesis of hemoglobin Alc. *FEBS Lett* 1976;71:356–360.
217. Koenig RJ, Peterson CM, Kilo C, Cerami A, Williamson JR: Hemoglobin Alc as an indicator of the degree of glucose intolerance in diabetes. *Diabetes* 1976;25:230–232.
218. Koenig RJ, Peterson CM, Jones RL, et al: Correlation of glucose regeneration and hemoglobin Alc in diabetes mellitus. *N Engl J Med* 1976;295:417–420.
219. Gabbay KH, Hasty K, Breslow JL, et al: Glycosylated hemoglobins and long-term blood glucose control in diabetes mellitus. *J Clin Endocrinol Metab* 1977;44:859–864.
220. Gonen B, Rubenstein AH, Rochman H, Tanega SF, Horwitz DL: Hemoglobin A1: An indicator of the metabolic control of diabetic patients. *Lancet* 1977;2:734–737.
221. Tze WJ, Thompson KH, Leichter J: HbA1c: An indication of diabetic control. *J Pediatr* 1978;93:13–16.
222. Ditzel J, Kjaergaard J: Hemoglobin Alc concentrations after initial insulin treatment for newly discovered diabetes. *Br Med J* 1978;1:741–742.
223. Goldstein DE, Parker KM, England JD, et al: Clinical application of glycosylated hemoglobin measurements. *Diabetes* 1982;31(suppl 3):70–78.
224. Duncan BB, Heiss G: Nonenzymatic glycosylation of proteins: A new tool for assessment of cumulative hyperglycemia in epidemiologic studies, past and future. *Am J Epidemiol* 1984;120:169–189.
225. Nelson DM, Barrows HJ, Clapp DH, Orthman-Nabi J, Whitehurst RM: Glycosylated serum protein levels in diabetic and nondiabetic pregnant patients: An indication of short-term glycemic control in the diabetic patient. *Am J Obstet Gynecol* 1985;151:1042–1047.
226. Albutt EC, Nattrass M, Northam BE: Glucose tolerance test and glycosylated haemoglobin measurement for diagnosis of diabetes mellitus—an assessment of the criteria of the WHO Expert Committee on Diabetes Mellitus 1980. *Ann Clin Biochem* 1985;22:67–73.
227. Lester E, Frazer AD, Shepherd CA, Woodroffe FJ: Glycosylated haemoglobin as an alternative to the glucose tolerance test for the diagnosis of diabetes mellitus. *Ann Clin Biochem* 1985;22:74–78.
228. Kilzer P: Glycated hemoglobin and diabetes: A case and an overview of the subject. *Clin Chem* 1985;31:1060–1067.
229. Maillard LC: Action des acides aminé's sur les sucres; formation des mélanoidines par voie méthodique. *CR Acad Sci* 1912;154:66–68.
230. Cerami A: Hypothesis: Glucose as mediator of aging. *J Am Geriatr Soc* 1985;33:626–630, and references cited.
231. Candiano G, Ghiggeri GM, Delfino G, et al: Reaction of lysine with aldoses. *Carbohydr Res* 1985;145:99–112.
232. Means GE, Chang MK: Nonenzymatic glucosylation of proteins. Structure and function changes. *Diabetes* 1982;31(suppl 3):1–4.
233. Shapiro R, McManus MJ, Zalut C, Bunn HF: Sites of non-enzymatic glycosylation of human hemoglobin A. *J Biol Chem* 1980;255:3120–3127.
234. Garlick RL, Mazer JS: The principal site of nonenzymatic glycosylation of human serum albumin in vivo. *J Biol Chem* 1983;258:6142–6146.

235. Guthrow CE, Morris MA, Day JF, Thorpe SR, Baynes JW: Enhanced nonenzymatic glycosylation of human serum albumin in diabetes mellitus. *Proc Natl Acad Sci* 1979; 76:4258–4261.
236. Cantor SM, Peniston QP: The reduction of aldoses at the dropping mercury cathode: Estimation of the aldehyo structure in aqueous solutions. *J Am Chem Soc* 1940; 62:2113–2121.
237. Bunn HF, Higgins PJ: Reaction of monosaccharides with protein: Possible evolutionary significance. *Science* 1981;213:222–224.
238. Dolhofer R, Wieland OH: In vitro glycosylation of hemoglobins by different and sugar phosphates. *FEBS Lett* 1978;85:86–90.
239. Spicer KM, Allen RC, Hallet D, Buse MG: Synthesis of hemoglobin Alc and related minor hemoglobins by erythrocytes. *J Clin Invest* 1979;64:40–48.
240. Urbanowski JE, Cohenford, MA, Dain JA: Nonenzymatic glycosylation of human serum albumin. *J Biol Chem* 1982;257:111–115.
241. Monnier VM, Stevens VJ, Cerami A: Nonenzymatic glycosylation, sulfhydryl oxidation, and aggregation of lens proteins in experimental sugar cataracts. *J Exp Med* 1979;150:1098–1107.
242. Chiou S, Chylack LT Jr, Bunn HF, Kinoshita JH: Role of nonenzymatic glycosylation in experimental cataract formation. *Biochem Biophys Res Comm* 1980;95:894–901.
243. Powell HC, Ivor L, Costello ML, Wolf PL: Elevated hemoglobin A1 in streptozotocin diabetic rats and in rats on sucrose and galactose-enriched diets. *Clin Biochem* 1982;15:133–137.
244. Ivor LP, Wolf PL, Costello ML, Powell HC: Elevated hemoglobin A1c in experimental galactosemia. *Clin Chem* 1979;25:1076.
245. Mortensen HB, Christophersen C: Glucosylation of human haemoglobin in red blood cells studied in vitro. Kinetics of the formation and dissociation of haemoglobin A1c. *Clin Chim Acta* 1983;134:317–326.
246. Goldstein DE, Peth SB, England JD, Hess RL, Da Costa J: Effect of acute changes in blood glucose on HbA. *Diabetes* 1980;29:623–628.
247. Acharya AS, Sussman LG: The reversibility of the ketoamine linkages of aldoses with proteins. *J Biol Chem* 1984;259:4372–4378.
248. Stevens VJ, Monnier VM, Cerami A: Hemoglobin glycosylation as a model for modification of other proteins. *Tex Rep Biol Med* 1980;40:387–396.
249. Cerami A: Aging of proteins and nucleic acids: what is the role of glucose? *TIBS* 1986;11:311–314.
250. Proceedings of a conference on nonenzymatic glycosylation and browning reactions: Their relevance to diabetes mellitus. *Diabetes* 1982;31(suppl 3):V–VI, 1–82.
251. Wieland OH, Dolhofer R, Schleicher E, et al: Nonenzymatic glucosylation (glycation) of proteins — possible relevance to diabetic complications. *Int Congr Ser* 1985; 681:361–369.
252. Cohen MP: *Diabetes and protein glycosylation.* New York, Berlin, Heidelberg, Tokyo, Springer-Verlag, 1986.
253. Ditzel J: Oxygen transport impairment in diabetes. *Diabetes* 1976;25(suppl 2):832–838.
254. McDonald MJ, Bleichman M, Bunn HF, Noble RW: Functional properties of the glycosylated minor components of human adult hemoglobin. *J Biol Chem* 1979;254:702–707.
255. Samaja M, Melotti D, Carenini A, Pozza G: Glycosylated hemoglobins and the oxygen affinity of whole blood. *Diabetologia* 1982;23:399–402.
256. Ditzel J, Standl E: The problem of tissue oxygenation in diabetes mellitus. II. Evidence of disordered oxygen release from the erythrocytes of diabetics in various conditions of metabolic control. *Acta Med Scand* 1975;578(suppl):49–58.

257. Bunn HF, Gabbay KH, Gallop PM: The glycosylation of hemoglobin: Relevance to diabetes mellitus. *Science* 1978;200:21–27.
258. Bailey AJ, Robins SP, Tanner MJA: Reducible components in the proteins of human erythrocyte membrane. *Biochim Biophys Acta* 1976;434:51–57.
259. Miller JA, Gravallese E, Bunn HE: Non-enzymatic glycosylation of erythrocyte membrane proteins; relevant to diabetes. *J Clin Invest* 1980;65:896–901.
260. Schleicher E, Scheller L, Wieland OH: Quantitation of lysin-bound glucose of normal and diabetic erythrocyte membranes by HPLC analysis of furosine. *Biochem Biophys Res Com* 1981;99:1011–1019.
261. McMillan DE, Utterback NG, La Puma J: Reduced erythrocyte deformability in diabetes. *Diabetes* 1978;27:895–901.
262. McMillan DE, Utterback NG, Sparks LL, Bramwell PC: Impaired doublet formation in diabetes. *Diabetologia* 1981;21:575–578.
263. Baba Y, Motoaki K, Kamada T, Setoyama S, Otsuji S: Higher levels of erythrocyte membrane microviscosity in diabetes. *Diabetes* 1979;28:1138–1140.
264. Mortensen HB, Brahm J: Glucose transport in erythrocytes of diabetic and healthy children as related to hemoglobin A1c. *Clin Chem* 1985;31:1387–1389.
265. Williamson JR, Gardner RA, Boylan CW, et al: Microrheologic investigation of erythrocyte deformability in diabetes mellitus. *Blood* 1985;65:283–288.
266. Juhan-Vagua I, Vague P: Properties of erythrocytes and platelets and degree of diabetic control. *Nouv Rev Fr Haematol* 1982;24:191–195.
267. Watala C, Zawodniak M, Bryszewska M, Nowak S: Non-enzymatic protein glycosylation. I. Lowered erythrocyte membrane fluidity in juvenile diabetes. *Ann Clin Res* 1985;107:327–330.
268. Day JF, Thrope SR, Baynes JW: Nonenzymatically glucosylated albumin. *J Biol Chem* 1979;254:595–597.
269. Mereish KA, Rosenberg H, Cobby J: Glycosylated albumin and its influence on salicylate binding. *J Pharm Sci* 1982;71:235–238.
270. McFarland KF, Catalano EW, Day JF, Thorpe SR, Baynes JW: Non-enzymatic glycosylation of serum proteins in diabetes mellitus. *Diabetes* 1979;28:1011–1014.
271. Yue DK, Morris K, McLennan S, Turtle JR: Glycosylation of plasma protein and its relation to glycosylated hemoglobin in diabetes. *Diabetes* 1980;29:296–300.
272. Dolhofer R, Wieland OH: Increased glycosylation of serum albumin in diabetes mellitus. *Diabetes* 1980;29:417–422.
273. Kennedy L, Mehl TD, Riley WJ, Merimee TJ: Non-enzymatically glycosylated serum protein in diabetes mellitus: An index of short-term glycemia. *Diabetologia* 1981;21:94–98.
274. Dolhofer R, Renner R, Wieland OH: Different behavior of hemoglobin A1c and glycosyl-albumin levels during recovery from diabetic ketoacidosis and non-acidotic coma. *Diabetologia* 1981;21:211–215.
275. Cecchini G, Calefatto V, Chiambretti A, et al: Glycosylated serum albumin; high performance liquid chromatography (HPLC) evaluation in normal and diabetic patients. *IRCS Med Sci* 1986;14:1027–1028.
276. Schleicher E, Wieland OH: Specific quantitation by HPLC of protein (lysine) bound glucose in human serum albumin and other glycosylated proteins. *J Clin Chem Clin Biochem* 1981;19:81–87.
277. Day JF, Thornburg RW, Thorpe SR, Baynes JW: Nonenzymatic glucosylation of rat albumin. *J Biol Chem* 1979;254:9344–9400.
278. Candiano G, Ghiggeri GM, Delfino G, et al: Glycosylation of human albumin in diabetes mellitus: extensive microheterogeneity of serum and urinary species as revealed by isoelectric focusing. *Electrophoresis* 1984;5:217–222.

279. Iberg N, Flückiger R: Nonenzymatic glycosylation of albumin in vivo. Identification of multiple glycosylated sites. *J Biol Chem* 1986;261:13,542–13,545.
280. Shaklai N, Garlick RL, Bunn HF: Nonenzymatic glycosylation of human serum albumin alters its conformation and function. *J Biol Chem* 1984;259:3812–3817.
281. Murtiashaw MH, Winterhalter KH: Nonenzymatic glycation of human albumin does not alter its palmitate binding. *Diabetologia* 1986;29:366–370.
282. Ghiggeri GM, Candiano G, Delfino G, Queirolo C: Conformational mediated renal selectivity towards albumin in diabetes mellitus. *Diab Metab* 1986;12:68–73.
283. Mahaffey EA, Buonanno AM, Cornelius LM: Glycosylated albumin and serum protein in diabetic dogs. *Am J Vet Res* 1984;45:2126–2127.
284. Morris MA, Preddy L: Glycosylation accelerates albumin degration in normal and diabetic dogs. *Biochem Med Metab Biol* 1986;35:267–270.
285. Rendell M, Nierenberg J: Aspirin inhibits galactosylation and fructosylation of protein as well as glycosylation. *Clin Res* 1985;33:65A.
286. Rendell M, Valentine J, Stephens P, Nierenberg J: Kinetics of inhibition of glycosylation by aspirin. *Clin Res* 1985;33:66A.
287. Hun-Opfer C, Mata-Segreda JF: Nonenzymatic acetylation of proteins by aspirin as protection against the secondary complications of diabetes mellitus. *Acta Physiol Pharmacol Latinoam* 1986;36:313–316.
288. Shaklai N, Garlick RL, Bunn HF: Tryptophan fluorescence and ligand binding properties of glycosylated human serum albumin. *Fed Proc* 1983;42:2098.
289. Tsuchiya S, Sakurai T, Sekiguchi S: Nonenzymatic glucosylation of human serum albumin and its influence on binding capacity of sulfonylureas. *Biochem Pharmacol* 1984;33:2967–2971.
290. Ruiz-Cabello F, Erill S: Abnormal serum protein binding of acidic drugs in diabetes mellitus. *Clin Pharmacol Ther* 1984;36:691–695.
291. Kearns GL, Kemp SF, Turley CP, Nelson D: Altered phenytoin protein binding in Type I diabetes mellitus. *Clin Res* 1986;34:237A.
292. Schleicher E, Duefel T, Wieland OH: Nonenzymatic glycosylation of human serum lipoproteins. *FEBS Lett* 1981;129:1–4.
293. Witztum JL, Mahoney EM, Branks MJ, et al: Nonenzymatic glucosylation of low-density lipoprotein alters its biologic activity. *Diabetes* 1982;31:283–291.
294. Lorenzi M, Cagliero E, Markey B, Henriksen T, Witztum JL: Interaction of human endothelial cells with elevated glucose concentrations and native and glycosylated low density lipoproteins. *Diabetologia* 1984;26:218–222.
295. Weisgraber KH, Innerarity TL, Mahley RW: Role of the lysine residues of plasma lipoproteins in high affinity binding to cell surface receptors on human fibroblasts. *J Biol Chem* 1978;253:9053–9062.
296. Steinbrecher UP, Witztum JL: Glucosylation of low-density lipoproteins to an extent comparable to that seen in diabetes slows their catabolism. *Diabetes* 1984; 33:130–134.
297. Witztum JL, Steinbrecher UP, Kasaniemi YA, Fisher M: Autoantibodies to glucosylated proteins in the plasma of patients with diabetes mellitus. *Proc Natl Acad Sci* 1984;81:3204–3208.
298. Curtiss LK, Witztum JL: A novel method for generating region-specific monoclonal antibodies to modified proteins. Application to the identification of human glucosylated low density lipproteins. *J Clin Invest* 1984;72:1427–1438.
299. Etchells E, Fong B, Angel A: Effect of nonenzymatic glycosylation of low density lipoprotein (LDL) on binding to purified human adipocyte plasma membranes. *Clin Invest Med* 1986;9:A35.
300. Schleicher E, Olgemoller B, Schon J, Durst T: Non-enzymatic glycosylation of LDL does not alter its recognition by the high affinity receptor. *Diabetologia* 1984;27:328A.

301. Curtiss LK, Witztum JC: Plasma apolipoproteins AI, AII, B, CI, and E are glycosylated in hyperglycemic diabetic subjects. *Diabetes* 1985;34:452–461.
302. Sampietro T, Lenzi S, Giampietro O, et al: Significance and clinical usefulness of low density lipoprotein electrophoretic mobility for the evaluation of nonenzymaic glycosylation. *Clin Physiol Biochem* 1986;4:125–129.
303. Jack CM, McAlister VP, Sheridan B, Stout RW, Kennedy L: Nonenzymatic glycosylation of low-density lipoprotein (LDL). *Diabetologia* 1986;29:552A.
304. Olgemoller B, Schleicher E, Wieland OH: Different effects of reductive and non-reductive glycosylation on LDL-catabolism. *Horm Metab Res* 1985;15:87–90.
305. Lyons TJ, Baynes JW, Patrick JS, Colwell JA, Lopes-Virella MF: Glycosylation of low density lipoprotein in patients with Type 1 (insulin-dependent) diabetes; correlations with other parameters of glycaemic control. *Diabetologia* 1986;29:685–689.
306. Cerami A, Vlassara H, Brownlee M: Role of nonenzymatic glycosylation in atherogenesis. *J Cel Biochem* 1986;30:111–120.
307. Barrett-Connor E, Criqui MH, Witztum JL, Philippi T, Zettner A: Population-based study of glycosylated hemoglobin, lipids, and lipoproteins in nondiabetic subjects. *Arteriosclerosis* 1987;7:66–70.
308. Dolhofer R, Siess EA, Wieland OH: Nonenzymatic glycation of immunoglobulins leads to an impairment of immunoreactivity. *Bibl Chem Hoppe-Seyler* 1985;366:361–266.
309. Brownlee M, Vlassara H, Cerami A: Trapped immunoglobulins on peripheral nerve myelin from patients with diabetes mellitus. *Diabetes* 1986;35:999–1003.
310. Ney KA, Pasqua JJ, Colley KJ, Guthrow CE, Pizzo SV: In vitro preparation of nonenzymatically glucosylated human transferrin, α_2-macroglobulin, and fibrinogen with preservation of function. *Diabetes* 1985;34:462–470.
311. Brownlee M, Vlassara H, Cerami A: Nonenzymatic glycosylation reduces the susceptibility of fibrin to degradation by plasmin. *Diabetes* 1983;32:680–684.
312. Kim HC, Heller I, Schneider SH, Avigad G, Saidi P: Functional alteration of fibrinogen by nonenzymatic glycosylation. *Thromb Haemostas* 1985;54:158.
313. Lutjens A, Te Velde AA, Van Den Veen EA, Van Den Meer J: Glycosylation of human fibrinogen in vivo. *Diabetologia* 1985;28:87–89.
314. Sampietro T, Lenzi S, Cecchetti P, et al: Nonenzymatic glycation of human platelet membrane proteins in vitro and in vivo. *Clin Chem* 1986;32:1328–1331.
315. Ducrocq R, Bachour H, Belkhodja R, Berriche S, Elion J: Evidence for nonenzymic glycation of antithrombin III in diabetic patients. *Clin Chem* 1985;31:338–339.
316. Brownlee M, Vlassara H, Cerami A: Inhibition of heparin-catalyzed human antithrombin III activity by nonenzymatic glycosylation. Possible role in fibrin deposition in diabetes. *Diabetes* 1984;33:532–535.
317. Ceriello A, Curcio F, Dello Russo P, Giugliano D: Nonenzymatic glycosylation reduces antithrombin III activity. *Thromb Haemostas* 1984:52:363.
318. Ceriello A, Giugliano D, Dello Russo P, et al: Metabolic control may alter antithrombin III activity but not its plasma concentration in diabetes: A possible role for nonenzymatic glycosylation. *Diabetes Care* 1986;9:32–35.
319. Hall P, Tryon E, Nikolai TF, Roberts RC: Functional activities and nonenzymatic glycosylation of plasma proteinase inhibitors in diabetes. *Clin Chim Acta* 1986;160:55–62.
320. McVerry BA, Hopp A, Fisher G, Huehns ER: Production of pseudodiabetic renal glomerular changes in mice after repeated injections of glycosylated proteins. *Lancet* 1980;1:738–740.
321. Jeraj KP, Michael AF, Mauer M, Brown DM: Glycosylated and normal human and rat albumin do not bind to renal basement membranes of diabetic and control rats. *Diabetes* 1983;32:380–382.

322. Ghiggeri GM, Candiano G, Delfino G, Bianchini F, Queirolo C: Glycosyl albumin and diabetic micro-albuminuria: Demonstration of an altered renal handling. *Kidney Int* 1984;25:565–570.
323. Gragnoli G, Signorini AM, Tanganelli I: Nonenzymatic glycosylation of urinary proteins in Type I (insulin-dependent) diabetes: Correlation with metabolic control and the degree of proteinuria. *Diabetologia* 1984;26:411–414.
324. Kowluru A, Kowluru RA, Johnson JD, Greenberg R, Bitensky MW: Preferential urinary excretion of glucosylated albumin in normal and diabetic individuals. *Diabetes* 1986;35(suppl 1):93A.
325. Pollak A, Coradello H, Leban J, et al: Inhibition of alkaline phosphatase activity by glucose. *Clin Chim Acta* 1983;133:15–24.
326. Pollak A, Schober E, Coradello H, et al: Influence of glucose fluctuations on alkaline phosphatase activity. *Acta Diab Lat* 1984;21:123–131.
327. Iberg N, Flückiger R: Nonenzymatic glycosylation (glycation) of proteins: The principal sites of in vitro glycation of RNase A. *Experientia* 1986;42:680.
328. Sharma C, Dalferes ER Jr, Radhakrishnamurthy B, Rosen EL, Berenson GS: Nonenzymatic glycosylation of proteins and protease activities in granulation tissues in experimental diabetes. *Inflammation* 1986;4:403–411.
329. Harding JJ, Dilley KJ: Structural proteins of the mammalian lens: A review with emphasis on changes in development, aging and cataract. *Exp Eye Res* 1976; 22:1–73.
330. Bloemendal H: The vertebrate eye lens. *Science* 1977;197:127–138.
331. Hoenders HJ, Bloemendal H: Lens protein and aging. *J Gerontol* 1983;38:278–286.
332. Pande A, Garner WH, Spector A: Glucosylation of human lens protein and cataractogenesis. *Biochim Biophys Res Comm* 1979;89:1260–1266.
333. Ansari NHM, Awasthi YC, Srivastava SK: Role of glycosylation in protein disulphide formation and cataractogenesis. *Exp Eye Res* 1980;31:9–19.
334. Chiou SH, Chylack LT Jr, Tung WH, Bunn HF: Nonenzymatic glycosylation of bovine lens crystallins. *J Biol Chem* 1981;256:5176–5180.
335. Monnier VM, Cerami A: Nonenzymatic glycosylation and browning in diabetes and aging. Studies on lens proteins. *Diabetes* 1982;31(suppl 3):57–63.
336. Kasai K, Nakamura T, Kase N, et al: Increased glycosylation of proteins from cataractous lenses in diabetes. *Diabetologia* 1983;25:36–38.
337. Mandel SS, Shin DH, Newman BL, et al: Glycosylation in vivo of human lens capsule (basement membrane) and diabetes mellitus. *Biochem Biophys Res Comm* 1983; 117:51–56.
338. Garlick RL, Mazer JS, Chylack LT Jr, Tung WH, Bunn HF: Nonenzymatic glycation of human lens crystallin. *J Clin Invest* 1984;74:1742–1749.
339. Lee JH, Shin DH, Lupovitch A, Shi DX: Glycosylation of lens proteins in senile cataract and diabetes mellitus. *Biochem Biophys Res Comm* 1984;123:888–893.
340. Liang JN, Hershorin LL, Chylack LT Jr: Nonenzymatic glycosylation in human diabetic lens crystalins. *Diabetologia* 1986;29:225–228.
341. Stevens VJ, Rouzer CA, Monnier VM, Cerami A: Diabetic cataract formation: Potential role of glycosylation. *Proc Natl Acad Sci* 1978;75:2918–2922.
342. Liang JN, Chylack LT Jr: Change in the protein tertiary structure with nonenzymatic glycosylation of calf-crystallin. *Biochem Biophys Res Comm* 1984;123:899–906.
343. Garlick RL, Mazer JS, Higgins PJ, Bunn HF: Characterization of glycosylated hemoglobins. *J Clin Invest* 1983;71:1062–1072.
344. Vlassara H, Brownlee M, Cerami A: Nonenzymatic glycosylation of peripheral nerve proteins in diabetes mellitus. *Proc Natl Acad Sci* 1981;78:5190–5192.
345. Vlassara H, Brownlee M, Cerami A: Excessive non-enzymatic glycosylation of peripheral and central nervous system myelin components in diabetic rats. *Diabetes* 1983;32:670–674.

346. Vogt BW, Schleicher ED, Wieland OH: ϵ-Amino-lysine-bound glucose in human tissues obtained at autopsy. Increase in diabetes mellitus. *Diabetes* 1982;31:1123–1127.
347. Scheinman JI, Fish AJ, Matas AJ, Michael AF: The immunohistopathology of glomerular antigens. *Am J Pathol* 1978;90:71–88.
348. Tarsio JF, Wigness B, Rhode TD, et al: Nonenzymatic glycation of fibronectin and alternations in the molecular association of cell matrix and basement membrane components in diabetes mellitus. *Diabetes* 1985;34:477–484.
349. Chang AY, Noble RE: 5-Hydroxymethylfurfural-forming proteins in the renal glomeruli of control and streptozotocin-diabetic rats. *Life Sci* 1980;26:1329–1333.
350. Uitto J, Perejda AJ, Grant GA, et al: Glycosylation of human glomerular basement membrane collagen: Increased content of hexose in ketoamine linkage and unaltered hydroxylysine-O-glycosides in patients with diabetes. *Conn Tis Res* 1982;10:287–296.
351. Li W, Shen S, Robertson GA, Khatami M, Rockey JH: Increased solubility of newly synthesized collagen in retinal capillary pericyte cultures by nonenzymatic glycosylation. *Ophthalmic Res* 1984;16:315–321.
352. Trueb B, Flückiger R, Winterhalter KH: Nonenzymatic glycosylation of basement membrane collagen in diabetes mellitus. *Collagen Rel Res* 1984;4:239–251.
353. Sasser BW, Poffenbarger PL: Nonenzymatic glycosylation of renal tubular basement membrane. *Diabetes* 1983;32:31A.
354. Bornstein P, Sage H: Structurally distinct collagen types. *Ann Rev Biochem* 1980;49:957–1003.
355. Uitto J, Ryhanen L, Tan EML: Collagen: Its structure, function, and pathology. *Progr Dis Skin* 1981;1:103–141
356. Rosenberg H, Modrak JB, Hassing JM, Al-Turk WA, Stohs SJ: Glycosylated collagen. *Biochem Biophys Res Comm* 1979;91:498–501.
357. Cohen MP, Urdanivia E, Surma M, Wu VY: Increased glycosylation of glomerular basement membrane collagen in diabetes. *Biochem Biophys Res Comm* 1980; 95:765–769.
358. Schnider SL, Kohn RR: Glucosylation of human collagen in aging and diabetes mellitus. *J Clin Invest* 1980;66:1179–1181.
359. Schnider SL, Kohn RR: Effects of age and diabetes mellitus on the solubility and nonenzymatic glucosylation of human skin collagen. *J Clin Invest* 1981;67: 1630–1635.
360. Kohn RR, Schnider SL: Glucosylation of human collagen. *Diabetes* 1982;31(suppl 3):47–51.
361. Hamlin CR, Kohn RR: Evidence for progressive, age-related structural changes in post-mature human collagen. *Biochim Biophys Acta* 1971;236:458–467.
362. Bailey AJ, Shimokomaki MS: Age-related changes in the reducible cross-links of collagen *FEBS Lett* 1971;16:86–88.
363. Hamlin CR, Kohn RR, Luschin JH: Apparent accelerated aging of human collagen in diabetes mellitus. *Diabetes* 1975;24:902–904.
364. Lyons TJ, Kennedy L: Effect of in vitro nonenzymatic glycosylation of human skin collagen on susceptibility to collagenase digestion. *Eur J Clin Invest* 1985;15: 128–131.
365. Kohn RR, Cerami A, Monnier VM: Collagen aging in vitro by nonenzymatic glycosylation and browning. *Diabetes* 1984;33:57–59.
366. Andreassen TT, Oxlund H: Thermal stability of collagen in relation to non-enzymatic glycosylation and browning in vitro. *Diabetologia* 1985;28:687–691.
367. Kent MJC, Light ND, Bailey AJ: Evidence for glucose-mediated covalent cross-linking of collagen after glycosylation in vitro. *Biochem J* 1985;225:745–752.

368. Guitton JD, Le Pape A, Muh JP: Influence of in vitro nonenzymatic glycosylation on the physicochemical parameters of Type I collagen. *Collagen Rel Res* 1984; 4:253–264.
369. Davis PF, Stehbens WE: Comparison of nonenzymatic glycosylation of arterial and venous collagens. *Biochem Med* 1984;32:15–21.
370. Le Pape A, Gutman N, Guitton JD, Legrand Y, Muh JP: Nonenzymatic glycosylation increases platelet aggregating potency of collagen from placenta of diabetic human beings. *Biochem Biophys Res Comm* 1983;111:602–610.
371. Monnier VM, Kohn RR, Cerami A: Accelerated browning of collagen in diabetic humans. *Diabetes* 1982;31(suppl 1): 28A.
372. Monnier VM, Kohn RR, Cerami A: Accelerated age-related browning of collagen in diabetes mellitus. *Proc Natl Acad Sci* 1984;81:583–587.
373. Monnier VM, Vishwanath V, Frank KE, et al: Relation between complications of Type I diabetes mellitus and collagen-linked fluorescence. *N Engl J Med* 1986;314: 403–408.
374. Vishwanath V, Frank KE, Elmets CA, Dauchot PJ, Monnier VM: Glycation of skin collagen in Type I diabetes mellitus. *Diabetes* 1986;35:916–921.
375. Ahmed MU, Thorpe SR, Baynes JW: Identification of N^{ϵ}-carboxymethyllysine as a degradation product of fructoselysine in glycated protein. *J Biol Chem* 1986; 261:4889–4894.
376. Monnier VM, Elmets CA, Frank KE, Vishwanath V, Yamashita T: Age-related normalization of the browning rate of collagen in diabetic subjects without retinopathy. *J Clin Invest* 1986;78:832–835.
377. Jones AF, Jennings PE, Wakefield A, et al: Collagen-linked fluorescence in diabetes mellitus. *N Engl J Med* 1986;315:323–324.
378. Jones AF, Jennings PE, Wakefield A, Winkles JW, Lunec J, et al: Protein browning and diabetic complications. *Lancet* 1986;2:459.
379. Monnier VM, Cerami A: Non-enzymatic browning in vivo: possible process for aging of long-lived proteins. *Science* 1981;211:491–493.
380. Lunec J, Blake DR, McCleary SJ, Brailsford S, Bacon PA: Self-perpetuating mechanism of immunoglobulin G aggregation in rheumatoid inflammation. *J Clin Invest* 1985; 76:2084–2090.
381. Buckingham BA, Uitto J, Sandborg C, et al: Scleroderma-like changes in insulin-dependent diabetes mellitus: Clinical and biochemical studies. *Diabetes Care* 1984; 7:163–169.
382. Lyons TJ, Kennedy L: Nonenzymatic glycosylation of skin collagen in patients with Type 1 (insulin-dependent) diabetes mellitus and limited joint mobility. *Diabetologia* 1985;28:2–5.
383. Paisey RB, Clamp JR, Kent MJC, et al: Glycosylation of hair: Possible measure of chronic hyperglycemia. *Br Med J* 1984;288:669–671.
384. Thomas D, Delbridge L, Morris D, Howell M: Cyclohexanone extraction: An improvement on the thiobarbituric acid method for the determination of nonenzymatic glycosylation of epidermal keratin and hair. *Scand J Lab Clin Invest* 1984;44:451–461.
385. Delbridge L, Ellis ES, Robertson K, Lequesne LP: Nonenzymatic glycosylation of keratin from the stratum corneum of the diabetic foot. *Br J Dermatol* 1985;112: 547–554.
386. Oimomi M, Nishimoto S, Kitamura Y, et al: Increased fructose-lysine of hair protein in diabetic patients. *Klin Wochenschr* 1985;63:728–730.
387. Oimomi M, Maeda Y, Hata F, et al: Glycosylation levels of nail proteins in diabetic patients with retinopathy and neuropathy. *Kobe J Med Sci* 1985;31:183–188.

388. Goldstein DE, Wiedmeyer HM, England JD, Little RR, Parker KM: Recent advances in glycosylated hemoglobin measurements. *CRC Crit Rev Clin Lab Sci* 1984;21:187–228.
389. Goldstein DE, Little RR, Wiedmeyer HM, England JD, McKenzie EM: Glycated hemoglobin: Methodologies and clinical applications. *Clin Chem* 1986;32:B64–B70.
390. Dolhofer R, Wieland OH: Improvement of the thiobarbituric acid assay for serum glycosylprotein determination. *Clin Chim Acta* 1981;112:197–204.
391. Gallop PM, Flückiger R, Hanneken A, Mininsohn MM, Gabbay KH: Chemical quantitation of hemoglobin glycosylation: Fluorimetric detection of formaldehyde released upon periodate oxydation of glycoglobin. *Anal Biochem* 1981;117:427–432.
392. Johnson RN, Metcalf PA, Baker JH: Fructosamine: A new approach to the estimation of serum glycosylprotein. An index of diabetic control. *Clin Chim Acta* 1982;127:87–95.
393. Baker JR, O'Connor JP, Metcalf PA, Lawson MR, Johnson RN: Clinical usefulness of estimation of serum fructosamine concentration as a screening test for diabetes mellitus. *Br Med J* 1983;287:863–867.
394. Baker JR, Metcalf PA, Holdaway IM, Johnson RN: Serum fructosamine concentration as measure of blood glucose control in Type I (insulin dependent) diabetes mellitus. *Br Med J* 1985;290:352–355.
395. Hindle EJ, Rostron GM, Gatt JA: The estimation of serum fructosamine: An alternative measurement to glycated haemoglobin. *Ann Clin Biochem* 1985;22:84–89.
396. Caines PSM, Thibert RJ, Draisey TF: Colorimetric determination of non-enzymatically glycated albumin. *Clin Biochem* 1985;18:209.
397. Johnson RN, Baker JR: The alkaline reducing activity of glycated serum proteins and its relevance to diabetes mellitus. *Clin Chem* 1986;32:368–370.
398. Caines PSM, Thibert RJ, Draisey TF: Colorimetric determination of nonenzymatically glycated albumin. *Clin Biochem* 1986;19:26–30.
399. Acharya AS, Manning JM: Amadori rearrangement of glyceraldehyde-hemoglobin Schiff-base adducts. *J Biol Chem* 1980, 255:7218–7224.
400. Sagniez M, Krempf M, Le Bastard N: Corrélation entre le dosage de l' hémoglobine glycosylée A1c et celui de la fructosamine chez des diabétiques soumis à une visite de contrôle systématique. *Path Biol* 1985;33:914–916.
401. Hindle EJ, Rostron GM, Clark SA, Gatt JA: Serum fructosamine and glycated haemoglobin measurements in diabetic control. *Arch Dis Child* 1986;61:113–117.
402. Collins ACG, Weekes RA, Mattock MB, Mather HM, Keen H: Fructosamine in serum and plasma as an integrating index of diabetic control: Relationship with glucosylated haemoglobin (HbA) and plasma glucose in diabetics. *Diabetes* 1986:35(suppl 1):95A.
403. Furrer J, Brogli S, Gautschi K: Glycosylated serum proteins (fructosamine) for diabetic control. *Diabetes* 1986;35(suppl 1):95A.
404. Klenk DC, Hermanson GJ, Krohn RI, et al: Determination of glycosylated hemoglobin by affinity chromatography: Comparison with colorimetric and ion-exchange methods, and effects of common interferences. *Clin Chem* 1982;28:2088–2094.
405. Hall PM, Cook JGH, Gould RJ: An inexpensive, rapid and precise affinity chromatography method for the measurement of glycosylated haemoglobins. *Ann Clin Biochem* 1983;20:121–135.
406. John WG, Albutt EC, Handley G, Richardson RW: Affinity chromatography for the measurement of glycosylated haemoglobin: Comparison with two methods in routine use. *Clin Chim Acta* 1984;136:257–262.
407. Yatscoff RW, Tevaarwerk GJM, MacDonald JC: Quantification of nonenzymically glycated albumin and total serum protein by affinity chromatography. *Clin Chem* 1984;30:446–449.

408. John WG, Jones AE: Affinity chromatography: A precise method for glycosylated albumin estimation. *Ann Clin Biochem* 1985;22:79–83.
409. Gould BJ, Flatt PR, Kotecha S, Collett S, Swanston-Flatt SK: Measurement of glycosylated haemoglobins and glycosylated plasma proteins in animal models with diabetes and inappropriate hypoglycemia. *Horm Metab Res* 1986;18:795–799.
410. Brownlee M, Vlassara H, Cerami A: Measurement of glycosylated amino acids and peptides from urine of diabetic patients using affinity chromatography. *Diabetes* 1980;29:1044–1047.
411. Goldstein D, Soeldner S, Nathan D: Feasibility of long-term precise measurements of glycosylated hemoglobin for the diabetes control and complications trial (DCCT). *Diabetes* 1986;35(suppl 1):95A.
412. Shah SC, Malone JI, Harvey C: Glycosylated hemoglobin: colorimetric vs chromatographic measurement. *Diabetes Res* 1986;3:381–386.
413. Bunn HF, Shapiro R, McManus M, et al: Structural heterogeneity of human hemoglobin due to non-enzymatic glycosylation. *J Biol Chem* 1979;254:3892–3898.
414. Schmid R, Pollak A, Vycudilik W, et al: Determination of glucitollysine for the quantitation of nonenzymatic glucosylation by ion exchange chromatography and reverse phase liquid chromatography. *Clin Chim Acta* 1984;139:119–126.
415. Trueb B, Holenstein CG, Fischer RW, Winterhalter KH: Nonenzymatic glycosylation of proteins. A warning. *J Biol Chem* 1980;255:6717–6720.
416. Candiano G, Ghiggeri GM, Delfino G, Queirolo C, Ginevri F: Spectrophotometric determination of advanced products of nonenzymatic glycosylation of lysine by means of their reaction with diazonium salts. *Anal Chim Acta* 1986;184:323–327.
417. Nathan DM, Singer DW, Hurzthal K, Goodson JD: The clinical information value of the glycosylated hemoglobin assay. *N Engl J. Med* 1984;310:341–346.
418. Goldstein DE: Is glycosylated hemoglobin clinically useful? *N Engl J Med* 1984;310:384–385.
419. Spiro RG: Search for a basis of diabetic microangiopathy. *Diabetologia* 1976:12:1–14.
420. Woolley DW: Identification of the mouse antialopecia factor. *J Biol Chem* 1941;139:29–34.
421. Holub BJ: The natural significance, metabolism, and function of myo-inositol and phosphatidylinositol in health and disease. *Adv Nutr Res* 1982;4:107–141.
422. Holub BJ: 1982 Borden Award Lecture: Nutritional, biochemical, and clinical aspects of inositol and phosphatidylinositol metabolism. *Can J Physiol Pharmacol* 1984;62:1–8.
423. Michell RH: Phosphatidylinositol turnover in signal transduction. *Neurosci Res Prog Bull* 1982;20:338–350.
424. Agranoff BW: Biochemical mechanism in the phosphatidylinositol effect. *Life Sci* 1982;32:2047–2054.
425. Berridge MJ, Dawson RMC, Downes CP, Heslop JP, Irvine RF: Changes in the levels of inositol phosphates after agonist-dependent hydrolysis of membrane phosphoinositides. *Biochem J* 1983:212:473–482.
426. Hokin LE: Receptors and phosphoinositide-generated second messengers. *Ann Rev Biochem* 1985;54:205–235, and references cited.
427. Strep H, Irvine RF, Berridge MJ, Schultz I: Release of Ca from a nonmitochrondrial intracellular store in pancreatic acinar cells by inositol-1,3,5-triphosphate. *Nature* 1983;306:67–69.
428. Nishizuka Y: Calcium, phospholipid turnover and transmembrane signalling. *Phil Trans R Soc Lond B* 1983;302:101–112.
429. Nairn AC, Hemmings HC Jr, Greengard P: Protein kinases in the brain. *Ann Rev Biochem* 1985;54:931–976, and references cited.

430. Holub BJ: Metabolism and function of myo-inositol and inositol phospholipids. *Ann Rev Nutr* 1986;6:563–597.
431. Berridge MJ: Intracellular signaling through inositol trisphosphate and diacylglycerol. *Biol Chem Hoppe-Seyler* 1986;367:447–456.
432. Eagle H, Oyama VI, Levy M, Freeman AE: Myo-inositol as an essential growth factor for normal and malignant human cells in tissue culture. *J Biol Chem* 1957;226: 191–205.
433. Clements RS Jr, Diethelm AG: The metabolism of myo-inositol by the human kidney. *J Lab Clin Med* 1979;93:210–219.
434. Clements RS Jr, Reynertson R: Myoinositol metabolism in diabetes mellitus. Effect of insulin treatment. *Diabetes* 1977;26:215–221.
435. Hauser G: The formation of free and lipid myo-inositol in the intact rat. *Biochim Biophys Acta* 1963;70:278–289.
436. Dawson RMC, Freinkel N: The distribution of free mesoinositol in mammalian tissues, including some observations in the lactating rat. *Biochem J* 1961;78:606–610.
437. Greene DA, De Jesus PV Jr, Winegrad AI: Effects of insulin and dietary myoinositol on impaired peripheral motor nerve conduction velocity in acute streptozotocin diabetes. *J Clin Invest* 1975;55:1326–1336.
438. Palmano KP, Whiting PH, Hawthorne JN: Free and lipid myo-inositol in tissues from rats with acute and less severe streptozotocin-induced diabetes. *Biochem J* 1977;167:229–235.
439. Benjamins JA, Agranoff BW: Distribution and properties of CDP-diglyceride:inositol transferase from brain. *J Neurochem* 1969;16:513–527.
440. Takenawa T, Egawa K: CDP-diglyceride:inositol transferase from rat liver. *Biol Chem* 1977;252:5419–5423.
441. Simmons DA, Winegrad AI, Martin DB: Significance of tissue myo-inositol concentrations in metabolic regulation in nerve. *Science* 1982;217:848–851.
442. Winegrad AI: Banting Lecture 1986. Does a common mechanism induce the diverse complications of diabetes? *Diabetes* 1987;36:396–406.
443. Van Heyningen R: Mesoinositol in the lens of mammalian eyes. *Biochem J* 1957;65:24–27.
444. Oliver GL, Gardiner RJ, Rossiter RJ: Inositol in normal lenses and cataracts. *Can J Ophthalmol* 1968;3:266–269.
445. Wada E, Tsumita T: Ageing and compositional changes of rat lens. *Mech ageing & develop* 1984;27:287–294.
446. Cotlier E: Characteristics of an active transport system for inositol in the lens. *Invest Ophthalmol* 1968;7:118–119.
447. Cotlier E: Myo-inositol: Active transport by the crystalline lens. *Invest Ophthalmol* 1970;9:681–691.
448. Varma SD, Chakrapani B, Reddy VN: Intraocular transport of myoinositol. II. Accumulation in the rabbit lens in vitro. *Invest Ophthalmol* 1970;9:794.
449. Stewart MA, Kurien MM, Sherman WR, Cotlier EV: Inositol changes in nerve and lens of galactose fed rats. *J Neurochem* 1968;15:941–946.
450. Broekhuyse RM: Changes in myo-inositol permeability in the lens due to cataractous conditions. *Biochim Biophys Acta* 1968;163:269–272.
451. Hutton JC, Schofield PJ, Williams JF, Hollows FS: Sorbitol metabolism in the retina: Accumulation of pathway intermediates in streptozotocin induced diabetes in the rat. *Austr J Exp Biol Med Sci* 1974;52(pt 2):361–373.
452. Kinoshita JH, Barber GW, Merola LO, Tung B: Changes in the levels of free amino acids and myo-inositol in the galactose-exposed lens. *Invest Ophthalmol* 1969;8:625–632.

453. Kinoshita JH, Dvornik D, Kraml M, Gabbay KH: The effect of an aldose reductase inhibitor on the galactose-exposed rabbit lens. *Biochim Biophys Acta* 1968;158:472–475.
454. Kawaba T, Cheng HM, Kinoshita JH: The accumulation of myoinositol and rubidium ions in galactose-exposed rat lens. *Invest Ophthalmol Vis Sci* 1986;27:1522–1526.
455. Cook L, Freinkel N: "Free" myoinositol in diabetic cataracts. *Clin Res* 1980;28:398A.
456. Hutson NJ, Yeh LA, Rafford CE, Goddu KJ, Beyer TA: The effects of diabetes and the aldose reductase inhibitor sorbinil on lens metabolism in the rat. *Diabetes Res Clin Pract Suppl* 1985;1:S-253.
457. Bucci F, Chan P, Cruz E, Beyer-Mears A: Myo-inositol diminution of diabetic cataract. *Invest Ophthalmol Vis Sci* 1985;26(suppl):118.
458. MacGregor LC, Rosencan LR, Laties AM, Matschinsky FM: Microanalysis of total lipid, glucose, sorbitol, and glucose, sorbitol, and myoinositol in individual retinal layers of normal and alloxan diabetic rabbits. *Diabetes* 1984;33(suppl 1):89A.
459. Clements RS Jr: Review of myo-inositol and sorbinil studies. *Clin Physiol* 1985;5(suppl 5):90–93.
460. Clements RS Jr: Peripheral nerve biochemistry in diabetes. *Clin Physiol* 1985;5(suppl 5):19–22.
461. Greene DA: Sorbitol, myo-inositol and sodium-potassium ATPase in diabetic peripheral nerve. *Drugs* 1986;32(suppl 2):6–14.
462. Greene DA, Lattimer SA: Biochemical alterations and complications in diabetes. *Clin Chem* 1986;32:B42–B47.
463. Greene DA, Lattimer SA, Sima AAF: Sorbitol, phosphoinositides, and sodium-potassium-ATPase in the pathogenesis of diabetic complications. *N Eng J Med* 1987;316:599–606.
464. Stewart MA, Passonneau JV: Identification of fructose in mammalian nerve. *Biochem Biophys Res Comm* 1964;17:536–541.
465. Sherman WR, Stewart MA: Identification of sorbitol in mammalian nerve. *Biochem Biophys Res Comm* 1966;22:492–497.
466. Stewart MA, Sherman WR, Anthony S: Free sugars in alloxan diabetic rat nerve. *Biochem Biophys Res Comm* 1966;22:488–491.
467. Stewart MA, Sherman WR, Kurien MM, Moonsammy GI, Wisgerhof M: Polyol accumulations in nervous tissue of rats with experimental diabetes and galactosemia. *J Neurochem* 1967;14:1057–1066.
468. Kador PF, Kinoshita JH: Role of aldose reductase in the development of diabetes-associated complications. *Am J Med* 1985;79(suppl 5A):8–12.
469. Nishimura C, Kinoshita JH: Aldose reductase and myo-inositol in sciatic nerve. *Diabetes* 1986;35(suppl 1):198A.
470. Mizisin AP, Myers RR, Powell HC: Endoneurial sodium accumulation in galactosemic rat nerves. *Muscle Nerve* 1986;9:440–444.
471. Clements RS: Diabetic neuropathy: new concepts of its etiology. *Diabetes* 1979; 28:604–611.
472. Greene DA, Lattimer SA: Sodium- and energy-dependent uptake of myo-inositol by rabbit peripheral nerve. Competitive inhibition by glucose and lack of insulin effect. *J Clin Invest* 1982;70:1009–1018.
473. Clements RS Jr, De Jesus PV Jr, Winegrad AI: Raised plasma-myoinositol levels in uremia and experimental neuropathy. *Lancet* 1973;1:1137–1141.
474. De Jesus PV Jr, Clements RS Jr, Winegrad AI: Hypermyoinositolemia polyneuropathy in rats: A possible mechanism for uremic polyneuropathy. *J Neurol Sci* 1974; 21:237–249.

475. Reznek RH, Salway JG, Thomas PK: Plasma-myoinositol concentrations in uremic neuropathy. *Lancet* 1977;1:675–676.
476. Jeffreys JGR, Palmano KP, Sharma AK, Thomas PK: Influence of dietary myoinositol on nerve conduction and inositol phospholipids in normal and diabetic rats. *J Neurol Neurosurg Psychiatry* 1978;41:333–339.
477. Clements RS Jr, Vourganti B, Kuba T, Oh SJ, Darnell B: Dietary myo-inositol intake and peripheral nerve function in diabetic neuropathy. *Metabolism* 1979; 28(suppl 1):477–483.
478. Thomas PK, Jeffreys JGR, Sharma AK, Bajada S: Nerve conduction velocity in experimental diabetes in the rat and rabbit. *J Neurol Neurosurg Psychiatry* 1981;44:233–238.
479. Greene DA, Lewis RA, Lattimer SA, Brown MJ: Selective effects of myo-inositol administration on sciatic and tibial motor nerve conduction parameters in the streptozotocin-diabetic rats. *Diabetes* 1982;31:573–578.
480. Greene DA, Lattimer SA, Sima AAF: Acute paranodal nerve fiber swelling and conduction slowing in the insulin-deficient BB rat reflects myo-inositol depletion and Na/K-ATPase deficiency rather than sorbitol accumulation. *Clin Res* 1986;34:683.
481. Whiting PH, Palmano KP, Hawthorne JN: Enzymes of myo-inositol and inositol lipid metabolism in rats with streptozotocin-induced diabetes. *Biochem J* 1979; 179:549–553.
482. Hothersall JS, McLean P: Effect of experimental diabetes and insulin on phosphatidylinositol synthesis in rat sciatic nerve. *Biochem Biophys Res Comm* 1979; 88:477–484.
483. Clements RS Jr, Stockard CR: Abnormal sicatic nerve myo-inositol metabolism in the streptozotocin-diabetic rat. *Diabetes* 1980;29:227–235.
484. Simmons DA, Winegrad AI, Martin DB: Significance of myo-inositol concentrations in metabolic pathways. *Trans Assoc Am Phys* 1982;95:292–298.
485. Kai M, Hawthorne JN: Physiological significance of polyphosphoinositides in brain. *Ann NY Acad Sci* 1969;165:761–773.
486. Charalampous FC: Metabolic functions of myo-inositol. VIII. Role of inositol in Na^+-K^+ transport and in Na^+- and K^+-activated adenosine triphosphatase in KB cells. *J Biol Chem* 1971;246:455–460.
487. Bell ME, Eichberg J: Decreased incorporation of [^{3}H]inositol and [^{3}H]glycerol into glycerolipids of sciatic nerve from the streptozotocin diabetic rats. *J Neurochem* 1985;45:465–469.
488. Berti-Mattera L, Peterson R, Bell M, Eichberg J: Effect of hyperglycemia and its prevention by insulin treatment on the incorporation of 32p into polyphosphoinositides and other phospholipids in peripheral nerve of the streptozotocin diabetic rat. *J Neurochem* 1985;45:1692–1698.
489. Ward JD, Baker RWR, Davis BH: Effect of blood sugar control on the accumulation of sorbitol and fructose in nervous tissues. *Diabetes* 1972;21:1173–1178.
490. Greene DA, Lattimer SA: Impaired rat sciatic nerve sodium-potassium adenosine triphosphatase in acute streptozotocin diabetes and its correction by dietary myo-inositol supplementation. *J Clin Invest* 1983;72:1058–1063.
491. Finegold D, Lattimer SA, Nolle S, Bernstein M, Greene DA: Polyol pathway activity and myo-inositol metabolism: A suggested relationship in the pathogenesis of diabetic neuropathy. *Diabetes* 1983;32:988–992.
492. Greene DA, Lattimer SA: Action of sorbinil in diabetic peripheral nerve: Relationship of polyol (sorbitol) pathway inhibition to a myo-inositol-mediated defect in sodium-potassium ATPase activity. *Diabetes* 1984;33:712–716.

493. Mayer JH, Tomlinson DR: Slow orthograde axonal transport in experimental diabetes in the rat: Effects of an aldose reductase inhibitor. *J Physiol* 1984;351:16P.
494. Yue DK, Hanwell MA, Satchell PM, Handelsman DJ, Turtle JR: The effects of aldose reductase inhibition on nerve sorbitol and myoinositol concentrations in diabetic and galactosemic rats. *Metabolism* 1984;33:1119–1122.
495. Kemper C, Dvornik D: Prevention of neural myoinositol depletion in diabetic rats by aldose reductase inhibition with tolrestat. *Proc Soc Exp Biol Med* 1986;182:505–510.
496. Okuda J, Yashima K, Inagakai K, Miwa I: Effects of an aldose reductase inhibitor, 1-[(p-bromophenyl)-sulfonyl] hydantoin, on cataract formation and tissue polyol levels in galactosemic rats. *Chem Pharm Bull* 1985;33:2990–2995.
497. Greene DA, Winegrad AI: In vitro studies of the substrates for energy production and the effects of insulin on glucose utilization in the neural components of peripheral nerve. *Diabetes* 1979;28:878–887.
498. Greene DA, Winegrad AI: Effects of acute experimental diabetes on composite energy metabolism in peripheral nerve axons and Schwann cells. *Diabetes* 1981;30:967–974.
499. Das PK, Bray GM, Aguayo AJ, Rasminsky M: Diminished ouabain-sensitive, sodium-potassium ATPase activity in sciatic nerves of rats with streptozotocin-induced diabetes. *Exp Neurol* 1976;53:285–288.
500. Greene DA, Lattimer SA: Impaired energy utilization and Na,K ATPase in diabetic peripheral nerve. *Am J Physiol* 1984;246:E311–E318.
501. Greene DA: Metabolic abnormalities in diabetic peripheral nerve: Relation to impaired function. *Metabolism* 1983;32(suppl 1):118–123.
502. Greene DA, Yagikashi S, Lattimer SA, Sima AAF: Nerve NA^+-K^+ ATPase, conduction and myo-inositol in the insulin-deficient BB rat. *Am J Physiol* 1984;247: E534–E539.
503. Green RJ, King RHM, Thomas PK, Baron DN: Sodium-potassium ATPase activity in the dorsal root ganglia of rats with streptozotocin-induced diabetes. *Diabetologia* 1985;28:104–107.
504. Greene DA, Lattimer SA: Protein kinase C agonists acutely normalize decreased ouabain-inhibitable respiration in diabetic rabbit nerve. Implications for (Na,K)-ATPase regulation and diabetic complications. *Diabetes* 1986;35:242–245.
505. Ochs S: Systems of material transport in nerve fibers (axoplasmic transport) related to nerve function and trophic control. *Ann NY Acad Sci* 1974;228:202–223.
506. Brismar T, Sima AAF: Changes in nodal function in nerve fibers of the spontaneously diabetic BB-Wistar rat. Potential clamp analysis. *Acta Physiol Scand* 1981; 113:499–506.
507. Sima AAF, Lattimer SA, Yagihashi S, Greene DA: Axoglyal dysjunction. A novel structural lesion that accounts for poorly reversible slowing of nerve conduction in the spontaneously diabetic Bio-Breeding rat. *J Clin Invest* 1986;77:474–484.
508. Sima AAF, Brismar T: Reversible diabetic nerve dysfunction: Structural correlates to electro physiological abnormalities. *Ann Neurol* 1985;18:21–29.
509. Gillon RW, Hawthorne JN: Transport of myo-inositol into endoneurial preparations of sciatic nerve from normal and streptozotocin-diabetic rats. *Biochem J* 1983;210: 775–781.
510. Sima AAF, McEwen TAJ, Chakrabarti S: The effect of statil on early nerve dysfunction. *Diabetes* 1986;35(suppl 1):206A.
511. Greene DR, Lattimer SA, Finegold DN, Tamres LK: Impaired Na-dependent amino acid uptake in diabetic peripheral nerve: Correction by aldose reductase inhibition or myo-inositol supplementation. *Clin Res* 1985;33:431A.
512. Simmons DA, Kern EFO, Winegrad AI, Martin DB: Basal phosphatidylinositol turnover controls aortic Na^+-K^+- ATPase activity. *J Clin Invest* 1986;77:503–513.

513. Clements RS Jr, Stockard CR; Neural abnormalities in myoinositol metabolism in the streptozotocin-diabetic rats, in Shafrir E, Renold AE (eds): *Lessons from animal diabetes.* London, Libbey, 1984, pp 460–464.
514. Cameron NE, Leonard MB, Ross IS, Whiting PH: The effects of sorbinil on peripheral nerve conduction velocity, polyol concentrations and morphology in the streptozotocin-diabetic rat. *Diabetologia* 1986;29:168–174.
515. Dvornik D, Sredy J, Hicks D, Sawicki D, Ackerman D: Polyol pathway and myoinositol (MI) content in peripheral nerve of long-term streptozocin (STZ) diabetic rats. *Diabetes*, 1987;36(suppl):185A.
516. Cohen AM, Teitelbaum A: Effect of different levels of protein in "sucrose" and "starch" diets on the glucose tolerance and growth. *Metabolism* 1966;15:1034–1038.
517. Boot-Handford R, Heath H: Identification of fructose as the retinopathic agent associated with the ingestion of sucrose-rich diets in the rat. *Metabolism* 1980;29: 1247–1252.
518. Poulsom R, Boot-Handford RP, Heath H: The effects of long-term treatment of streptozotocin-diabetic rats with an aldose reductase inhibitor. *Exp Eye Res* 1983; 37:507–515.
519. Greene DA, De Jesus PV, Winegrad AI: Motor nerve conduction velocity (MNCV) in acute and chronic streptozotocin diabetes (SD). *Diabetes* 1974;23:357.
520. Llewelyn JG, Simpson CMF, Thomas PK, King RHM, Hawthorne JN: Changes in sorbitol myo-inositol and lipid inositol in dorsal root and sympathetic ganglia from streptozotocin-diabetic rats. *Diabetologia* 1986;29:876–881.
521. Winegrad AI, Greene DA: Diabetic polyneuropathy: The importance of insulin deficiency, hyperglycemia and alterations in myoinositol metabolism in its pathogenesis. *N Engl J Med* 1976;295:1416–1421.
522. Vohl H: Ueber das Auftreten des Inosits im Harn bei Nierenkrankheiten und die Verwandlung des Diabetes mellitus in Diabetes inositus. *Arch Physiol Heilkunde* 1958;2:410–412.
523. Daughaday WH, Larner J, Houghton E: The renal excretion of inositol in normal and diabetic human beings. *J Clin Invest* 1954;33:326–332.
524. Perles R, Colas MC: Détermination microbiologique du mésoinositol sanguin. *Clin Chim Acta* 1960;5:95–99.
525. Pitkanen E: The serum polyol pattern and the urinary polyol excretion in diabetic and uremic patients. *Clin Chim Acta* 1972;38:221–230.
526. Aloia JF: Monosaccharides and polyols in diabetes mellitus and uremia. *J Lab Clin Med* 1973;82:809–817.
527. Pitkanen E: Changes in serum and urinary myo-inositol levels in chronic glomerulonephritis. *Clin Chim Acta* 1976;71:461–468.
528. Melmed S, Lewin LM, Bank H: Myoinositol clearance in renal failure and in patients with normal renal function. *Am J Med Sci* 1977;274:55–59.
529. Gregersen G, Borsting H, Thiel P: Influence of myo-inositol on human diabetic nerve and retina. *Diabetologia* 1977;13:397.
530. Gregersen G, Borsting H, Thiel P, Servo C: Myoinositol and function of peripheral nerves in human diabetics. *Acta Neurol Scand* 1978;58:241–248.
531. Salway JG, Whitehead L, Finnegan JA, et al: Effect of myoinositol on peripheral-nerve function in diabetes. *Lancet* 1978;2:1282–1284.
532. Dyck PJ, Sherman WR, Hallcher LM, et al: Human diabetic endoneurial sorbitol, fructose, and myo-inositol related to sural nerve morphometry. *Ann Neurol* 1980;8:590–596.

533. Greene DA, Brown MJ, Braunstein SN, et al: Comparison of clinical course and sequential electrophysiological tests in diabetics with symptomatic polyneuropathy and its implications for clinical trials. *Diabetes* 1981;30:139–147.
534. Gregersen G, Bertelsen B, Harbo H, et al: Oral supplementation of myoinositol: Effects on peripheral nerve function in human diabetics and on the concentration in plasma, erythrocytes, urine and muscle tissue in human diabetics and normals. *Acta Neurol Scand* 1983;67:164–172.
535. Mayhew JA, Gillon KRW, Hawthorne JN: Free and lipid inositol, sorbitol and sugars in sciatic nerve obtained post-mortem from diabetic patients and control subjects. *Diabetologia* 1983;24:13–15.
536. Sherman WR, Dyck PJ: Free inositol, sorbitol and fructose levels in sciatic nerve. *Diabetologia* 1983;25:452–453.
537. Hale PJ, Nattrass M, Sennit C, et al: Sorbitol, fructose, glucose and myoinositol concentrations in nerve biopsies taken at amputation in diabetic patients and normal subjects. *Diabetologia* 1986;29:545A.
538. Ewing DJ, Clarke BF: Diabetic autonomic neuropathy: present insights and prospects. *Diabetes Care* 1986;9:648–665.
539. Ulbrecht JS, Bensen JT, Greene DA: Sodium-dependent myo-inositol uptake in isolated renal glomeruli: Possible inhibition by glucose. *Diabetes* 1985;34(suppl 1): 13A.
540. Ulbrecht JS, Olszowy MW: Effects of sorbinil and sorbitol on Na-dependent myoinositol uptake in isolated renal glomeruli. *Diabetes* 1986;35(suppl 1):102A.
541. Cohen MP, Dashmahapatra A, Shapiro E: Reduced glomerular sodium/potassium adenosine triphosphatase activity in acute streptozocin diabetes and its prevention by oral sorbinil. *Diabetes* 1985;34:1071–1074.
542. Cohen MP, Klepser H, Cua E: Effect of diabetes and sorbinil treatment on phospholipid metabolism in rat glomeruli. *Biochim Biophys Acta* 1986;876:226–232.
543. Goldfarb S, Simmons DA, Kern E: Amelioration of glomerular hyperfiltration in acute experimental diabetes by dietary myoinositol and by an aldose reductase inhibitor. *Clin Res* 1986;34:725A.
544. Servo C, Bardy A, Pasternack A, Pitkanen E: Plasma, red cell and cerebrospinal fluid concentrations of myoinositol in patients with severe chronic renal failure. *Ann Clin Res* 1976;8:374–377.
545. Servo C: Accumulation of myoinositol in plasma and red cells of diabetic patients. *Acta Med Scand* 1977;201:59–62.
546. Malone JI, Harvey RC, Putnam JC: Sorbitol, inositol and phosphatidylinositol (PI) elevated in diabetic red cells. The influence of sorbinil. *Diabetes* 1983;32:161A.
547. Malone JI, Leavengood H, Peterson MN, et al: Red blood sorbitol as an indicator of polyol pathway activity. Inhibition by sorbinil in insulin-dependent diabetic subjects. *Diabetes* 1984;33:45–49.
548. Malone JI, Knox G, Benford S, Tedesco TA: Red cell sorbitol. An indicator of diabetic control. *Diabetes* 1980;29:861–864.
549. Peterson MJ, Page MG, Just LJ, Aldinger CE, Malone JI: Applicability of red blood cell sorbitol measurements to monitor the clinical activity of sorbinil. *Metabolism* 1986;35(suppl 1):93–95.
550. Malone JI, Lowitt S, Harvey HC, Mandlow S: The effect of sorbinil (an aldose reductase inhibitor) upon red cell sorbitol and inositol. *Diabetes* 1984;33(suppl 1):172A.
551. Popp-Snijders C, Lomecky-Janousek MZ, Schouten JA, Van Der Veen EA; Myo-inositol and sorbitol in erythrocytes from diabetic patients before and after sorbinal treatment. *Diabetologia* 1984;27:514–516.

552. Wright J, Passas R, Stevenson D, Collier J: The effect of oral sorbinil at two doses on erythrocyte sorbitol and myoinositol concentration in diabetes. *Diabetes Res Clin Pract* 1985;1(suppl):S-609.
553. Martyn CN, Matthews DM, Popp-Snijders C, et al: Effects of sorbinil treatment on erythrocytes and platelets of persons with diabetes. *Diabetes Care* 1986;9:36–39.
554. Broadstone VL, Pfeifer MA: Lack of correlations between RBC-sorbitol levels and diabetic neuropathy. *Clin Res* 1985;33:839A.
555. Dasmahapatra A, Cohen MP, Robey C: Dichotomous changes in erythrocyte ATPase activities in diabetes and their normalization by sorbinil. *Clin Res* 1985;33:427A.
556. Morrison AD: Aortic smooth muscle metabolism: Effect of polyol pathway inhibition. *Clin Res* 1984;32:851A.
557. Hod M, Star S, Passonneau JV, Unterman TG, Freinkel N: Effect of hyperglycemia on sorbitol and myo-inositol content of cultured rat conceptus: failure of aldose reductase inhibitors to modify myo-inositol depletion and dysmorphogenesis. *Biochem Biophys Res Comm* 1986;140:974–980, and references cited.

Chapter 3

Animal Models of Diabetic Complications and Their Relation to Aldose Reductase Inhibition

by Dushan Dvornik, D.Sc.

SYNOPSIS

Ever since Banting and Best's work with dogs, animal models have proved indispensable for understanding the etiology and pathophysiology of diabetes mellitus. Such research has provided much of the evidence underlying our present understanding of this manifold metabolic disorder.

Since sudden death from diabetic ketoacidosis declined after the introduction of insulin into clinical medicine, the focus of animal research has shifted to the neurologic and vascular complications of long-term diabetes. This chapter reviews the three animal models of human diabetes and discusses the applicability of these models to the ocular, neural, and renal complications. The animal models discussed are those involving spontaneous diabetes, those with chemically induced diabetes, and two in which diabetes is induced nutritionally. Because aldose reductase activity becomes evident only in the presence of high ambient sugar levels, these models are studied when persistently high systemic sugar levels are attained experimentally.

Spontaneous diabetes occurs in both mice and rats. Because of their short life span and their tendency to infertility, these inbred spontaneously diabetic rodents present practical problems for the study of diabetic complications resulting from long duration of the disease. For this reason, there is still interest in other methods of producing diabetes in longer-lived species.

Diabetes can also be induced in rodents and other laboratory animals by destroying pancreatic beta-cells; the β-cytotoxicants alloxan and streptozocin have been employed effectively to produce hyperglycemic states similar to those occurring in diabetes mellitus.

Of the nutritional animal models used in the study of diabetic complications, one is based on the feeding of excess galactose, resulting in severe galactosemia, and the other, on the feeding of excess sucrose. Galactosemia in rats and dogs provides important animal models for studying the role of aldose reductase in the pathogenesis of diabetic complications.

Animal models are of great assistance to research in the diabetic ocular complications in two ways: by enabling the production of lesions at all stages of the complication and in all forms, including in situ and in tissue culture, and by providing animal subjects for therapeutic trials impossible or impractical in human subjects. Experiments have produced cataracts, retinal abnormalities, and corneal lesions similar to those in humans and have demonstrated the activation of aldose reductase in long-term experimental diabetes.

Although studies of diabetic neuropathy in laboratory animals have been useful, extrapolation of their observations to humans has been difficult, in part because animal models cannot mimic the subjective end-points of pain and paresthesia. Nevertheless, prevention of neural impairment in rats has been accomplished by aldose reductase inhibition in the presence of severe systemic glycemia and galactosemia.

Animal models develop a broad spectrum of diabetic nephropathy, from early renal hypertrophy to late lesions of glomeruli and other structures. Recent studies in animals with experimentally induced diabetes have identified microalbuminuria as a marker for renal dysfunction occurring well before overt proteinuria, hitherto the first clinically apparent sign of diabetic nephropathy, has been observed. Studies in galactosemic rats have also demonstrated the presence of aldose reductase in the kidney, and aldose reductase inhibition has been found to prevent renal polyol accumulation.

Contents

INTRODUCTION

Diabetes mellitus is not one disease, but a complex of symptoms resulting from a variable interplay of genetic and environmental factors. The diabetic syndrome is characterized by elevated plasma glucose levels, by abnormal insulin action and/or secretion, and by a variety of metabolic, vascular, and other pathologic manifestations. Because it is nearly always associated with fasting hyperglycemia, diabetes mellitus is perceived in the context of this monograph as a readily detectable abnormality in metabolism resulting in hyperglycemia.

Diabetes has been classified into two major types. Insulin-dependent diabetes mellitus (juvenile-onset, Type I, ketosis-prone) is characterized by an almost total lack of insulin and the dependence on exogenous insulin for the maintenance of life. While the causes of insulin-dependent diabetes mellitus (IDDM) are not clear, destruction of the beta-cell by chemical toxins, virus, or auto-immune mechanisms is implicated. The susceptibility of the beta-cells to such damage appears to be dependent on the genetics and the metabolic state. Immune and auto-immune phenomena may be involved either as etiological or as amplifying factors.[1]

In non-insulin-dependent diabetes mellitus (Type II, maturity-onset, non-ketosis-prone), insulin is produced, albeit in quantities that are not adequate to maintain glucose homeostasis; in addition, target-organ resistance to insulin is present and plays an important pathophysiological role. Non-insulin-dependent diabetes mellitus (NIDDM) has a strong genetic basis, but its onset can be exacerbated by obesity, by diet, and by endocrine or autonomic nervous system factors.[1]

Spontaneous diabetes is relatively common in a variety of animal species and occurs occasionally in cats, dogs, tree shrews, ground squirrels, foxes, dolphins, hippopotami, antelope, and most farm animals.[2] Diabetes can also be induced experimentally, particularly in rodents, by appropriate chemical agents or other procedures. The use of animals as models of diabetes in humans has proved invaluable for our understanding of the etiology and pathophysiology of the disease and has contributed greatly to the development of therapy with insulin.

In 1981, the Diabetes Coordinating Committee of the National Institutes of Health convened a task force to explore the appropriateness of existing and new animal models for studying problems concerning the etiology, pathogenesis, and underlying mechanisms of chronic diabetes and its complications. The task force thoroughly evaluated six types of diabetic complications, i.e., metabolic, cardiovascular, ocular, renal, central and peripheral nervous system, and those of pregnancy and fetal development, and prepared a comprehensive report, published in 1982.[3]

The purpose of this chapter is to describe those animal models that have been found useful in studying the involvement of aldose reductase in the pathogenesis of chronic diabetic complications.

Because the activity of aldose reductase becomes evident only after it is increased by high ambient sugar levels, the laboratory animals used in aldose reductase research must have persisting high systemic sugar levels.

In general, animals used as models of human diabetes can be separated into three types: animals with spontaneously occurring diabetes mellitus, animals with chemically induced diabetes, and animals with nutritionally induced diabetic-like complications.

ANIMALS WITH SPONTANEOUSLY OCCURRING DIABETES

The available animals with spontaneous diabetes can be distinguished by leanness or obesity. The lean animals have little or no peripheral resistance to insulin; their capacity for insulin secretion is low, varying from modest secretion to virtually none. The obese highly inbred animals, e.g., ob/ob and db/db obese mice, are particularly useful for studying the genetics of obesity. They rarely develop ketosis and usually have high levels of insulin and insulin resistance. A detailed description and comprehensive bibliography on animals with spontaneous diabetes has been provided by Grodsky et al.[1] In 1982, the Juvenile Diabetes Foundation organized a workshop on the spontaneously diabetic BB rat and its potential for insight into human diabetes. The presentations were published in 1983.[4]

The currently available animals with spontaneous diabetes are listed in Table 1. However, some practical problems are associated with these animals. Most of the large animal species, such as the Keeshond dog, the golden retriever, the miniature pig, and some of the monkeys, are not readily available. With the rodents, inbreeding to attain genetic homogeneity often leads to infertility. In most instances, their life-span is too short for far-advanced complications to develop. In addition, diet plays a vital part in the manifestation of spontaneous diabetes: high-fat hypercaloric diets can exacerbate diabetes, while dietary restriction may decrease or prevent hyperglycemia. The diet can also affect beta-cell proliferation and degeneration.

ANIMALS WITH CHEMICALLY INDUCED DIABETES

The chemical agents producing diabetes can be separated into three categories[1]: beta-cytotoxic agents,[12] causing a primary insulin deficiency state; agents causing transient inhibition of insulin biosynthesis or insulin secretion; and agents increasing the endogenous insulin requirements, thus stressing the pancreas and producing diabetes secondarily.

Agents in the first category are of particular interest, because they can be used to produce variable degrees of hyperglycemia similar to those occurring with the severe insulin deficiency of IDDM or the stable hyperglycemia of NIDDM, thus presenting a relatively permanent experimentally induced diabetes suitable for chronic studies. Two of the most extensively used agents in this group are alloxan and streptozocin.

Table 1. Animals with spontaneous diabetes. (Adapted from Grodsky et al.[1])

Animal	Obesity	Plasma glucose	Plasma insulin	Insulin resistance	Ref
Single gene mutants					
Obese mouse (C57BL/6J, ob/ob)	+ +	↑,n	↑,n	+	5
Diabetic mouse (C57BL/KsJ, db/db)	+ +	n,↑	↑↓	+	5
Zucker fatty rat	+ +	n,(↑)	↑	+	6
Inbred strains					
NZO obese mouse	+ +	(↑)	↑	+	6
KK mouse	+	(↑)	(↑)	+	6
Chinese hamster	n	↑	n,↓	?	7
Impure strains					
Spiny mouse	+	↑	n,↓	?	
Sand rat	+	(↑)	(↑)	?	
BB-Wistar rat	n	↑↑	↓	n	8,9
Non-obese diabetic rat	n	↑	↓	n	6
Djungarian hamster	+	n,(↑)	↑	?	
South-African hamster	n	↑	?	?	
Guinea pig	n	↑	?	?	
NZ white rabbit	n	↑	↓	?	
Dog (Keeshond, golden retriever)	n	(↑)	↓	?	10
Macaca nigra	n	↑	↓	n	11

+ = present; n = normal; (↑) = slightly elevated; ↑ = high; ↓ = low; ? = unknown.

Alloxan

The diabetogenic activity of alloxan was first described in 1943 by Dunn et al,[13] who observed necrosis of pancreatic islets in rabbits given alloxan by intravenous injection. The subsequent finding that alloxan produces a diabetic state marked the beginning of intense research on "chemical diabetes," which supplemented the already known types of experimental diabetes induced by either pancreatectomy[14] or growth hormone.[15]

Because of its high affinity for the islet-cell membranes, alloxan binds very rapidly to the membranes and inhibits the secretion of insulin. The earliest structural alterations observed in the beta-cells of alloxan-treated animals are mitochondrial swelling and disruption of the inner membranes. Later, many mitochondria are disintegrated, and the endoplastic reticulum and Golgi complex are disorganized.[16]

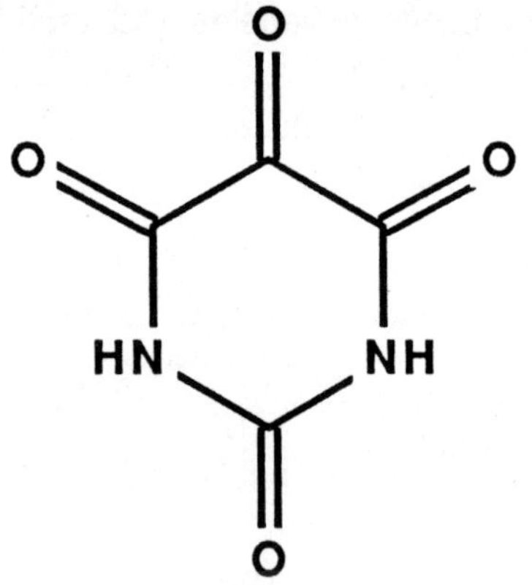

Alloxan

In vivo, the effect of alloxan is characteristically triphasic: the initial one- to four-hour interval of acute hyperglycemia is followed by severe hypoglycemia and insulin release lasting up to 48 hours, resulting in convulsions and death unless prevented by administration of glucose. Chronic hyperglycemia develops after one to two days. The toxicity of alloxan is thus produced within the first few minutes of exposure, though its final effect may take many hours to be established.

There are many factors known to increase or inhibit the diabetogenic action of alloxan.[12] Protection from alloxan is afforded by pretreatment with D-glucose or 3-0-methyl-D-glucose. The much smaller protective effect of mannose and fructose[17] may be due to their limited conversion to glucose.[18]

According to Malaisse,[19] the selective toxicity of alloxan to the pancreatic beta-cell is essentially attributable to the coincidence of a rapid accumulation of the drug in islet cells and to the exquisite sensitivity of the beta-cells to peroxides, particularly the hydroxyl radical. The postulate is supported, first, by the protective effect in vivo of a number of hydroxyl radical scavengers such as dimethylsulfoxide,[20] N,N'-dimethylurea,[21] thiourea,[22] short-chain aliphatic alcohols, e.g., n-butanol,[22] and butylated hydroxyanisole.[23] Sakurai et al[24] repeated the work and concluded that hydroxyl radicals initially damage the beta-cell membranes by acting at a site involved in insulin release, and subsequently damage the intracellular components. Second, it is supported by the protective action of D-glucose, its isomer, anomers, and epimers, which can be accounted for by the sugar-induced increase in reducing equivalents, particularly NADPH, in the islet cells.[19] Incidentally, the protective effect of mannoheptulose is attributed to its inhibition of glucose phosphorylation, and that of 3-0-methyl-D-glucose, to interference with alloxan uptake by the islet cells.[19]

The guinea pig was found to be relatively insensitive to alloxan; since its beta-cells lack zinc, it may be that alloxan's beta-cytotoxicity is due to interference with zinc metabolism. The cat is also resistant to the diabetogenic effect of alloxan but is susceptible to its toxic effects on the kidney.[25]

In addition to pancreatic lesions, alloxan also produces renal tubular damage,[26] the severity of which varies from hydropic degeneration to necrosis. Both the incidence and the severity of the renal lesions have been shown to be dose-dependent.[27] The alloxan-induced glycogen nephrosis is a reversible lesion.[28]

Streptozocin

The diabetogenic action of streptozotocin,* an antibiotic produced by *Streptomyces achromogenes*,[29] was described in 1963 by Rakieten et al.[30] Chemically, streptozocin (STZ) is the N-methyl-N-nitrosourea derivative of 2-deoxy-D-glucopyranose.[31]

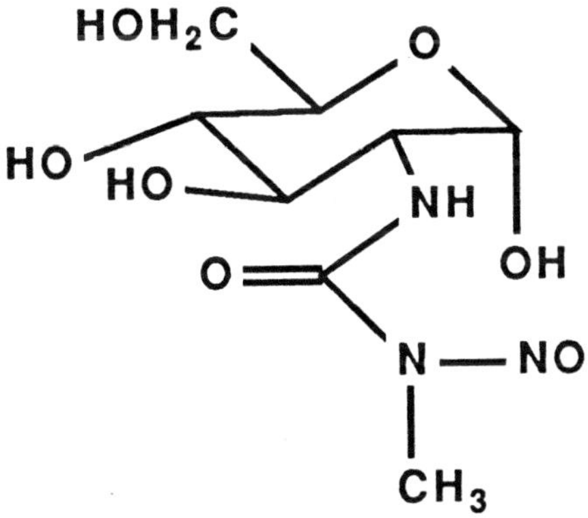

Streptozocin

The finding that the α-anomer of the glucosamine moiety is more cytotoxic than the β-anomer suggests that the damaging mechanism to the beta-cell is stereospecific.[2] The beta-cytotoxicity is presumably provided by the nitrosourea moiety, possibly through a process of methylation.[32] It is of interest that exchange of the methyl group on the nitrosourea moiety for a 2-chloroethyl group to give the anti-cancer drug chlorozocin[33] resulted in a diabetogenic agent with different species specificity and alternative mechanisms of beta-cytotoxicity.[34]

Because removal of the glucose fragment renders STZ much less beta-cytotoxic,[2] the glucose moiety may act as a carrier, thereby facilitating the transport of STZ.[35] Compared with that of alloxan, STZ damage is generally more predictable.[36,37]

Streptozocin interferes with NAD formation in the beta-cell, which may be the event initiating beta-cell necrosis, an effect abolished by pretreatment with nicotinamide.[38,39] NAD is the specific substrate for the synthesis of the chromosomal polymer, poly(ADP-ribose), which may be involved in the mutagenic or cytotoxic effects of alkylating agents. The STZ-induced decrease in NAD levels was reflected in a three-fold increase in activity of the poly(ADP-ribose)polymerase.[40]

This interference with poly(ADP-ribose)polymerase formation may lead to changes in the regulation of DNA synthesis, DNA repair, and cell differentiation, and may participate in beta-cell necrosis.[1] Streptozocin-induced activation of

*The abbreviated generic name, streptozocin, will be used in this book.

poly(ADP-ribose)synthetase and subsequent NAD depletion in isolated rat islet can be prevented by thymidine.[41] 3-Aminobenzamide, an inhibitor of poly(ADP-ribose)synthetase, was found to prevent the inhibition of glucose-stimulated insulin release induced by STZ in vitro, as well as protecting the rats from the diabetogenic effect of STZ administered in vivo.[42] Quantitatively, the protective action of 3-aminobenzamide appeared to be comparable to that of nicotinamide.

Protection of the beta-cell from STZ is also afforded by a variety of sugars, notably by 3-0-methyl-D-glucose, which protects the beta-cell from both alloxan and STZ. It is unknown whether this protective effect reflects an interaction with glucoreceptors involved in insulin secretion[1] or with glucose transport and metabolism.[18] Modification of STZ-induced diabetes by protective agents was reviewed recently by Preston.[43]

The effective dose of STZ depends on the age, sex, and nutritional state of the animal.[44] The greater susceptibility to STZ-induced hyperglycemia of male as compared with female mice, first observed by Rossini et al,[45] has been attributed to testosterone, since the hyperglycemic response to STZ in males was decreased by castration and restored with testosterone administration. Treatment with testosterone also enhanced the response in both normal and castrated females. Maclaren et al[46] confirmed the finding in normal and inbred mice of the DBA/2J strain. Subsequently, Paik et al[47] demonstrated that the susceptibility of mice to STZ is determined by the relative overall excess of androgens over estrogens rather than by the absolute concentration of androgens. The protective effect of estrogens in diabetic animals[48] was attributed to inhibition of STZ uptake by beta-cells.[47] Interestingly, in male rats treated with STZ intravenously (60 mg/kg), a 93% reduction in serum testosterone was observed after 21 days.[49]

The fact that in rodents a single high dose of STZ impairs the amino acid-induced glucagon release suggests nonspecific alpha-cell damage.[50,51]

Streptozocin is not diabetogenic in cats,[52] but causes permanent diabetes in 9- to 12-week-old pigs upon intravenous injection at doses of 100 to 150 mg/kg.[53]

The strain-related resistance to STZ-induced diabetes, observed in the C3H/HeJ and C3H/eb mice, may be mediated at the level of the beta-cell's responsiveness to the cytotoxic action of the drug.[54]

Depending on dosage, three types of diabetic syndrome can be induced with STZ. First, a single large dose produces acute beta-cell necrosis, depletion of insulin, and marked hyperglycemia within 24 to 48 hours. Like alloxan, STZ produces a characteristic triphasic sequence of blood glucose levels, corresponding to an initial inhibition of insulin release, followed within a few hours by massive release of insulin from the necrotizing cells, followed by cell necrosis.[37,38] Thus, in neonatal rats given STZ intraperitoneally (90 mg/kg) two days after birth, a transient hyperglycemic phase is followed by a recovery phase and a subsequent deterioration to a chronic diabetic state.[55]

The second type of diabetic syndrome is produced by multiple sub-diabetogenic doses of STZ.[56] In mice, such treatment results in sub-clinical chemical beta-cell destruction followed by pancreatic insulitis. In time, this auto-immune process leads to further beta-cell destruction and diabetes. Upon induction of hyperglycemia, the pancreatic islets are infiltrated by large numbers of mononuclear inflammatory cells (lymphocytes and macrophages), resulting in insulitis, which may be analogous to that reported in IDDM patients. This model is of particular interest, since cell-mediated immunity may be involved. However, this progression of events develops only in specific strains of mice, and the same experimental conditions have failed to produce similar lesions in rats.

The third type of diabetic syndrome, representing a milder degree of diabetes that progresses over a period of up to 60 days, can be induced by a single low dose of STZ.[1,57] For example, stable mild diabetes in male Wistar rats was induced by a single intraperitoneal injection of STZ at a dose of 35 mg/kg.[58] Irreversible damage to the beta-cells was complete by three days, and plasma insulin was undetectable throughout the 12-week period of investigation. In contrast to severe diabetes, plasma fatty acids rose only gradually, ketone bodies were only slightly elevated, and liver glycogen was maintained at about 30% of the normal value.

Iwase et al[59] have found that administration of STZ to 2-day-old male spontaneously hypertensive rats does not affect the development of hypertension, and hence represents a model of IDDM associated with persisting hypertension.

In rats, STZ-induced diabetes resulted in rapid atrophy of the thymus, the weight of which was reduced to one-fifth of its original weight within three weeks.[60] Histologically, the atrophy was associated with a great loss of cortical thymocytes and a marked increase in most cells in the thickened fibrous tissue. The finding may have a bearing on the state of immune deficiency observed in animals with STZ-induced diabetes. That STZ is toxic for rapidly proliferating cells of primary lymphoidal tissues in mice was shown by Wellhausen.[61] A single non-diabetogenic dose (50 mg/kg) of STZ administered intravenously in mice depleted thymocytes and depressed the ratio of circulating lymphocytes to neutrophils. It was concluded that STZ-induced diabetes is an inappropriate model for studies of the immune system in diabetes.

Comparison of alloxan and streptozocin

Streptozocin is particularly toxic to the beta-cells by inducing lesions in the DNA[62] while alloxan appeared to destroy the beta-cells by an extracellular process that results in enhanced permeability of the membranes.[63] Although alloxan and STZ may act by different molecular mechanisms, both drugs induced an increase in vascular permeability in the pancreatic islets,[64,65] possibly by a secondary release of vasoactive substances from the islets during beta-cell destruction.[65] The nitrosoureas are cytotoxic because they cross-link DNA molecules and may act on the bone marrow.[66] Alloxan appears to be diabetogenic without such effects on the DNA.[61] It is of interest that alterations in lymphoid tissues observed in STZ-treated animals far exceeded those in alloxan-treated animals.[61]

While both alloxan and streptozocin are beta-cytotoxic, and therefore produce similar end-effects on blood glucose,[67] the two diabetogenic agents differ in their toxicity and general metabolic effects.[68] In rats injected intravenously with equimolar doses of the beta-cytotoxicants, the 40% mortality after alloxan (40 mg/kg) was ten times greater than the 4% mortality observed after STZ (65 mg/kg).[67] The values are similar to those reported earlier for alloxan[28] and STZ.[69] In rats unprotected by clamping the renal vessels against high initial alloxan concentrations in the blood, alloxan caused tubular atrophy and interstitial fibrosis.[26] In contrast, no renal injury was detected at eight weeks in rats administered STZ at a diabetogenic dose of 60 mg/kg.[70] According to Jensen et al,[71] STZ is not nephrotoxic. However in mice, dogs, and rhesus monkeys, STZ caused lesions in the proximal convoluted tubules of the kidney.[72]

The metabolic patterns found in the blood and hearts of rats with alloxan-induced diabetes differ markedly from those with STZ-diabetes.[73] Alloxan increased plasma free fatty acids and ketone bodies and cardiac glycogen levels at intravenous doses of 65 mg/kg, while STZ had no significant effect on either plasma free fatty acid or ketone levels and lowered the glycogen content in the heart. Ketosis was, however, reported in rats injected with STZ intravenously at a dose of 50 mg/kg, but not at a dose of 35 mg/kg.[74] While perfused hearts from STZ-treated rats had normal concentrations of glycolytic intermediates, alloxan caused a marked elevation of all these constituents. In a comprehensive study of the gluconeogenic and glycolytic capacities and metabolic zonation in rat liver, Miethke et al[75] demonstrated that intravenously administered STZ (75 mg/kg) caused a non-ketotic, and intravenously administered alloxan (60 mg/kg) a severely ketotic, form of diabetes. While STZ increased blood glucose to about 450% with ketone bodies in the normal range, alloxan increased blood glucose, acetoacetate, and β-hydroxybutyrate well over 500%. This difference in the metabolic state was attributed to differences in the hormonal state; while the decrease in circulating insulin was clearly less pronounced after STZ than after alloxan, the increase in glucagon levels was more pronounced after STZ than after alloxan.

Because many subjects with diabetes are hyperglycemic but not ketotic, their patterns of tissue metabolism may resemble more closely those found in the STZ-diabetic animal models than in the alloxan-diabetic animal models.[73]

An interesting difference between alloxan and STZ was revealed by differences in beta-cell protection afforded by pretreatment with D-glucose, D-mannose, 2-deoxy-D-glucose, and 3-0-methyl-D-glucose.[17,18,39,76–78] The findings summarized in Table 2 suggest, first, that the beta-cytotoxic effects of alloxan and STZ may not be intracellular, since they were prevented by 3-0-methyl-D-glucose, a

Table 2. Agents protective against beta-cytotoxicity of alloxan and streptozocin.

Agent	Protection afforded from	
	Alloxan	**Streptozocin**
D-Glucose	+	0
D-Mannose	+	0
2-Deoxy-D-glucose	0	+
3-0-Methyl-D-glucose	+	+
D-Mannoheptulose	0	0
3-0-Methyl-D-glucose + D-mannoheptulose	0	+
Nicotinamide	+	+

+ = protected; 0 = not protected

non-metabolizable and non-insulinogenic analogue of glucose[18,79]; the protective effect of the α-anomer of 3-0-methyl-D-glucose appeared to be even greater.[18,80] Second, the failure of mannoheptulose to alter the protective action of 3-0-methyl-D-glucose against STZ but not against alloxan indicates that the two agents probably act at different sites of the beta-cell surface.[79]

NUTRITIONAL ANIMAL MODELS OF DIABETIC COMPLICATIONS

Two nutritional models have been used to study the development of diabetic complications in laboratory animals.[81] One is based on the feeding of excess galactose, which results in severe galactosemia, and the other on the feeding of excess sucrose. Experimental galactosemia in rats is of particular interest because it represents an important animal model for studying the role of aldose reductase.[81] Recently, experimental galactosemia in dogs has been used as a model for studying diabetic retinopathy[82] and kidney morphology.[83]

Experimental galactosemia

Metabolic disposition of galactose

D-Galactose is an epimer of D-glucose and differs in the configuration of the hydroxyl and hydrogen on the carbon 4:

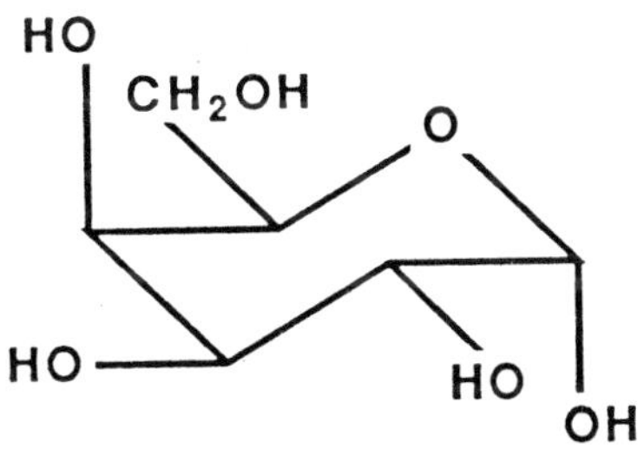

α-D-Galactose

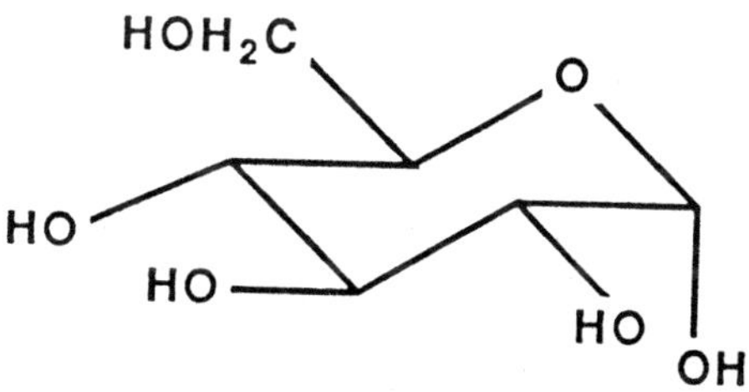

α-D-Glucose

The major dietary source of galactose is lactose (milk sugar), a unique constituent of milk. Lactose is a disaccharide in which D-galactose is joined by a 1,4-glycosidic bond to carbon 4 of D-glucose. Ingested lactose is gradually hydrolyzed into its constituents by the enzyme lactase, present in the brush border of the mucosal epithelial cells.[84] If the amount of ingested lactose exceeds the capacity of available lactase, the unhydrolyzed lactose draws water into the intestinal lumen and is fermented by the gut flora, thus producing symptoms ranging from a mild bloated feeling to severe diarrhea.

Absorption and elimination

Galactose and glucose are absorbed by a common carrier; however, galactose is absorbed at a slightly faster rate than glucose.[85] Sodium ions are essential for the active transport of sugars across the intestine,[86,87] and a sodium-dependent carrier, present in the brush border of the intestinal mucosa, is shared by galactose and glucose.[88] An interaction between the carrier and a localized sodium pump allows the hexose to be actively concentrated within the cell.

In rats, galactose administered by gavage at doses of 0.5 to 1.2 mg/kg[89,90] or ingested with the diet is rapidly and well absorbed.[91,92] The serum galactose concentration/time curves obtained in rats given single oral doses of galactose, ranging from 1 to 10 mg/kg, indicate that the rate of absorption is dose-dependent, since similar peak concentrations were attained with doses of 5 and 10 mg/kg (Fig 1). However, the systemic availability of galactose, expressed as the area under the serum galactose concentration/time curves (AUC), increases in proportion to the dose.[93]

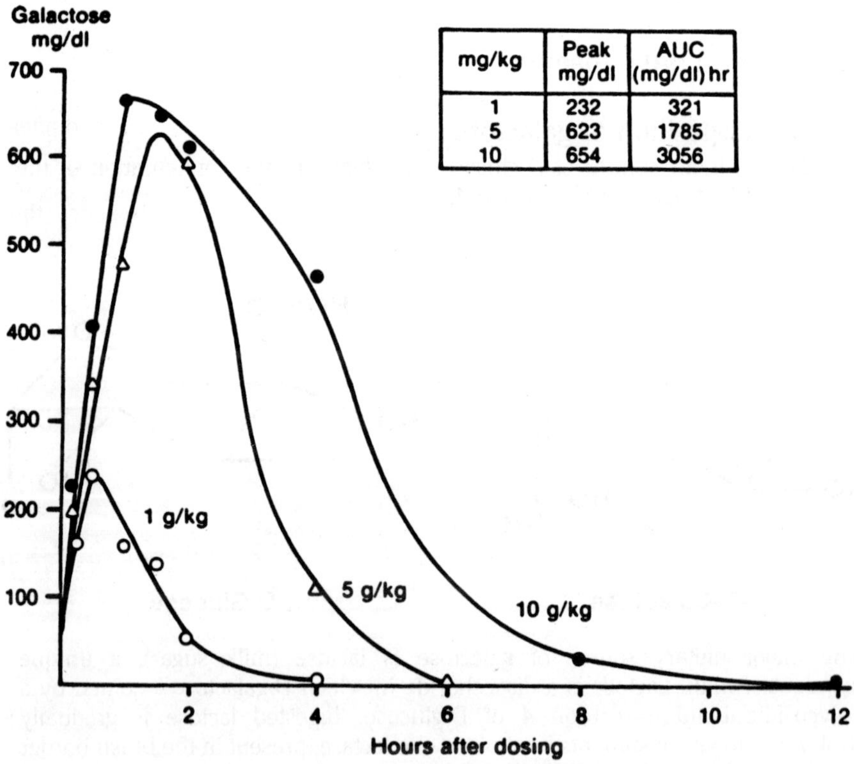

Figure 1. Serum galactose concentration/time curves in rats given galactose by gastric intubation. (From Dvornik et al.[93])

The rat can absorb considerable amounts of orally administered galactose, particularly if it is ingested with the diet.

In rats given access to a 60% galactose diet, a peak reducing sugar level of at least 530 mg/dL (29.4 mM) was attained within approximately 1.5 hours, then disappeared with a half-life of about 2 hours.[94] A similar mean peak plasma galactose concentration of 600 ± 58 mg/dL (33.3 ± 3.2 mM) (±SE) was found in rats trained to consume in 30 minutes a ration containing 40% galactose.[92] In rats given access to galactose at 20% or 50% of the diet for four days, we have found peak serum galactose concentrations of 262 ± 19 mg/dL (14.5 ± 1.1 mM) (±SE) and 910 ± 14.5 mg/dL (50.5 ± 0.8 mM), respectively.[95]

Galactose is rapidly phosphorylated in the liver to galactose-1-phosphate. Because it does not pass through cell membranes, galactose-1-phosphate does not re-enter the circulation.[96] This large extraction of galactose has been used to estimate hepatic blood flow and liver-cell function.[97]

In the rat, the rate of galactose elimination follows saturation kinetics, with an estimated maximal elimination rate of 630 μmol/hr/kg body weight.[98] Galactose seems to equilibrate in the available volume of distribution in less than 30 minutes.[98] In rats, the half-life of galactose elimination from serum varied from 1.3 to 1.6 hours.[95]

In dogs given 50% galactose in the diet, the absorption is slower, peak serum galactose concentrations of 458 ± 47 mg/dL (25.4 ±2.6 mM) being attained after four hours.[95]

A substantial portion of the ingested galactose is excreted unchanged in the urine[91,99] (Table 3). In young inbred albino rats fed on 35% galactose diet, the urinary concentration of glucose (505 ± 68 μmol/hr) was twice that of galactose (250 ± 59 μmol/hr),[100] thus suggesting that galactose may compete for the transport of glucose in the kidney. As shown in Table 4, rats given access to a 40% galactose diet for up to eight months excreted in the urine about 25% of the ingested galactose (2.0 g/day); the difference was regarded as the amount of galactose that the rats were able to metabolize.[101] About 3% of the ingested galactose was excreted as galactitol.

In rats, prolonged feeding on a diet rich in galactose is accompanied by increased water consumption and increased urine output[102] while the food intake and body weight gain are usually not affected[103]; however, in long-term studies the body weight gain was decreased.[99,100,102] In dogs fed for five years on a diet containing

Table 3. Urinary excretion of galactose in rats fed 70% galactose with the diet. (From Cryer and Bartley.[99])

Days	Daily excretion of galactose	
	g	Percentage of ingested galactose
2–3	3.15	36.5
6–7	4.41	22.7
9–10	4.73	21.2
13–14	4.81	20.5

Table 4. Urinary excretion of galactose and galactitol in rats fed 40% galactose with the diet. (From Poiffait et al.[101])

Duration of feeding	Excreted in urine in % of galactose ingested	
	Galactose	**Galactitol**
1 day	21.8 ± 3.0	0.6 ± 0.1
4 days	23.4 ± 5.4	2.0 ± 0.2
1 month	23.5 ± 2.0	2.7 ± 0.3
3 months	22.7 ± 1.3	2.7 ± 0.3
8 months	21.3 ± 1.8	3.9 ± 0.3

30% galactose, food consumption was about 30% greater than in age-matched normal dogs; the increase was regarded as compensation for the galactose added to the diet.[83]

In adult rats, ingestion of 40% galactose with the diet had no effect on blood glucose levels either acutely,[92] or after five months of feeding on the galactose-containing diet.[104] In young rats fed on a 70% galactose diet, the initially decreased blood glucose returned to normal levels by 14 days.[99] However, in inbred albino rats fed on a 35% galactose diet, plasma glucose levels increased from 141 to 331 mg/dL in the presence of galactose (250 mg/dL).[100]

In rats fed on a galactose-rich diet, insulin had no effect on plasma galactose concentrations.[91] In fact, galactose exerts little if any insulinotropic action, and feeding a galactose-rich diet does not induce secretory responsiveness to galactose in the pancreatic beta-cell.[105] The poor insulinotropic activity of galactose is attributed mainly to low galactokinase activity in the beta-cell. Feeding of rats and dogs on diets containing 50% galactose had no significant effect on their glucose tolerance.[106]

Regarding the possible interaction between galactose and glucose during transport from blood to brain, Gjedde[107] found no substantial change in glucose transport across the cerebral capillary endothelium in adult rats fed for three weeks on a diet containing 40% galactose. At 10 mM galactose in plasma (180 mg/dL), the apparent inhibition of glucose transport corresponded to a moderate reduction (20%) in plasma glucose; in suckling rats, however, the inhibition corresponded to 50%. It has been shown earlier that in suckling rats the influx of glucose into the brain is reduced in dose-related fashion by galactose in the blood.[108]

Metabolic transformation

The main pathway of galactose metabolism is named for Leloir.[109] As shown in Fig 2, the Leloir pathway consists of four enzymes that convert galactose to glucose-1-phosphate, which can be converted to glucose. While the major site of the pathway is the liver, the pathway is also present in the kidney and in erythrocytes. The amount of galactose that is metabolized via the Leloir pathway depends on the activity of the galactokinase, the excess of the galactose being distributed throughout the organism. According to Mangeot et al,[102] in rats fed on a 50% galactose diet for five weeks, the activities of hepatic galactokinase and

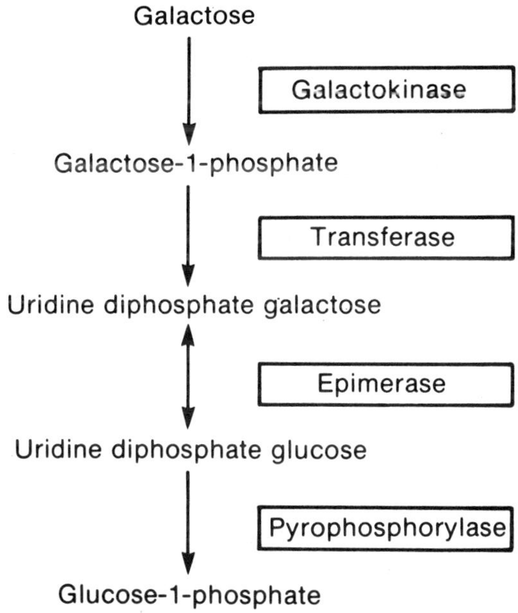

Figure 2. Leloir pathway of galactose metabolism.

galactose-1-phosphate uridyl (GPU)-transferase were increased. Interest in the disposition of such excessive amounts of galactose was stimulated by the observations of Van Heyningen[110] that the lenses of galactose-fed rats contained a considerable amount of galactitol (110 nmol/mg) formed enzymatically from galactose by the action of the enzyme aldose reductase. Galactitol was also detected in the heart and leg muscle, but at lower concentrations than in the lens. Subsequently, galactitol was identified by Wells et al[111] in the urine of two infants with galactosemia. Since in a galactosemic patient given orally [1-^{14}C]galactose 27% of the radioactivity found in the urine was due to [1-^{14}C]galactitol,[112] the authors concluded that in man the reduction of galactose to galactitol may be more significant than the conversion to glucose.

These observations, along with the finding of sorbitol in clear lenses and cataracts from diabetic patients by Pirie and Van Heyningen,[113] represent the first indication that in man, as in the rat, an excess of systemically available glucose or galactose can be metabolized by aldose reductase. According to Williamson et al,[114] the activity of the aldose reductase in rats is modulated by sex hormones.

Prompted by the detection of significant amounts of galactitol in the urine of galactosemic rats, Quan-Ma and Wells[115] found readily detectable levels of galactitol in a variety of rat tissues. As shown in Table 5, the highest relative concentrations of galactitol were present in the lens (44.4 nmol/mg), followed by the skeletal (22.3 nmol/mg) and cardiac muscles (18.1 nmol/mg). Lesser amounts

Table 5. Galactitol levels in tissues of weanling male Holtzman rats fed 35% galactose with the diet for 16 days. (From Quan-Ma and Wells.[115])

Tissue	Galactitol nmol/mg ± SD
Lens	44.4
Skeletal muscle	22.3 ± 2.8
Cardiac muscle	18.1 ± 3.7
Brain	5.2 ± 0.6
Kidney	3.2 ± 0.9
Small intestine,	
proximal ⅓	2.0 ± 0.3
distal ⅔	1.2 ± 0.4
Blood cells, packed	0.7 ± 0.1*

*μmol/mL

were found in the brain, kidney, and red blood cells; the galactitol levels in the liver and plasma were below the limit of detection.[116] The authors regarded the tissue accumulation of galactitol as a strong indication that it was synthesized from galactose in situ. The alternative, namely that preformed galactitol was taken up by a given tissue, was dismissed in view of the low permeability of cellular membranes to polyols.[117,118]

The presence of galactitol in tissues of galactosemic rats was corroborated and expanded by Stewart et al.[119,120] The levels found in rats fed on a 40% galactose diet for one month (Table 6) were similar to those reported earlier by Quan-Ma and Wells.[115] The very pronounced accumulation of galactitol in the lens and sciatic nerve was associated with a marked fall in myoinositol content: in the sciatic nerve, from 3.7 ± 0.6 to 1.2 ± 0.2 nmol/mg; and in the lens, from 1.6 ± 0.1 to 0.16 ± 0.08 nmol/mg (±SE). The similar galactitol levels found in the sciatic nerve after five weeks of 40% galactose feeding (Table 7)[120] were associated with similar depletion of myoinositol, i.e., from 4.1 ± 0.3 to 1.0 ± 0.1 nmol/mg (±SE). In rats

Table 6. Galactitol levels in tissues of adult female Holtzman rats fed 40% galactose with the diet for one month. (From Stewart et al.[119])

Tissue	Galactitol nmol/mg ± SE
Lens	41.1 ± 20.7
Heart	29.1 ± 4.7
Sciatic nerve	22.3 ± 1.5
Forebrain	10.4 ± 1.1
Cerebellum	8.6 ± 0.5
Small intestine	6.6 ± 0.2
Ovary	3.3 ± 1.3
Kidney	2.5 ± 0.2
Lung	2.5 ± 0.8
Pancreas	0.9 ± 0.2
Liver	0.7 ± 0.1
Serum	0.7 ± 0.0

Table 7. Galactitol levels in tissues of adult female Holtzman rats fed 40% galactose with the diet for five weeks. (From Stewart et al.[120])

Tissue	Galactose nmol/mg ± SE	Galactitol nmol/mg ± SE
Nerve	5.2 ± 0.5	17.4 ± 1.5
Brain	4.8 ± 0.7	9.3 ± 0.5
Cord	5.2 ± 0.5	4.5 ± 0.5
Kidney	16.7 ± 2.8	4.4 ± 0.5
Serum	10.6 ± 1.1*	0.9 ± 0.1*

*μmol/mL ± SE

fed on a 40% galactose diet for 120 to 140 days, galactitol accumulation (0.65 ± 0.11 nmol/mg) in the liver was associated with unchanged myoinositol levels (0.89 ± 0.19 nmol/mg compared with 0.76 ± 0.09 nmol/mg in normal controls).[121] The level of galactose in the kidney (16.7 ± 2.8 nmol/mg), which was about three times higher than the level of glucose (3.6 ± 0.2 nmol/mg), was attributed to urine in the kidney.[85] Feeding rats on a 40% galactose diet for five months did not produce a further increase of galactitol levels in the brain and nerves (Table 8).[120] In rats with free access to diets containing different amounts of admixed galactose, the concentrations of galactitol in the diaphragm, sciatic nerve, and lens were dependent upon the amount of ingested galactose, the highest levels occurring in the lens[93] (Fig 3).

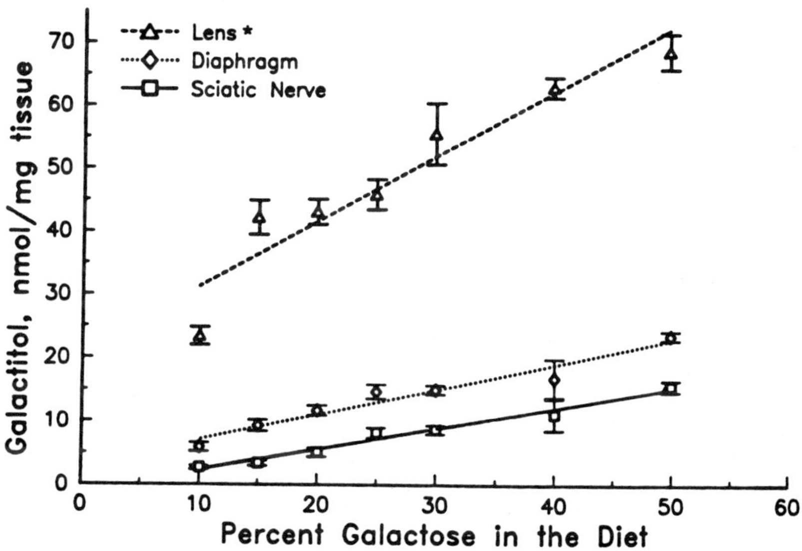

*The determinations were made while the functional integrity of the lens was not affected by galactitol accumulation.

Figure 3. Tissue galactitol accumulation in rats fed a galactose diet for four days. (From Dvornik et al.[93])

Table 8. Galactitol levels in tissues of adult female Holtzman rats fed 40% galactose with the diet. (From Stewart et al.[120])

Duration of feeding on galactose	Galactose nmol/mg ± SE		Galactitol nmol/mg ± SE	
	Brain	Nerve	Brain	Nerve
5 months	6.7 ± 1.5	10.9 ± 1.0	6.5 ± 0.3	19.3 ± 0.7
5 months + 4 days on regular diet	—	0.5 ± 0.2	0.1 ± 0.0	1.4 ± 0.1

In rats fed for four days on a diet containing 20% galactose, upon removal of galactose from the diet, the galactitol concentrations in the sciatic nerves decreased with a half-life of ten hours.[93]

Galactitol also accumulates in tissues of dogs fed galactose.[93] As shown below, in dogs administered galactose by gastric intubation once daily at a dose of 15 g/kg for four days, readily detectable levels of galactitol were found in several tissues known to contain aldose reductase.

Tissue	Galactitol nmol/mg ± SE
Diaphragm	38.6 ± 0.8
Kidney medulla	28.6 ± 3.1
Lens	26.2 ± 1.0
Aorta	8.8 ± 1.6
Sciatic nerve	8.3 ± 0.9
RBC	717 ± 82 nmol/mL blood

Galactosemia in man

In 1945, cataract was reported as a complication of galactosemia in human subjects.[122,123] The two types of galactosemia occurring in human subjects are caused by congenital deficiency of enzymes needed for galactose metabolism (Fig 2).

Classic galactosemia is due to the absence of GPU-transferase, occurring in about one of 60,000 births.[124] The defect causes accumulation of galactose-1-phosphate, which, in turn, inhibits the galactokinase, thus producing increased systemic galactose levels and, eventually, cataract. In addition, the accumulated galactose-1-phosphate interferes with the glycolytic pathway, the hexose monophosphate shunt, and the formation of glycogen; by depleting the liver of inorganic phosphate it also leads to liver failure and its sequelae. However, GPU-transferase is usually present in excess, and reductions up to 50% may not cause clinical manifestation of the disease.[125]

The second type of galactosemia in man is due to deficiency of galactokinase, which causes accumulation of galactose and results in rapid cataract development.[126] Galactokinase deficiency is present in approximately 1.9% of persons with cataract occurring within the first year of life.[127] The incidence of galactokinase-deficiency-induced galactosemia is believed to be 1:40,000.[84]

The usefulness of the galactose-fed rat as a comprehensive model of GPU-transferase deficiency in man is questionable, even though it invariably develops bilateral cataracts.[128] Because of its much lower tolerance to galactose,[89,129] the galactose-fed rat is not a good model for extrapolation to man. In addition, the rate of galactose utilization by the rat liver is one-half that of the human liver,[130] and in contrast to man,[84] glucose does not reduce plasma galactose levels in the rat.[90]

As mentioned earlier, galactitol was isolated and identified in the brain of deceased human subjects with galactosemia.[131] Subsequently, Quan-Ma et al[132] have determined post mortem the distribution of galactitol in the tissues of a 23-day-old infant presumed to be galactosemic. As shown in Table 9, the highest levels of galactitol were found in the brain (22.2 nmol/mg) and skeletal muscle (16.2 nmol/mg). In contrast to rats fed on a 35% galactose diet for 16 days and showing the relatively highest galactitol level in the lens (44.4 nmol/mg),[115] the lens of the infant contained a much lower level of galactitol (2.6 nmol/mg). Later, Gitzelmann et al[133] detected post mortem a galactitol level of 4 nmol/mg in the lens of a 15-day-old galactosemic infant.

Table 9. Galactitol levels in the tissues of a galactosemic child. (From Quan-Ma et al.[132])

Tissue	Galactitol nmol/g
Brain	22.18
Skeletal muscle	16.24
Diaphragm muscle	11.46
Kidney	5.60
Pancreas	4.55
Heart	4.47
Liver	3.90
Spleen	3.45
Small intestine	3.38
Lung	3.01
Thymus	2.59
Lens	2.56
Spinal cord	2.10
Serum (post mortem)	5.30*
Aqueous + vitreous humors	1.16*
Urine	11.05*

*nmol/mL

The biochemistry, genetics, pathophysiology, and developmental aspects of galactosemia in man were reviewed by Kalckar et al.[134]

Sucrose-fed rats

Sucrose, a disaccharide, is hydrolyzed by the enzymes in the brush-border membrane of the gut into its constituents D-glucose and D-fructose.[135] Fructose is readily absorbed by a specific carrier-mediated transport mechanism not involving an active pump. Liver cells are freely permeable to fructose.[136,137] As shown in Fig 4, fructose is metabolized by a specific pathway involving fructokinase, which converts fructose to its 1-phosphate.[138] Fructokinase has a very high affinity (low Km) for fructose and is not affected by glucose or insulin. Thus, neither the entry of fructose into liver cells nor the first step in its metabolism depends on insulin. The insulin secretory response to fructose is significantly lower than to glucose or sucrose. The diabetic organism can, therefore, rapidly start to metabolize fructose, even if glucose utilization is impaired.[139] Fructose-1-phosphate is subsequently split by aldolase B into the trioses dihydroxyacetone phosphate and glyceraldehyde. The further metabolism of these trioses is, however, insulin-dependent: in the presence of insulin, the trioses enter the glycolytic pathway and are oxidized to pyruvate, which enters the citric acid cycle. In insulin deprivation, the fructose-derived trioses are converted to glucose.[139,140] In man, the metabolism of fructose is very rapid, its half-life being approximately 18 minutes.[141]

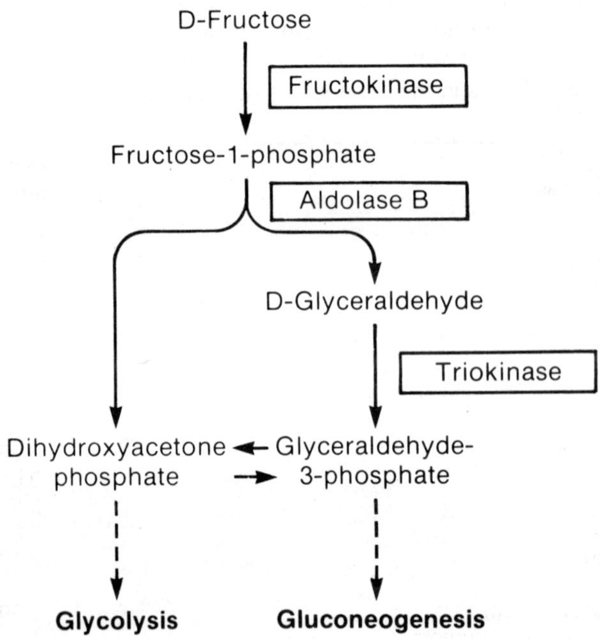

Figure 4. Metabolism of fructose.

Interest in rats fed on a sucrose-rich diet was prompted by the observation that such animals showed impaired glucose tolerance.[142] The impairment was enhanced when the sucrose content was increased to 79%.[143] Subsequently, diffuse intercapillary[144] and exudative glomerulosclerosis with marked proteinuria[145] were produced in rats fed for nine to 18 months on a 79% sucrose diet ("Cohen diabetic rat"). The observation was corroborated by Taylor et al,[146] who also found a two-fold increase in glucosyl-transferase activity in kidney supernatants prepared from sucrose-fed rats. Kidney enlargement and increased urinary excretion of N-acetyl-β-glucosaminidase were also observed in sucrose-fed rats.[147]

Characterization and prevention of nephropathy in Cohen's diabetic rat was reviewed by Rosenmann and Cohen.[148]

In the genetically selected (for low glucose tolerance), sucrose-fed rat, ovariectomy caused a 16% decrease ($p<0.01$) in the incidence of nephropathy, while estradiol treatment of ovariectomized animals increased the incidence by 44% ($p<0.02$); orchidectomy had no significant effect.[149] In accordance, long-term treatment of female Cohen diabetic rats with the estrogen antagonist tamoxifen caused a 12.5% decrease ($p<0.01$) in the incidence of glomerulosclerosis.[150] The only common denominator that could be related to the reduced incidence of glomerulosclerosis in the ovariectomized[149] and tamoxifen-treated[150] animals was the decrease in plasma estradiol levels.

In later investigations, in 31% of genetically selected (for low glucose tolerance)[151] and sucrose-fed rats, a retinopathy was observed resembling human diabetic retinopathy, particularly in the loss of intramural pericytes.[152,153]

The observation that feeding on a 68% sucrose diet for six to 11 months resulted in retinal microangiopathy was confirmed by light microscopy in rats with streptozocin-induced diabetes.[154] Addition of sucrose to the diet of the diabetic rats accelerated the appearance of retinal alterations, which were indistinguishable in frequency, nature, and severity from lesions produced in normal rats fed on the high-sucrose diet. It is peculiar that the retinopathy produced in normal sucrose-fed rats was not associated with elevated blood glucose levels.

Based on results reported in a 15-day feeding experiment,[155] Papachristodoulou et al[154] speculated that the observed retinopathic changes may not be due to increased sorbitol levels in the retina. However, it is very likely that the retinal sorbitol levels and fructose levels measured after 15 days of sucrose feeding[155] were not representative of the levels accumulating during six to 11 months of sucrose feeding.[154] However, even in the short-term experiment,[155] the retinal sorbitol and fructose levels in the diabetic animals rose by 255% and 203% in the sucrose-fed group as compared with 153% and 120% in the starch-fed group used as control. The mean retinal sorbitol (2.4 nmol/mg) and fructose (approximately 2.5 nmol/mg) concentrations were, in fact, higher than those usually found in the nerves of streptozocin-induced diabetic rats (see Chapter 4, Table 16, page 246). Because aldose reductase is not evenly distributed thoughout the retina,[156] damage may occur at sites of its localization and sorbitol accumulation.[157] Of relevance is the finding of Pocknee et al[158] that the rat retina has no protective barrier against high systemic sugar concentrations: in both non-diabetic and diabetic rats, retinal glucose and sorbitol concentrations were correlated with plasma glucose ($p<0.001$), with higher concentrations occurring in the diabetic retina ($p<0.001$).

Examination of retinal segments of sucrose-fed rats by electron-microscopy revealed ultrastructural differences between the non-diabetic and streptozocin-induced diabetic rats maintained for six to 11 months on a diet containing 68% sucrose.[159] The main difference was in the retinal capillary basement membrane thickening, which was present only in the diabetic animals. Since the thickening was not related to either blood glucose or the severity of retinopathy, the authors attributed the development of retinopathy to the deposition of material within the membrane (observed in non-diabetic rats fed on the sucrose diet) rather than to capillary basement membrane thickening (observed only in diabetic rats fed on the sucrose diet).

Retinal vascular changes occurring in Cohen's diabetic rat were reviewed by Yanko and Cohen.[160]

Prominent thickening of retinal capillary basement membranes in diabetic rats fed fructose with the diet was also reported by Kojima et al[161]; the development of diabetic microangiopathy was attributed to activation of the polyol pathway.

Boot-Handford and Heath established that the sucrose-induced retinopathy[162] and glomerulosclerosis[163] are due to fructose liberated in vivo from sucrose. Feeding normal rats on a diet containing 50% fructose resulted in increased sorbitol and fructose levels in the kidney.[164]

APPLICABILITY OF ANIMAL MODELS OF DIABETIC COMPLICATIONS

Ocular complications

Animal models of diabetic ocular complications can be of substantial assistance in research. First, they can provide lesions at all stages of the development of such complications, either as tissue samples or for study in situ. Second, animals that develop ocular complications of diabetes can be used for therapeutic trials conducted under conditions impracticable or impossible in man.[165]

Cornea

The corneal epithelium of streptozocin-induced diabetic rats has been found to become thickened and excessively laden with glycogen. Upon experimental removal of the corneal epithelium in such rats, the rate of re-epithelialization was slower than normal.[166] The abnormalities observed during corneal re-epithelialization in diabetic rats were duplicated in rats fed on a galactose-rich diet.[167] The involvement of aldose reductase (AR) in the process of corneal re-epithelialization was demonstrated by the use of AR inhibitors in vitro[168] and in vivo[166,168] as well as in man.[169]

In alloxan-induced diabetic rabbits, metabolic abnormalities, including elevated tissue levels of sorbitol, fructose, and glycogen, have been identified in the corneal epithelium, but the healing rate of the epithelium did not seem to be affected.[170]

Dogs with alloxan-induced diabetes of 28 to 59 months' duration showed corneal endothelial changes similar to those seen in diabetic patients,[171] suggesting that these animals can be a useful model for studying diabetic corneal endothelium.[172]

Lens

Cataracts have been reported in diabetic animals of all species examined, except the mouse, with the clinical stages of diabetic cataract being similar in most species.[165] Clinical and histologic changes in the lens are similar in all sugar cataracts,[173] galactosemic or diabetic. Because the role of aldose reductase in the initiation of a diabetic complication was first demonstrated in sugar cataract formation, the galactosemic and diabetic cataract are discussed in more detail.

Galactosemic cataract

The use of galactose to induce cataract formation in laboratory animals was derived from investigations of the nutritional cataract in rats. In 1934, Mitchell and Dodge[174] made the accidental observation of mature cataracts in the first three rats given a 70% lactose ration. The observation was promptly confirmed by the finding of mature or markedly advanced cataracts in all rats fed on a 70% lactose diet.[175] The authors have provided the first description of ophthalmoscopically detectable lenticular changes progressing to cataract and have shown that the rate of cataract development depends on the amount of lactose ingested (Table 10), and that it is slower in older animals.

Table 10. Rate of cataract development in rats fed lactose with the diet. (From Mitchell and Dodge.[174])

Lactose in the diet	First appearance of lenticular changes after	Mature cataract in
70%	9 days	68%/10 weeks
50%	17 days	27%/17 weeks
30%	25 days	0%

Subsequently, both Mitchell[176] and Yudkin and Arnold[177] demonstrated that similar lenticular changes can be induced in rats fed diets containing galactose instead of lactose. The finding was corroborated by Day,[94] who showed that rats given 60% galactose with the diet developed cataract after 11 days. He linked the rapid rate of cataract development to the high systemic availability of galactose and was the first to suggest that the diabetic and galactosemic cataract may share a common mechanism of formation. That the rate of development of lenticular changes depends on the age of rats fed on a 50% galactose diet was documented by Sasaki,[178] who also provided the first detailed description of the changes monitored by slit-lamp.

According to Mitchell,[179] reduction of protein content from 15% to 5% of the diet accelerated galactosemic cataract development from 26 to 15 days; conversely, high protein rations tended to delay cataract formation. Addition of various fats (up to 46%) to the galactose-containing diet had no effect on production of cataract; an apparent delay with high fat rations fed ad libitum proved to be caused by differences in galactose intake. Later, retardation in the rate of cataract formation was reported in rats given access to a 35% galactose diet and, on alternate days, to a diet containing fat and casein or glucose[180]; however, no difference in lens galactitol levels was recorded.[181]

While cataract formation in galactose-fed rats is associated with high systemic galactose levels,[91,94] the excess of galactose in the lens does not interfere with glucose utilization[182] or lactate production.[183] In addition, no significant change in lens ATP levels occurs at the time when the opacities first become visible. The ATP levels are markedly decreased only in the later stages of cataract development when a lack of ATP-derived energy may become a contributing factor.[184]

The degree of susceptibility to galactosemic cataract depends on the age of the animal: while rats aged 28 to 32 days and placed on a 60% galactose diet develop dense lenticular opacification in 12 to 18 days, animals aged 85 to 100 days require about 70 days for cataract to occur.[185] Lerman[185] attributed the difference to a decrease in hexose monophosphate shunt activity in the rat lens as the animal ages.

That the rate of cataract development in rats depends on the amount of ingested galactose was first reported by Patterson,[186] who correlated the time required for cataract formation with the blood sugar level. This relationship was corroborated by Keiding and Mellemgaard[187] in female rats given access to liquid diets containing various amounts of galactose and ethanol, which was expected to decrease the elimination of galactose.[188] All rats fed 15% of the calories as galactose developed cortical cataract, but none progressed to the nuclear cataract after 75 days of access to the galactose-containing diet. This amount of galactose may thus represent the threshold for the development of nuclear cataract. According to Ribaya-Mercado and Gershoff,[189] upon feeding on a diet containing 25% galactose, only one of six rats had visible cataracts after 34 days, and two of six rats had cataracts after 49 days. Feeding on 15% galactose diets did not result in visible lenticular opacities even after 49 days.

We have investigated the relationship between the rate of cataract development and the amount of galactose ingested by monitoring the progression of lenticular changes by slit-lamp microscopy[190] using a modification[191] of the classifications of Cotlier[192] and Sippel.[193] As shown in Table 11, in male rats weighing 80 to 90 g fed on diets containing 30% to 50% galactose, the rate of cataract development depended upon the amount of galactose ingested and upon the duration of access to the galactose-containing ration. With a fixed amount of galactose added to the diet, the rate of cataract development was time-dependent, while with a fixed time period of galactose feeding, the rate of cataract development depended upon the amount of galactose ingested.[190] Thus, similar lenticular changes were found in rats fed for 14 days on a diet containing 30% galactose or for six days on a diet containing 50% galactose.

The development of nuclear cataract in rats fed on a 35% galactose diet was accelerated by supplementing the diet with 1.6% magnesium oxide.[189] The effect was attributed to increased aldose reductase activity.

Based on the postulate of Kinoshita et al[194] that the process of cataractogenesis is triggered by elevated lenticular polyol concentrations, we have investigated the relationship between ingested galactose and lenticular galactitol levels. As shown in Table 12, in rats fed for four days on diets containing 10% to 50% galactose, the concentration of galactitol in the lens is proportional ($r = 0.954$, $p < 0.0008$) to the amount of ingested galactose.[190]

The galactitol concentration/time curve in the lenses of galactose-fed rats

Table 11. Rate of cataract development in galactose-fed rats as dependent on galactose intake and duration of exposure. (From Simard-Duquesne et al.[190])

Galactose in diet (%)	Day	Percentage of lenses at stage I	II	III	IV
30	6	92	8		
	8	67	33		
	10	58	42		
	14		75	25	
	16		50	50	
	20		25	75	
40	6	17	58	25	
	8		42	58	
	10		50	50	
	14		8	75	17
	16			50	50
	20			17	83
50	6		75	25	
	8		42	58	
	10		25	75	
	14			33	67
	16			33	67
	20			25	76

Table 12. Galactitol accumulation in the lenses of galactose-fed rats as dependent on galactose intake. (From Simard-Duquesne et al.[190])

Galactose In diet (%)	Galactose Ingested (g/kg/day)	Galactitol accumulation in lens (nmol/mg ± SE)*
10	13.0	23.4 ± 1.4
15	20.6	42.2 ± 2.7
20	29.5	43.1 ± 2.0
25	34.0	45.8 ± 2.4
30	43.7	55.4 ± 4.9
40	65.0	62.8 ± 1.6
50	71.5	68.8 ± 2.8

*There were 6 rats per group.

displays a characteristic profile. As illustrated in Figs 5 and 6, the galactitol concentrations rise very rapidly, attain a peak after ten to 12 days, then decrease relatively rapidly.[191,195–199] Comparison of the results obtained in the lenses of galactosemic rats by different groups of investigators demonstrates first, the parallel relationship between the levels of galactitol and water,[193,195,196,200] and second, the more or less inverse relationship between galactitol and the lenticular contents of

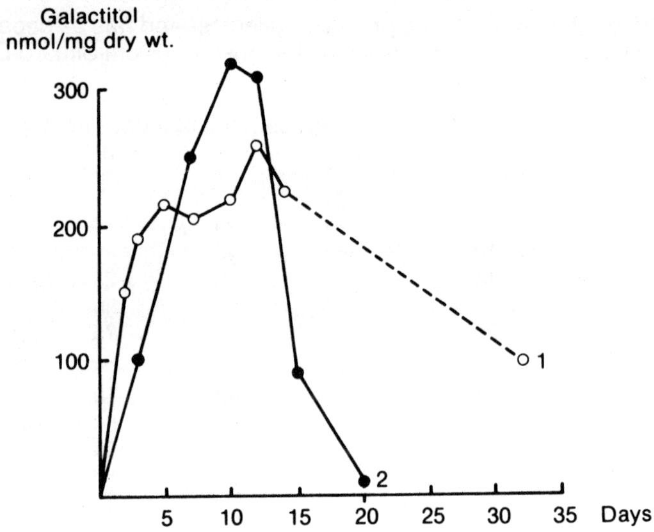

1:In 100-g rats (from Kinoshita et al [195])
2:In 50- to 60-g female rats (from Reddy et al[196])

Figure 5. Galactitol concentration/time curves in lenses of Sprague-Dawley rats fed galactose with the diet; expressed in nmol/mg dry lens weight.

glutathione[193,196] and its synthesis,[196] of protein[193,201] and amino acids,[196] of sodium and potassium,[196,200] of the cation pump,[200] and of ATP.[187]

The progression of lenticular changes leading to sugar cataract has been arbitrarily divided into three different stages.[200] The first stage represents the initial vacuole formation due to osmotic swelling produced by the very rapid accumulation of galactitol formed from galactose by the action of aldose reductase. The rat lens is particularly prone to galactitol accumulation because the activity of the competing galactokinase is sluggish[184] and because galactitol is practically not metabolized by the sorbitol dehydrogenase.[202–204] The second stage represents the time period between the initial vacuolar stage and the late vacuolar stage, preceding the appearance of nuclear opacity. The relevant changes result from increases in galactitol and electrolyte concentrations. The third stage is characterized by the breakdown of lenticular permeability,[205–207] resulting in a fall in galactitol levels, the breakdown of the cation pump, a marked increase in cellular hydration, and the appearance of a dense nuclear opacity.

Experimental results suggest that the vacuolar phase is associated with galactitol levels of about 40 nmol/mg lens (wet wt.), attained in four[190] to six[191] days in young rats fed on a diet containing 15% to 25% galactose.[190,191] Similarly, a

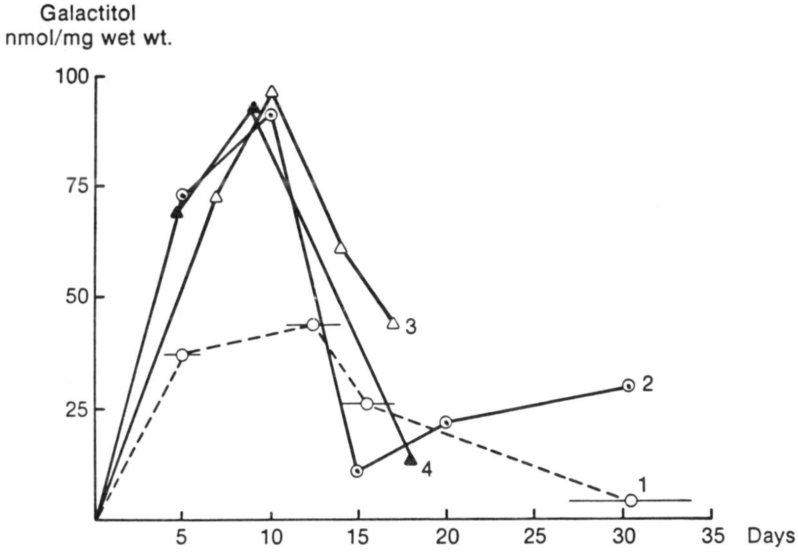

1:In male rats weighing 50 to 60 g and fed on 25% galactose (from Simard-Duquesne and Dvornik[191])
2:In rats weighing 50 g and fed on 50% galactose (from Hu et al[197])
3:In female rats weighing about 60 g and fed on 50% galactose (from Beyer-Mears et al[198])
4:In female rats weighing 45 to 60 g and fed on 50% galactose (from Okuda et al[199])

Figure 6. Galactitol concentration/time curves in lenses of Sprague-Dawley rats fed on a galactose diet; expressed in nmol/mg wet lens weight.

galactitol level of 37.0 ± 2.4 nmol/mg lens was found in rats fed for seven days on a diet containing 30% galactose.[208]

By comparing the relationship between the amount of ingested galactose, the rate of progression of lenticular changes (Table 11), and the lenticular galactitol levels (Table 12), it appears that a galactitol level of at least 50 nmol/mg lens is associated with the appearance of cortical changes. The point of irreversibility, on the other hand, seems to be associated with a peak galactitol level of about 75 nmol/mg lens.[195,197,209] In young rats fed on a 50% galactose diet, the appearance of dense nuclear cataract (usually after ten days) is preceded by galactitol levels above 90 nmol/mg lens.[197–199,210] It is pertinent that once formed a mature nuclear cataract will not completely disappear upon placing the cataractous rat on a galactose-free diet.[179,196,206,211–217]

The progression of galactose-induced cataractogenesis is accompanied by a significant increase of the lysosomal hydrolases, acid phosphatase, and the arylsulfatases.[218,219] A similar increase was observed in senile cataracts of rats.[220] A correlation appears to exist between the extent of galactose-induced lenticular damage and arylsulfatase activity; it is of interest that on day 12 of feeding on a

50% galactose diet, i.e., when the point of irreversibility was attained, a rapid and significant increase in arylsulfatase activity was observed.[221] Addition to the diet of the AR inhibitor sorbinil, at a dose of 50 mg/kg/day, inhibited the galactose-induced lenticular damage and prevented the increase in lysosomal activity.

Diabetic cataract

The development of diabetic cataracts was first described in dogs with pancreatic [222] or hypophyseal diabetes,[223] in depancreatized rats,[224] and subsequently in rabbits and rats[225] with diabetes produced by alloxan.[13] In alloxan-diabetic rats, the rate of cataract development was age-dependent, ranging from 58 days in animals with an initial body weight of about 100 g, to 104 days in rats initially weighing 280 to 300 g. Within a group, the rate of cataract development was correlated ($r = 0.912 \pm 0.235$) to the degree of glycosuria.[226] The inverse relationship between the time required for the occurrence of cataract and the extent of hyperglycemia was confirmed by Patterson[227,228] in rats made hyperglycemic with dehydroascorbic acid and related substances. The minimal blood sugar level associated with cataract formation was approximately 225 mg/dL, and at least 36 days were required for mature cataract formation. A blood glucose level of around 300 mg/dL was found to be critical for cataract development in STZ-induced diabetic rats.[229] The dependence of cataract development on the degree of hyperglycemia was also shown by the absence of cataract in partially pancreatectomized or alloxan-treated rats (fed on a high-fat diet) that did not have pronounced hyperglycemia.[230]

After the initial finding of bilateral cataracts in rats given STZ,[12,231] the first detailed study of the relevant lenticular changes was reported by Von Sallmann and Grimes.[232] In male rats, weighing 155 to 180 g and given STZ intravenously at a dose of 65 mg/kg, the onset of lenticular changes was noted after ten to 28 days, with 70% of the animals showing incipient opacities after ten to 15 days, and complete lens opacification by three months. Weanling rats appeared to be less sensitive to STZ.

The much slower rate of cataract development in rats made diabetic with alloxan or STZ, as compared with rats fed galactose, is associated with a slower rate of polyol accumulation in the lens. The concentrations of lens sorbitol usually range from 12.2 to 45.4 nmol/mg lens (Table 13) and are generally higher with diabetes of longer duration. While the values vary between laboratories, reflecting the differences in the experimental conditions used, including strain and age of the animals, usually at least three weeks of diabetes are required to accumulate lens sorbitol levels that correspond to those of galactitol produced in rats fed on a 15% galactose diet for four days, i.e., approximately 40 nmol/mg lens (Table 12). However, the increased levels of fructose may also contribute to the osmotic stress created in the lens of diabetic rats. The rate of cataract development was shown to depend on the carbohydrate content in the diet. According to Schmidt et al,[240] in rats with STZ-induced diabetes and fed on diets containing 5% to 27% carbohydrate, cataract development was delayed because of decreased blood glucose concentrations. By slit-lamp examination, Lee et al[241] detected thin equatorial cataracts in about one-half of young rats after only three days of feeding on 50%

Table 13. Sorbitol and fructose concentrations in the lens of experimentally diabetic rats, as dependent on duration of diabetes.

Strain (sex, body wt)	Diabetes inducer (mg/kg)	Duration of diabetes (days)	Group	nmol/mg ± S.E. Sorbitol	Fructose	Authors
Wistar (Male, 250 g)	Alloxan (200,s.c.)	6	ND	0.33 ± 0.03	0.55 ± 0.05	Gonzalez et al[233]
			D	12.20 ± 0.52	3.20 ± 0.10	
Sprague Dawley (Male, 150-240 g)	STZ (85, i.v.)	14	ND	0.15 ± 0.03	—	Malone et al[234]
			D	18.8 ± 1.3	—	
Charles River (80 g)	STZ (100, i.v.)	14	ND	0.90 ± 0.29	0.40	Fukushi et al[235]
			D	27.70 ± 2.40	8.90 ± 1.50	
Sprague Dawley (Male, 150 g)	STZ (55, i.v.)	21	ND	0.52 ± 0.05	—	Simard-Duquesne et al [236]
			D	37.22 ± 2.51	—	
Wistar (Male, 250 g)	STZ (75, i.v.)	22	ND	0.36 ± 0.05	0.78 ± 0.07	Poulsom, Heath[237]
			D	27.35 ± 2.18	9.64 ± 0.85	
Charles River (Male, 200–250 g)	STZ (85, i.v.)	22	D	25.60 ± 2.37	—	Peterson et al[238]
Sprague Dawley (Female, 60 g)	STZ (65, i.v.)		ND	0.28 ± 0.05	—	Beyer-Mears, Cruz[239]
		10	D	36.74 ± 5.76	—	
		16	D	21.01 ± 1.05	—	
		21	D	31.30 ± 1.98	—	
		30	D	45.35 ± 4.79	—	
Sprague Dawley (100 g)	Alloxan (100)	28	ND	1.5 ± 0.6	0.7 ± 0.08	Kinoshita et al[195]
			D	31.3 ± 3.0	16.3 ± 0.30	

ND = non-diabetic; D = diabetic; STZ = streptozocin

galactose, or nine days after STZ-induced diabetes. The changes were accompanied by a fall in NADPH levels and an increase in $NADP^+$ levels.

A comprehensive study of the course of cataract development in STZ-induced diabetic rats was carried out at the Kanazawa University. Based on examination by photoslit lamp, the lenticular changes were classified into six stages. While similar to the classification of changes occurring in the lenses of galactosemic rats described by Sippel,[193] the classification of Sasaki et al[242] differed in the characterization of two early vacuolar changes, Types A and B. Upon disappearance of the vacuoles, differences between Types A and B were no longer apparent. The time course and incidence of lenticular opacifications observed by Sasaki et al[242] are shown in Fig 7. It is likely that differentiation of the early lenticular changes was possible because of the considerably slower rate of cataract development in STZ-diabetic rats as compared with galactose-fed rats, particularly when a 50% galactose diet is used. The concomitant changes in lenticular glucose, sorbitol, fructose, and myoinositol concentrations are shown in Fig 8. Sorbitol levels increased relatively rapidly until the third week after induction of diabetes (Stages I to III) and decreased gradually thereafter. At Stage V, when opacities appeared near the central part of the lens, a marked increase in the Na/K ratio was accompanied by a rise in lens hydration (Fig 9), and significant differences between Types A and B were no longer detectable.[243]

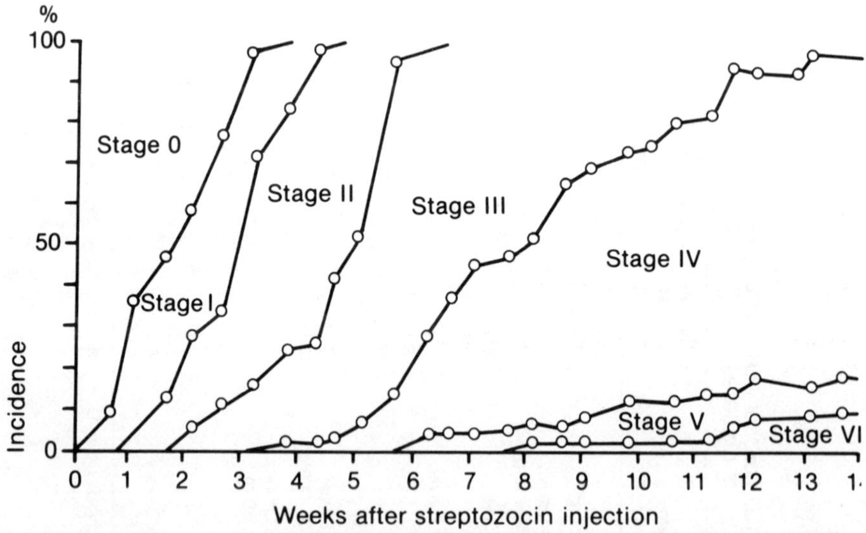

Figure 7. Rate of development of lenticular changes in rats with streptozocin-induced diabetes. (From Sasaki et al.[242])

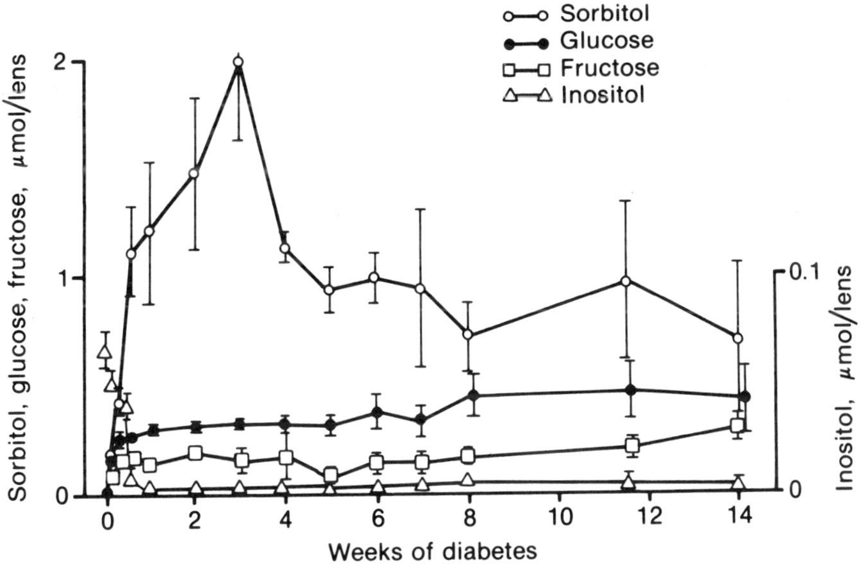

Figure 8. Lenticular glucose, sorbitol, fructose, and myoinositol levels in rats with streptozocin-induced diabetes. (From Kuriyama et al.[243])

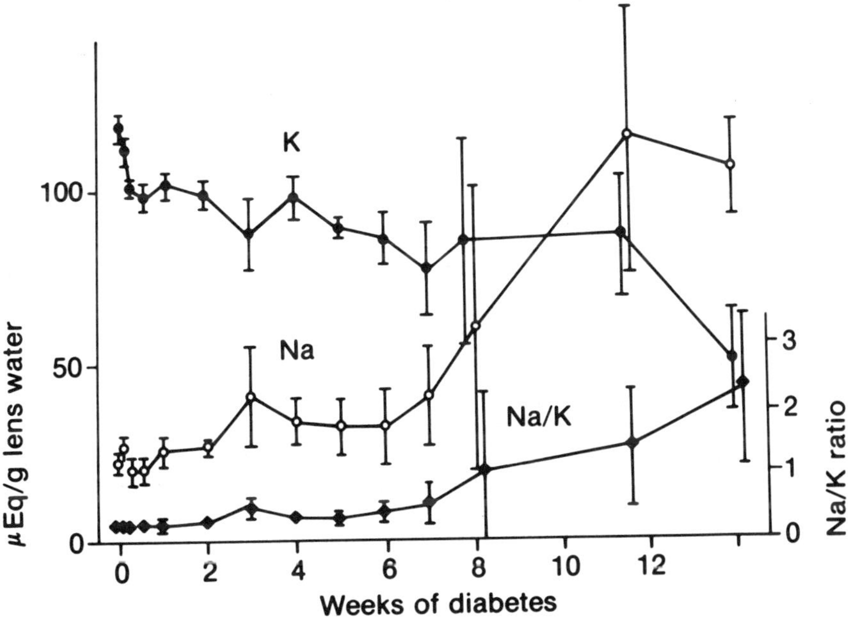

Figure 9. Sodium and potassium levels in the lenses of streptozocin-diabetic rats. (From Kuriyama et al.[243])

Retina

The morphological abnormalities of retinal vessels occurring in human diabetes mellitus include capillary basement membrane thickening, formation of capillary aneurysms, disappearance of pericytes, atrophy of capillaries, and extravascular changes such as hemorrhages and exudates. New vessels may eventually appear on the surface of the retina or in the vitreous humor, presumably because of the preceding "background" abnormalities.[165]

There are two types of animal models that are available for the investigation of diabetic retinal lesions.[173] In the first type, the ocular changes observed are identifiable with the metabolic or genetic characteristics of diabetes, or both. Retinal abnormalities reported recently in diabetic animals are listed in Table 14. In the second type, the animal is not diabetic, but the lesions occurring in the retina are morphologically similar to those of diabetes. Of particular interest among the second type[244] are the nutritional models, such as the galactose-fed rat and dog, and the sucrose-fed rat.

A hypothesis relating diabetic capillary disease of the retina to enhanced activity of aldose reductase and the ensuing osmotic damage resulting from sorbitol accumulation was originally proposed by Beaumont et al.[267] The same investigators demonstrated the presence of the polyol pathway by the accumulation of sorbitol (approximately 80 nmol/mg protein) and fructose (approximately 20 nmol/mg protein) in the retina of rats with STZ-induced diabetes.[157] In view of the relatively low retinal sorbitol accumulation,[268] Hutton et al[157] modified their hypothesis by suggesting that sorbitol accumulation may be of osmotic significance, provided that it is localized within a small cellular compartment of the retina. Their view is supported by the localization of aldose reductase in the Müller cells of rat[156] and human retina.[269] Accumulation of sorbitol and fructose in the retina of rats with STZ-induced diabetes was corroborated by Poulsom et al[270–272] (Chapter 4, Tables 32 and 33, pages 260, 261) and by Stribling et al[273] (Chapter 4, Table 34, page 261).

According to Engerman[246] and Engerman et al,[165] in spite of a number of retinal lesions reported in diabetic animals, "an unequivocal saccular capillary aneurysm has never been encountered among the many non-diabetic or diabetic rats, mice and hamsters which have been studied. . . ."[244] The apparent absence of these aneurysms might be attributable to the brevity of diabetes in these short-lived species, or alternatively, to some fundamental biological difference between these rodents and man.[165]

Retinal lesions morphologically similar to those in humans were found to develop only in dogs and, possibly, in monkeys. The first canine diabetic retinopathy was observed in 1962 by Patz and Maumenee[257] in a spontaneously diabetic cocker spaniel. Subsequently, retinopathy was shown to develop in dogs with spontaneous or experimentally induced diabetes.[261] According to Engerman and Kern,[274] in alloxan-induced diabetic dogs, retinopathy may be prevented by good glycemic control, but may be resistant to arrest or reversal even in its incipient stages, before more than the first few aneurysms are formed.

Basement membrane thickening was found to occur in retinal capillaries of

Table 14. Retinal angiopathy reported recently in rats, dogs, and monkeys.

Species	Status of the animal	Retinal abnormality	Ref.
Rat	Pancreatectomy	Aneurysm of small arterioles	245
	Alloxan-diabetes	Intravitreal new vessels	246
	Alloxan-diabetes	Ultrastructural disorders of the vessels and basement membrane	247
	Sucrose-fed	Loss of intramural pericytes or endothelial cells, occurrence of capillary strands and microaneurysms	153
	Alloxan-diabetes	Retinal atrophy and new vessels	248
	Alloxan-diabetes and iminodipropionitrile	Vessel atrophy and aneurysms	249
	Streptozocin-diabetes	Microaneurysms or basement membrane changes	250, 251
	Streptozocin-diabetes	Vasodilatation	252
	Sucrose-fed with streptozocin diabetes	Microaneurysms, loss of pericytes, endothelial proliferation, strand formation, acellularity, basement membrane thickening	154, 159, 162
	Streptozocin-diabetes	Proliferation of basement membrane-like material into Müller cells; accumulation of electron-dense bodies in Müller cell cytoplasm	253
	Galactose-fed	Capillary basement membrane thickening	254–256
Dog	Spontaneous diabetes	Microaneurysms, loss of pericytes, acellular capillaries	257, 258
	Spontaneous diabetes	Microaneurysms, acellular capillaries	259
	Spontaneous diabetes	Microaneurysms	260
	Alloxan-diabetes	Microaneurysms, loss of pericytes, acellular capillaries	261
	Metapituitary diabetes	Microaneurysms	262
	Metapituitary diabetes	Microaneurysms, loss of perictyes, acellular capillaries	261, 263, 264
	Galactose-fed	Saccular capillary aneurysms, hemorrhages, accellular vessels, hypertrophic capillaries, loss of pericytes	82

Table 14. (continued)

Species	Status of the animal	Retinal abnormality	Ref.
Monkey	Alloxan-diabetes	Microaneurysms	265
	Alloxan-diabetes	Microaneurysms, acellular capillaries, cotton wool spots, maculopathy	266

rats[158,251] and dogs[83,275] with experimentally induced diabetes. Since in dogs such thickening was prevented by improved control of diabetes,[275] the thickening was attributed to uncontrolled hyperglycemia rather than to the diabetogenic agent.

Of particular importance were the observations made in galactosemic dogs and rats. In dogs fed on a diet containing 30% galactose, Engerman and Kern[82,83,276] found after three to five years retinal lesions that were morphologically similar to those occurring in diabetic dogs and diabetic patients. The authors concluded that the morphological similarity between the diabetic and galactosemic retinopathy suggests that these microvascular abnormalities are produced by a common final pathway. The diabetic-like retinal changes in galactose-fed dogs occurred in the presence of insulin, thus supporting the view that increased systemic sugar levels are an important determinant of retinopathy.[82]

Marked thickening of the retinal capillary basement membranes also occurs in rats fed on a 50% galactose diet.[103,254–256,277–279] Pertinently, the thickening was prevented by treatment with AR inhibitors.[254–256,277–279]

Retinal pigmented epithelium, which forms the outer component of the blood-retinal barrier, partly determines the composition of the retinal interstitial fluid; it also generates the c-wave component of the electroretinogram. As reported by MacGregor and Matschinsky,[280] the amplitude of the c-wave in pigmented rats decreased progressively upon induction of diabetes with streptozocin. The decline was arrested by treatment with the AR inhibitor sorbinil, or by myoinositol supplementation. The pigmented epithelium of the retina may therefore provide a useful model for studying the pathogenesis of diabetic retinal complications.

Progressive ultrastructural changes in the retinal pigmented epithelium have also been observed in the spontaneously diabetic BB rat.[281] Immunohistochemical staining demonstrated aldose reductase in the retinal pigmented epithelium, ciliary epithelium, and vascular endothelium in diabetic human and rat eyes, but not in the eyes of non-diabetic rats, rabbits, and humans. The finding suggests that aldose reductase is induced in diabetes and that activation of the polyol pathway in retinal pigmented cells may lead to progressive damage.

Nervous system complications

The cellular and molecular mechanisms underlying peripheral nerve degeneration in human diabetic neuropathy are at present unknown,[282] and progress in the understanding of nerve damage in diabetes is slowed by the difficulty in carrying out studies directly on human tissue.[283] While studies of diabetic neuropathy in laboratory animals can be very useful, their application to the human condition remains uncertain because better characterization of human diabetic neuropathy is needed for the elaboration of animal models that completely mimic the changes occurring in man.[282] In addition, animal models cannot mimic the subjective end-points of pain and paresthesia.

Clinical studies and experimental data suggest that diabetic polyneuropathy is related to metabolic abnormalities and that such abnormalities may underlie the neuropathy.[282] Abnormalities in motor nerve conduction velocity occurring in newly diagnosed diabetic patients and in laboratory animals soon after the induction of diabetes, coupled with the demonstration that treatment with insulin (or oral anti-hyperglycemic agents) results in general improvement of nerve function, support the concept that the early reversible nerve dysfunction may be caused by metabolic derangements preceding the structural alterations of the nerve.[282] In a recent extensive review of neuropathy, Brown and Asbury[284] reiterate the view that hyperglycemia appears to be the major factor involved in the metabolic derangements of the nerve.

The metabolic pathway receiving most in-depth study is the polyol pathway for the disposition of excess intracellular glucose occurring in tissues not in need of insulin for their uptake of glucose (see Chapter 4 for a more extensive discussion of the polyol pathway and aldose reductase). Originally it was postulated[285] that in the Schwann cells, hyperglycemia increased the activity of aldose reductase, the first enzyme of the polyol pathway, causing accumulation of sorbitol (and fructose) as a direct function of the plasma glucose level. Since aldose reductase is localized in the Schwann cells of the myelin sheath,[286] the accumulation of sorbitol in these cells was postulated to cause a localized osmotic effect, resulting in cytotoxic Schwann cell edema and subsequent demyelination.[287] However, findings in laboratory animals[288] indicate that it is the endoneurial space rather than the Schwann cell that is expanded by fluid under high pressure[289–293] and the edema is formed by the osmotic pressure of the accumulated products of the polyol pathway.

The role of the polyol pathway in the pathogenesis of diabetic neuropathy can be investigated in laboratory animals only in the presence of high systemic sugar concentrations occurring in spontaneously diabetic animals. Experimentally, such a condition is produced either by inducing diabetes, usually with the administration of the β-cytotoxicant streptozocin, or by inducing galactosemia in animals fed on a diet rich in galactose.

The alterations observed in nerve tissues from STZ-induced diabetic rats include electrophysiological abnormalities,[294–303] axonal dwindling,[304,305] decreased myelinated fiber size,[302,306,307] endoneurial edema,[289] ischemia,[308] susceptibility of peripheral nerves to compression,[309] myelinated nerve fiber degeneration,[310] delayed peripheral nerve regeneration,[311] and decreased axonal transport,[283,312,313] as well as ultrastructural alterations.[314–316] Because the slowing in nerve conduction is prevented by insulin treatment,[305,307,310] it is likely that the electrophysiological abnormality is caused by hyperglycemia rather than by an independent toxic effect of streptozocin on peripheral nerve. It is pertinent that prompt continuous subcutaneous insulin infusion normalized neural sorbitol, fructose, and myoinositol levels, and prevented a decrease in myelinated fiber diameter in 8-week STZ-induced diabetic rats.[317]

The galactosemic rat possesses many clinical and pathological features of diabetes mellitus,[282] and is characterized by increased glycated hemoglobin concentrations,[318] galactitol accumulation and myoinositol depletion in peripheral nerves,[119,120,199,319] increased endoneurial sodium accumulation,[320] increased hydration of nerve tissue,[119,321] progressive elevation of endoneurial fluid pressure,[290–292] decreased endoneurial blood flow[322,323] and hypoxia,[323] decreased nerve conduction velocity,[324] and demyelination.[293]

Because the activity of aldose reductase and the resulting accumulation of galactitol may have a direct effect on the fluid environment surrounding the nerve fiber, the galactosemic rat is an attractive model for studying diabetic neuropathy.[282,292] The relatively greater severity of such changes in experimental galactosemia enhances its value as an animal model of neuropathy.[1]

According to Powell et al,[291] endoneurial fluid pressure was also increased in rats fed on a diet containing 68% sucrose.

The finding of Greene et al[310] that the decrease in nerve conduction velocity in STZ-induced diabetic rats is associated with a decrease in nerve myoinositol levels and that both defects can be restored by adding 1% myoinositol to the diet provoked considerable interest in the potential role of myoinositol in the development of diabetic neuropathy.[283] As discussed more extensively in Chapter 2, a decrease of about 25% in neural myoinositol levels of diabetic rats was considered to be sufficient to affect the small, rapidly turning-over neural pools of phosphatidylinositol postulated to be involved in the control of nerve metabolism.[325,326] Subsequently it was found that the depletion of neural myoinositol levels, linked with the decrease in nerve conduction velocity (see Chapter 2, Table 2, page 114), is also associated with decreases in orthograde axonal transport[327–330] and Na/K-dependent ATPase activity.[331–333] All of these impairments were prevented by oral administration of myoinositol to the diabetic animals.

Several fundamental studies on the pathogenesis of diabetic neuropathy were carried out in the spontaneously diabetic BB rat,[9,334–336] the animal model that most closely simulates IDDM in man. Investigations were done on the correlations between hyperglycemia, the myoinositol-related Na/K-dependent ATPase defect, and the reversible component of nerve conduction slowing,[333] nodal function[337] and axo-glial junction complexes.[338] According to Greene et al,[339] axo-glial dysfunction, a structural abnormality that characterizes the peripheral nerve nodes of Ranvier in human and murine diabetes, is preceded by paranodal swelling. Based on observations in spontaneously diabetic BB rats, the authors believe that paranodal fiber swelling is due to myoinositol depletion and an associated Na/K-ATPase defect rather than to a direct osmotic effect of sorbitol accumulation.

A particularly important finding first reported in 1983 by the Nottingham group of investigators[327,340] was that in acutely diabetic rats, inhibition of aldose reductase prevented both the depletion of neural myoinositol and the impairment in motor nerve conduction velocity (MNCV). The involvement of aldose reductase in the control of neural myoinositol availability in acutely diabetic rats was rapidly corroborated by several groups of investigators using several structurally distinct AR inhibitors.[273,327–329,341–344] The work has culminated in the finding that AR inhibitors also prevent the diabetes-induced impairment of the Na/K-dependent ATPase[345] and axonal transport.[327–329] The metabolic abnormalities and impaired functions in the diabetic nerve were thus linked with the increased flux of glucose through the polyol pathway. As shown by Carroll et al,[346] altered glutathione redox state plays no detectable role in the pathogenesis of the Na/K-ATPase defect in diabetic peripheral nerves. Relevantly, in diabetic rats, prevention of these impairments with either myoinositol or an AR inhibitor is achieved in the presence of high systemic glucose concentrations.

It is interesting that myoinositol depletion is readily detectable in rats with spontaneous[333] or experimental diabetes of three months' duration but not of six months' duration.[347,348] According to Cameron et al,[347] the findings suggest that the myoinositol deficit may be transient.

The measurement of motor or sensory nerve conduction velocity in the sciatic or tail nerves of rats is a relatively simple procedure; however, in order to stimulate and record from the nerve, the animal is usually anesthetized, giving rise to hypothermia, which can impair transmission. Furthermore, the assessment of peripheral nerve conduction velocity requires the precise measurement of the distance between the stimulating and recording electrodes, and of the latency of the evoked electrical response. To avoid these potential sources of error, open-field auditory-evoked brainstem responses (ABR) have been measured in conscious unrestrained non-diabetic and STZ-induced diabetic rats.[349] After two weeks of diabetes, the distal nerve transmission time of the auditory pathway (peak II latency of the ABR), which includes conduction along the VIII cranial nerve, was significantly prolonged ($p<0.05$). The impairment of the auditory pathway in diabetic rats is similar to changes reported for the ABR of diabetic patients.[350] That aldose reductase is involved in this model of diabetic cranial nerve neuropathy was shown by preventing the diabetes-induced deficit with the AR inhibitor tolrestat.[351]

In the urinary bladder base region of STZ-induced diabetic rats, a 39% increase in response to acetylcholine was detected at six weeks after induction of diabetes; the responsiveness increased to 66% above control after 11 months of diabetes. The response to α- and β-adrenergic agonists was smaller and regionally specific.[352]

Kudlacz et al[353] have compared the urinary bladder function in 4-week STZ-induced diabetic rats and in rats fed for four weeks on a 60% galactose diet. While bladder elasticity was altered in both groups of animals, the galactosemic rats differed from the diabetic rats by the two-fold increase in the volume of fluid needed to elicit first micturition. While in vivo the bladder contractions were similar in both groups, the frequency and duration of contraction were reduced in diabetic animals, possibly because of parasympathetic neuropathy. The observed differences appear to suggest that autonomic nerve function was affected by diabetes but not by galactosemia.

Structural and morphometric changes in visceral efferent and afferent fibers of predominantly parasympathetic nerves of the diabetic BB rat have been described by Yagihashi and Sima.[354] However, the changes are distinctly different from those occurring in the STZ-diabetic rat[298] and from the dystrophic axonal changes characteristic of the sympathic nerve of diabetic BB rats.[355]

Kidney complications

Diabetic nephropathy is defined as a multifaceted pathologic entity that spans the continuum from early renal hypertrophic changes to late changes of advanced structural distortion of glomeruli, renal vasculature, interstitium, and tubules.[356] A comprehensive review of renal diabetic complications and factors affecting their progression was presented by Steffes et al.[357]

Functional and structural renal changes have been recognized to occur soon after onset of IDDM.[358] Both in patients with diabetes[359–365] and in laboratory animals with experimentally induced diabetes,[366–373] kidney enlargement is noticeable shortly after the onset of hyperglycemia.[360,361,366,368,370,374–377] In diabetic rats, the increase in kidney weight in early diabetes is age-dependent and varies from 19 mg/day per g of kidney in the immature rat to 54 mg/day per g of kidney in the adult rat.[378] This rapid phase of kidney growth involves an admixture of cellular hypertrophy and hyperplasia.[368] In addition, both glomeruli and tubules are enlarged, with a 30% increase in total glomerular volume[370]; Na/K-dependent ATPase activity is increased along most of the length of the nephron so as to maintain electrolyte homeostasis,[379] but the activity was found to be decreased in isolated glomeruli preparations[380,381]; the glomerular filtration surface area is increased,[371,372] together with podocyte hypercellularity[382] and hypertrophy and hyperplasia of proximal and distal tubular cells.[383,384] Control of hyperglycemia by insulin prevented these changes in STZ-induced diabetic rats[385] and reversed them in diabetic patients.[360]

Hyperfunction of the kidney is well documented in early IDDM.[359–363] Glomerular filtration rate, renal plasma flow, and filtration fraction are increased in newly diagnosed diabetic patients before treatment with insulin.[360,363] The increased glomerular filtration rate is closely correlated with the enlarged kidney size.[359,360,364,365] However, the mechanism of renal hyperfunction in diabetes remains unclear.[358]

Glomerular hyperfiltration similar to that occurring in early human diabetes has also been demonstrated in pancreatectomized dogs,[385] in alloxan-[386] and STZ-induced diabetic rats,[387,388] and in two strains of spontaneously diabetic mice (C57BL/6J db/db and C57BL/KsJ db/db).[389] The available hemodynamic data suggest that the early hyperfiltration in diabetes is due to increased renal plasma flow associated with an increased transcapillary hydraulic pressure gradient.[390] The mechanism(s) of the altered renal resistances that underlie the increased plasma flow remain unknown.[390] Importantly, in rats with STZ-induced diabetes of 12 months' duration, dietary protein restriction limited both early elevations in glomerular pressures and flows and the subsequent development of glomerular structural injury.[391] Subsequently, glomerular hemodynamic alterations were also attenuated by converting enzyme inhibition with enalapril.[392] The finding that prevention of glomerular capillary hypertension protected the diabetic animals against the subsequent development of glomerular lesions and proteinuria despite persistent hyperglycemia supported the authors' view that hemodynamic rather than metabolic factors predominate in the pathogenesis of diabetic glomerulopathy.[392] That the increased glomerular filtration rate in early STZ-induced diabetic rats is caused mainly by an increased glomerular capillary pressure and a reduced pressure in the proximal tubule was demonstrated by Jensen et al.[71] Strict metabolic control prevented these changes, thus excluding a potential nephrotoxic effect of streptozocin per se. The pathogenesis of diabetic microangiopathy from a hemodynamic view was recently reviewed by Zatz and Brenner.[393]

Frank proteinuria has long been recognized as one of the characteristics of clinically apparent diabetic nephropathy. Classically, the appearance of protein in the urine is the first sign of this progressive condition. However, more recent studies have shown that microalbuminuria is detectable well before the stage of overt proteinuria.[394–396] The term "microalbuminuria"[397] was adopted to indicate an increase in urinary albumin excretion rate that is not detectable by Albustix.[358] That the increased excretion of albumin (and of immunoglobulin G) is of glomerular origin[398] was inferred from the lack of increase of β_2-microglobulin excretion,[390] a sensitive indicator of tubular function.[399]

Since, at the level of microalbuminuria, the charge- and size-selectivity of the glomerular membrane appears to be intact, the increased flux has been attributed to increased transglomerular pressure.[400] Supporting evidence was provided by the finding of an elevated transglomerular pressure-gradient in experimentally induced diabetic animals.[387] In studies on glomerular protein filtration function in STZ-induced diabetic rats, the excretion of albumin increased within 16 days [401] to two months after induction of diabetes,[402] then increased progressively over the next seven-month period.[402]

Cooper et al[403] have demonstrated that STZ-induced diabetes in 8- to 9-week-old spontaneously hypertensive (SH) rats resulted in a 100-fold increase in albuminuria and a two- to five-fold increase in total proteinuria over a period of six months. The finding suggests that there is a phase of "microalbuminuria" in the development of nephropathy in the diabetic SH rat and that hypertension may have a specific action on the acceleration of diabetic renal disease, independent of the glomerular filtration rate.

The increased rate of urinary albumin excretion in newly diagnosed IDDM patients is promptly reversed by insulin treatment.[404,405] However, in patients with established diabetes, the effect of strict metabolic control on urinary albumin excretion varies between studies, perhaps reflecting the degree of microalbuminuria at the outset.[406] While a positive effect was reported in the eight-month KROC study[407] and the two-year Steno study,[408] no reversal was detected by the Steno group in a one-year study.[406] The failure to reduce microalbuminuria by strict blood glucose control may, in part, be due to inclusion in such studies of diabetic patients with "intermittent clinical proteinuria,"[409] defined as a late phase of diabetic nephropathy when glomerular function is already declining. According to Bending et al,[409] the point of "metabolic no return" for the diabetic kidney lies at a phase preceding that of "intermittent nephropathy." In diabetic animals, albuminuria can be prevented with insulin treatment[410,411] or reversed by pancreatic islet transplantation.[402] Of importance is that albuminuria reversed to normal in the presence of continued thickening of the glomerular basement membrane. Therefore, per se, the thickened glomerular basement membrane does not appear to be directly related to albumin excretion in rats with long-term diabetes.[412]

Thickening of glomerular basement membrane and expansion of glomerular mesangium are characteristic of early diabetic glomerular pathology.[413] Renal changes similar in morphology and rate of development to those of mild to moderate diffuse diabetic glomerulosclerosis in humans were described by Stout et al[414] in female baboons with long-term diabetes induced by surgical total pancreatectomy. The glomerular basement membrane is a complex, charged, thin extracellular matrix that separates epithelial and endothelial cells and is rich in fixed anionic charges.[415] The porosity of the matrix and charge distribution along the constituent polypeptide chains are involved in the control of protein filtration from the serum into the urinary filtrate.[416] The glomerular basement membrane thus represents a size- and charge-selective barrier for macromolecular filtration.[415] The porosity of the glomerular membrane is determined by the nature of the polypeptides and the manner of their cross-linking. The major molecular species in the glomerular basement membrane is heparan sulfate. Studies carried out in rats with experimentally induced diabetes[417–421] suggest that both increased synthesis and decreased degradation may be involved in glomerular basement membrane thickening.[358] The thickened glomerular basement membranes of IDDM patients display a widespread decrease in sulfated proteoglycans (fixed anionic sites) as well as an irregular accumulation of anionic sites in the middle of the basement membrane.[415]

In human diabetes, immunohistopathologic studies have indicated a polyantigenic expansion of all the investigated components of the glomerular and tubular basement membranes and the mesangium during the early stages of nephropathy[422] Because of the complexity of the changes, not much is expected to be gained from biochemical studies on protein constituents of the glomerular basement membrane.[358,423]

While many compositional studies emphasize glomerular basement thickening as the central renal lesion in diabetes, Mauer et al[424] were unable to demonstrate the critical role of glomerular basement membrane in diabetic renal dysfunction. Rather, an important role in the functional deterioration was attributed to the mesangium,[424] thus supporting the much earlier observation by Gellman et al[425] that the salient clinical manifestations of diabetic nephropathy, i.e., proteinuria, hypertension, and, ultimately, decreased glomerular filtration rate, are better related to the severity of diffuse mesangial thickening than to any other single morphologic feature of diabetic nephropathy. Mauer et al[356] hypothesize that by restricting the glomerular capillary luminal space and the peripheral capillary filtration surface, mesangial expansion stimulates compensatory processes resembling those that result from a marked decrease in the number of nephrons. These compensatory mechanisms involve alterations in glomerular hemodynamics designed to maintain glomerular filtration, that, ultimately, injure the kidney.[356] This concept is known as "the remnant kidney hypothesis"[356] because of the remarkable similarities in alterations of the permselectivity characteristics of the glomerular filter in the remnant kidney model in rats[426] and in clinical diabetic nephropathy in man.[427,428] Supporting evidence for the remnant kidney hypothesis was obtained by the demonstration that in the rat, uninephrectomy, which accelerates diabetic lesions,[429] prevents the return of mesangial volume to normal upon establishment of normoglycemia by pancreatic islet transplantation.[430] According to Steffes et al,[357] the pathophysiological basis of the influence of the mesangium on renal function, particularly on the glomerular filtration rate, seems to be in its perturbation of other elements of glomerular structure that result in decreased volume of the glomerular capillaries and their corresponding surface available for filtration.

As mentioned earlier, islet transplantation-induced diabetes control in STZ-diabetic rats decreased albuminuria[402] and reversed the mesangial matrix and cell pathology,[431] despite persisting thickening of glomerular basement membranes.[412] A similar dissociation of diabetic mesangial and glomerular basement membrane pathology was found by Brown et al[432] in the spontaneously diabetic BB rat: despite thickened glomerular basement membranes, the BB rat lacked both glomerular mesangial pathology and increased urinary albumin. The finding demonstrates an association between the mesangial lesion and increased glomerular permeability, and indicates that the thickening of the glomerular basement membrane may not be associated with altered glomerular permeability to albumin.[412,432] These and other experiments[433] emphasize the reversibility of early lesions of diabetic nephropathy in the rat.[357]

According to Fine and Bradley,[434] the increase in kidney size that follows partial removal of kidney mass is mainly due to hypertrophy of the renal tubular cells, especially of the proximal tubule. The propensity of the proximal tubule to enlarge appears to be linked to increased glomerular filtration rate and to altered tubular fluid flow-rate, which, in turn, may induce an increase in Na/H-exchange (antiport). It was suggested that the latter may be the local stimulus that initiates hypertrophy and determines the organ specificity of the response.[435] It is unknown whether similar changes occur in the diabetic kidney.

The finding that improved diabetic control normalized urinary albumin excretion in patients without clinical nephropathy but not in patients with nephropathy[436] suggests that the functional manifestations of diabetic nephropathy can be influenced only before advanced renal lesions occur.[358] The finding supports the concept that the proteinuria of advanced diabetic nephropathology is independent of the diabetic state and may represent the establishment of new intraglomerular forces analogous to those of the remnant kidney.[358]

The presence of aldose reductase in the kidney was first suggested by the isolation of galactitol from the kidneys of galactosemic rats[115,119] and of a galactosemic child.[133] The findings were corroborated by Gabbay and O'Sullivan,[437] who measured polyol accumulation in diabetic and galactosemic rats and concluded that aldose reductase is localized in the kidney papilla. In rats fed for three weeks on a 50% galactose diet, the accumulation of galactitol amounted to 28.9 $\pm$ 8.4 nmol/mg ($\pm$SD). The presence of aldose reductase was also demonstrated in extracts of bovine kidney medullary and papillary tissue.[438]

Aldose reductase activity in monolayer cultures of monkey kidney epithelial cells was found by Hutton et al,[439] who detected sorbitol upon incubating the culture in glucose-rich medium and then prevented sorbitol formation by adding to the medium the AR inhibitor tetramethyleneglutaric acid.[440] Under similar experimental conditions, the formation of sorbitol was also prevented by three structurally distinct AR inhibitors, the oxyquinoline derivative ICI-105,552 and two flavonoids.[441]

Aldose reductase activity in the kidney was shown in vivo by Hutton et al,[442] who found increased polyol levels in the renal medulla but not in the glomeruli of 21-day STZ-induced diabetic rats:

	Polyol (nmol/mg protein ± SE)	
Renal tissue	**Non-diabetic**	**Diabetic**
Cortex	0.1 ± 0.02	0.3 ± 0.04
Cortical tubules	0.5 ± 0.06	3.1 ± 0.4
Medulla	1.0 ± 0.09	110 ± 10
Glomeruli	<0.1	<0.1

Similar results were obtained upon incubation of glomeruli in high-glucose medium.

Modest, albeit statistically significant increases in kidney sorbitol and fructose levels were also found in adult rats with 7-day alloxan-induced diabetes[376]:

Variable (±SE)	Non-diabetic	Diabetic
Body wt. (g)	319 ± 10	236 ± 5**
Kidney wt./100 g body wt.	0.86 ± 0.04	1.55 ± 0.07**
Blood glucose (nmol/L)	4.8 ± 0.4	30 ± 2**
Kidney: glucose (nmol/mg)	4.4 ± 0.2	28 ± 2**
sorbitol (nmol/mg)	0.26 ± 0.01	0.32 ± 0.02*
fructose (nmol/mg)	0.17 ± 0.01	0.26 ± 0.02**

*p<0.05; **p<0.01

Corder et al[443] found the highest AR activity in the medulla and lowest in the inner cortex of rat kidney, while the polyol dehydrogenase activity was diametrically different. Correspondingly, in the cortex of alloxan-induced diabetic rats, the increased glucose levels were not accompanied by increased sorbitol levels.

Aldose reductase was subsequently localized in the glomerular podocytes, Henle's loop, collecting tubules of the rat,[156] and cultured mesangial cells of rat glomeruli;[444] in the Henle's loop, collecting tubules, and interstitial cells of the dog;[445] and in human diabetic glomeruli.[446] Low AR activity was found in the kidneys of a strain of congenitally diabetic (NSY) mice possessing abnormally small vessels of the glomerulus.[447]

In a preliminary report, Bauman and Farnsworth[448] suggested that a sorbitol-dependent mechanism is involved in sodium reabsorption.

ICI-105,552, the first AR inhibitor tested in vivo for its effect on aldose reductase in the kidney of STZ-induced diabetic rats, had no detectable effect on renal sorbitol and fructose levels.[270–272] However, the more potent AR inhibitor sorbinil prevented renal polyol accumulation in both diabetic[449] and galactosemic rats.[450]

In contrast to the initial observation of Hutton et al,[442] sorbitol accumulation was reported to occur in the glomeruli of STZ-induced diabetic rats and to be prevented by sorbinil.[451]

The presence of aldose reductase in cultured mesangial cells of rat glomeruli was demonstrated by Kikkawa et al[444] by measuring polyol formation by the cells upon incubation with 55 mM (991 mg/dl) glucose or galactose. Polyol accumulation was arrested by the addition of an AR inhibitor, statil (1.3×10^{-5} M). It is tempting to link the loss of contractile properties of mesangial cells found in STZ-induced diabetic rats[452] with the capacity of mesangial cells to form and accumulate sorbitol, a process that, in turn, may result in deranged phosphoinositide metabolism.[444,453]

While according to Bauman and Farnsworth,[448] in either 2- to 4-week or 80- to 90-day[454] STZ-induced diabetic rats, the electrophoretic pattern of urinary protein is not different from that of age-matched controls, Beyer-Mears et al[455] reported that the urine of 4-week diabetic rats contained several proteins of molecular weight both above and below that of albumin. Since administration of sorbinil halted the progression of proteinuria and, after 13 weeks, restored the protein pattern toward the normal state, the authors concluded that aldose reductase was involved in the proteinuria. In contrast, while AR inhibition had no effect on protein excretion in diabetic rats, scanning electron microscopy indicated that the swelling of glomerular pedicles was prevented.[456] The finding was attributed to localized polyol accumulation due to the presence of aldose reductase in the podocytes.

The possible involvement of aldose reductase in diabetic renal hypertrophy is suggested by the following findings.

In rats, a 15% increase in kidney weight was observed after three to four days of STZ-induced diabetes[366,367]; the increase was 90%[367] after 42 days of diabetes. The protein content rose in parallel to the weight. Insulin treatment decreased the renal weight gain by about 67% during the first eight days of diabetes, but not after 25 days.[367] During the first seven days of diabetes the rate of kidney growth was correlated with the blood glucose concentration.[368] The free permeability of the kidney to glucose in the absence of insulin resulted in an approximately 15-fold increase in glucose levels in the kidney of diabetic rats.[457]

That the increases in weight and RNA content in the diabetic rat kidney are correlated with an increased flux of glucose through the hexose monophosphate shunt was demonstrated by Steer et al.[375] Based on the finding of sorbitol and fructose accumulation in diabetic rat kidneys,[457] the authors concluded that in the kidney, as in the lens, an increased flux of glucose through the polyol pathway could "drive" the hexose monophosphate shunt by reoxidation of the NADPH.[375] This concept was amplified by the finding of Sochor et al[378] that in comparison with the immature rat the adult rat responds to diabetes-induced hyperglycemia by increased kidney growth and increased flux of glucose through the hexose monophosphate shunt. Since the activity of the shunt in the kidney depends on the supply of $NADP^+$, and since aldose reductase is the major NADPH-utilizing system in the adult rat kidney that is dependent on high glucose concentrations, it is likely that, as shown originally in the lens,[202] the shunt is also linked to aldose reductase in the diabetic kidney. As the AR activity in the adult rat kidney is approximately two times higher than in the immature rat kidney, the authors suggested that the mechanism of the age-related growth responses in the diabetic kidney stems, in part, from the developmental pattern of aldose reductase.[378]

It is of interest that the renal hypertrophy produced in rats fed on a 50% galactose diet was diminished by adding to the diet the AR inhibitor sorbinil.[458] The cause of renal hypertrophy in galactosemic rats has not been established; it is pertinent, however, that the water intake of rats fed on a diet containing 50% galactose is about seven times higher than that of rats fed on a normal diet. Combined with the decreased body weight gain, galactosemic rats weighing about 70 g excreted 53 mL of urine.[211] Thus, in rats, galactose feeding appears to produce major changes in renal function that may be different from the diabetic state. Of particular interest is the unexpected finding of Kern and Engerman[83] that in dogs fed for five years on a diet containing 30% galactose, in contrast to dogs with five years of alloxan-induced diabetes, the kidney weight, the mesangial volume, and the prevalence of obliterated glomeruli, glomerular exudates, and mesangial nodules were comparable to those observed in age-matched normal dogs. However, as in diabetic dogs, the width of glomerular capillary basement membrane in the galactosemic dogs was significantly greater, i.e., 476 ± 104 nm ($\pm$SD), than in normal animals (316 ± 38 nm), though somewhat thinner than in diabetic dogs (618 ± 65 nm). While dog glomeruli have not been found to contain immunoreactive aldose reductase,[445] the finding in galactosemic dogs raises the possibility that the excessive flux of glucose through the polyol pathway may not be a major factor in the development of nephromegaly, mesangial expansion, and glomerular obliteration in diabetes.[83]

References

1. Grodsky GM, Anderson CE, Coleman DL, et al: Metabolic and underlying causes of diabetes mellitus. *Diabetes* 1982;31(suppl 1):45–53.
2. Mordes JP, Rossini AA: Animal models of diabetes. *Am J Med* 1981;70:353–360.
3. Proceedings of a Task Force on animals appropriate for studying diabetes mellitus and its complications, in Salans LB, Graham BJ (eds): *Diabetes* 1982;31(suppl 1): I–VIII,1–102.
4. The Juvenile Diabetes Workshop on the spontaneously diabetic BB rat: Its potential for insight into human juvenile diabetes. *Metabolism* 1983;32(suppl 1):1–166.
5. Coleman DL: Diabetes-obesity syndromes in mice. *Diabetes* 1982;31(suppl 1):1–6.
6. Coleman DL: Other potentially useful rodents as models for the study of human diabetes mellitus. *Diabetes* 1982;31(suppl 1):24–25.
7. Gerritsen GC: The Chinese hamster as a model for the study of human diabetes mellitus. *Diabetes* 1982;31(suppl 1):14–23.

8. Like AA, Butler L, Williams RM, et al: Spontaneous autoimmune diabetes mellitus in the BB rat. *Diabetes* 1982;31(suppl 1):7–13.
9. Sima AAF: The development and structural characterization of the neuropathies in the spontaneously diabetic BB Wistar rat. *Metabolism* 1983;32(suppl 1):106–111.
10. Engerman RL, Kramer JW: Dogs with induced or spontaneous diabetes as models for the study of human diabetes mellitus. *Diabetes* 1982;31(suppl 1):26–29.
11. Howard CF Jr: Nonhuman primates as models for the study of human diabetes mellitus. *Diabetes* 1982;31(suppl 1):37–42.
12. Rerup CC: Drugs producing diabetes through damage of the insulin secreting cells. *Pharmacol Rev* 1970;22:485–518.
13. Dunn JS, Sheehan HL, McLetchie NGB: Necrosis of islets of Langerhans produced experimentally. *Lancet* 1943;1:484–487.
14. Von Mering J, Minkowski O: Diabetes nach Pancreasextirpation. *Z Klin Med* 1889;10:393–394.
15. Young FG: Permanent experimental diabetes produced by pituitary (anterior lobe) injections. *Lancet* 1937;2:372–374.
16. Boquist L: The endocrine pancreas in early alloxan diabetes. *Acta Path Microbiol Scand*, 1977;85(Sect A):219–229.
17. Bhattacharya G: Protection against diabetes by mannose and fructose. *Science* 1953;117:230–231.
18. Rossini AA, Arcangeli MA, Cahill GF Jr: Studies on alloxan toxicity on the beta cell. *Diabetes* 1975;24:516–522.
19. Malaisse WJ: Alloxan toxicity to the pancreatic cell. A new hypothesis. *Biochem Pharmacol* 1982;31:3527–3534.
20. Heikkila RE: The prevention of alloxan-induced diabetes in mice by dimethyl sulfoxide. *Eur J Pharmacol* 1977;44:191–193.
21. Heikkila RE, Cabbot FS: Protection against alloxan-induced diabetes in mice by the hydroxyl radical scavenger dimethylurea. *Eur J Pharmacol* 1978;52:57–60.
22. Heikkila RE, Winston B, Cohen G, Barden H: Alloxan-induced diabetes-evidence for hydroxyl radical as a cytotoxic intermediate. *Biochem Pharmacol* 1976;25: 1085–1092.
23. Cowden WB, Lewis-Hughes PH, Clark IA: Protection against alloxan-induced diabetes in mice by the free radical scavenger butylated hydroxyanisole. *Biochem Pharmacol* 1985;34:3601–3603.
24. Sakurai K, Miura T, Ogiso T: Studies on biological damage by active oxygen. I. Protective effect of various hydroxyl radical scavengers against alloxan-induced diabetes. *Yakugaku Zasshi* 1986;106:1034–1039.
25. Hatchell DL, Reiser HJ, Bresnahan JF, Whitworth UG Jr: Resistance of cats to the diabetogenic effect of alloxan. *Lab Animal Sci* 1986;36:37–39.
26. Orskov H, Olsen TS, Nielson K, Rafaelsen OJ, Lundbaek K: Kidney lesions in rats with severe long-term alloxan diabetes . I. Influence of age, alloxan damage, and insulin administration. *Diabetologia* 1965;1:172–179.
27. Lazarow A, Palay SL: The production and course of alloxan diabetes in the rat. *J Lab Clin Med* 1946;31:1004–1015.
28. Curtis GW, Robbins SL, Glickman I: Studies on glycogen nephrosis in alloxan-treated diabetic rats. *J Exp Med* 1947;85:373–379.
29. Herr RR, Eble TE, Bergy ME, Jahnke HK: Isolation and characterization of streptozotocin. *Antiobiot Ann* 1959–1960;236–240.
30. Rakieten N, Rakieten MC, Nadkarni MV: Studies on the diabetogenic action of streptozotocin (NSC-37,917). *Cancer Chemother Rep* 1963;29:91–98.

31. Herr RR, Jahnke HK, Argoudelis AD: The structure of streptozotocin. *J Am Chem Soc* 1967;89:4808–4809.
32. Karunanayake EH, Baker JR, Christian AA, Hearse DJ, Mellows G: Autoradiographic study of the distribution and cellular uptake of [^{14}C]-streptozotocin in the rat. *Diabetologia* 1976;12:123–128.
33. Gralla RJ, Tan CTC, Young CW: Phase I trial of chlorozotocin. *Cancer Treat Rep* 1979;63:17–20.
34. Mossman BT, Wilson GL, Craigherd JE; Chlorozocin. A diabetogenic analogue of streptozocin with dissimilar mechanisms of action on pancreatic beta cells. *Diabetes* 1985;34:602–610.
35. Schein PS, Loftus S: Streptozotocin: Depression of mouse liver pyridine nucleotides. *Cancer Res* 1968;28:1501–1506.
36. Brosky G, Logothetopoulos J: Streptozotocin diabetes in the mouse and guinea pig. *Diabetes* 1969;18:606–611.
37. Junod A, Lambert AE, Orci L, et al: Studies of the diabetogenic action of streptozotocin. *Proc Soc Exp Biol Med* 1967;126:201–205.
38. Schein PS, Bates RW: Plasma glucose levels in normal and adrenalectomized mice treated with streptozotocin and nicotinamide. *Diabetes* 1968;17:760–765.
39. Dulin WE, Wyse BW: Studies on the ability of compounds to block the diabetogenic activity of streptozotocin. *Diabetes* 1969:18:459–466.
40. Whish WJD, Davies MI, Shall S: Stimulation of poly (ADP-ribose) polymerase activity by the anti-tumor antibiotic, streptozotocin. *Biochem Biophys Res Comm* 1975;65:722–730.
41. Bolaffi JC, Nagamatsu S, Grodsky GM: Thymidine, a novel inhibitor of streptozotocin damage to the B cell. *Diabetes* 1985;34(suppl 1):9A.
42. Masiello P, Locci-Cubeddu T, Frossina G, Bergamini E: Protective effect of 3-aminobenzamide, an inhibitor of poly(ADP-ribose) synthetase, against streptozotocin-induced diabetes. *Diabetologia* 1985;28:683–686.
43. Preston AM: Modification of streptozotocin-induced diabetes by protective agents. *Nutr Res* 1985;5:435–446.
44. Gold G, Manning M, Heldt A, et al: Diabetes induced with multiple subdiabetogenic doses of streptozotocin: Lack of protection by exogenous superoxide dismutase. *Diabetes* 1981;30:634–638.
45. Rossini AA, Williams RM, Appel MC, Like AA: Sex differences in the multiple-dose streptozotocin model of diabetes. *Endocrinology* 1978;103:1518–1520.
46. Maclaren NK, Neufeld M, McLaughlin JV, Taylor G: Androgen sensitization of streptozotocin-induced diabetes in mice. *Diabetes* 1980;29:710–716.
47. Paik SG, Michelis MA, Kim YT, Shin S: Induction of insulin-dependent diabetes by streptozotocin. *Diabetes* 1982:31:724–729.
48. Goodman MN, Hazelwood RL: Short-term effects of oestradiol benzoate in normal, hypophysectomized and alloxan-diabetic male rats. *J Endocrinol* 1974;62:439–449 and references cited.
49. Skett P, Cochrane RA, Joels LA: The role of androgens in the effect of diabetes mellitus on hepatic drug metabolism in the male rat. *Acta Endocrinol* 1984;107:506–512.
50. Pagliara AS, Stillings SN, Hover B, Martin DM, Matschinsky FM: Glucose modulation of amino acid-induced glucagon and insulin release in the isolated perfused rat pancreas. *J Clin Invest* 1974;54:819–832.
51. Gerich JE, Charles MA, Grodsky GM: Characterization of the effects of arginine and glucose on glucagon and insulin release from the in vitro perfused rat pancreas. *J Clin Invest* 1974;54:833–841.

52. Weinstein S, Gertner SB: The neurological and metabolic effects of streptozotocin in the cat. *Pharmacol* 1971;6:129–136.
53. Gabel H, Bitter-Suermann H, Henriksson C, et al: Streptozotocin diabetes in juvenile pigs. Evaluation of an experimental model. *Horm Metab Res* 1985;17:275–280
54. Abramovici Y, Agarwal MK: Prolonged refractoriness to the diabetogenic action of streptozotocin in mice. *Biochem Med* 1985;34:259–266.
55. Bonner-Weir S, Trent DF, Honey RN, Weir GC: Streptozotocin diabetes in neonatal rats: Recovery and subsequent deterioration. *Diabetes* 1979;28:383.
56. Like AA, Rossini AA: Streptozotocin-induced pancreatic insulitis: New model of diabetes mellitus. *Science* 1976;193:415–417.
57. Riley WJ, McConnell TJ, Maclaren NK, McLaughlin JV, Taylor G: The diabetogenic effects of streptozotocin in mice are prolonged and inversely related to age. *Diabetes* 1981;30:718–723.
58. Whiting PH, Middleton B, Thomas N, Hawthorne J: Studies on a stable, mild diabetes induced by streptozotocin in rats. *Br J Exp Path* 1982;63:408–413.
59. Iwase M, Kikuchi M, Nunoi K, et al: A new model of type 2 (non-insulin-dependent) diabetes mellitus in spontaneously hypertensive rats: diabetes induced by neonatal streptozotocin treatment. *Diabetologia* 1986;29:808–811.
60. Chatamra K, Daniel PM, Kendall MD, Lam DKC: Atrophy of the thymus in rats rendered diabetic by streptozotocin. *Horm Metab Res* 1985;17:630–632.
61. Wellhausen SR: Definition of streptozocin toxicity for primary lymphoidal tissues. *Diabetes* 1986;35:1404–1411.
62. Sandler S, Swenne I: Streptozotocin, but not alloxan induces DNA repair synthesis in mouse pancreatic islets in vitro. *Diabetologia* 1983;25:444–447.
63. Cooperstein SJ, Lazarow A: Distribution of alloxan C^{14} in islet and other tissues of the toadfish (*Opsanus tau*). *Am J Physiol* 1964;207:423–430.
64. Sandler S, Janson L: Vascular permeability of pancreatic islets after administration of streptozotocin. *Virchows Arch Path Anat* 1985;407:359–367.
65. Jansson L, Sandler S: Alloxan-induced diabetes in the mouse: Time course of pancreatic B-cell destruction as reflected in an increased islet vascular permeability. *Virchows Arch Path Anat* 1986;410:17–21.
66. Phillips FS, Sternberg SS, Schwartz HS, et al: Hydroxyurea. Acute cell death in proliferating tissues in rats. *Cancer Res* 1967;27:61–67.
67. Hoftiezer V, Carpenter AM: Comparison of streptozotocin and alloxan-induced diabetes in the rat, including volumetric quantitation of the pancreatic islets. *Diabetologia* 1973;9:178–184.
68. Rerup C, Tarding F: Streptozotocin- and alloxan-diabetes in mice. *Eur J Pharmacol* 1969;7:89–96.
69. Arison RN, Ciaccio EI, Glitzer MS, Cassaro JA, Pruss MP: Light and electron microscopy of lesions in rats rendered diabetic with streptozotocin. *Diabetes* 1967;16:51–56.
70. Evan AP, Mong SA, Gattone VH, et al: The effect of streptozotocin and streptozotocin-induced diabetes on the kidney. *Renal Physiol* 1984;7:78–89.
71. Jensen PK, Christiansen JS, Steven K, Parving HH: Strict metabolic control and renal function in streptozotocin diabetic rat. *Kidney Int* 1987;31:47–51.
72. Levine BS, Henry MC, Port CD, Rosen E: Toxicologic evaluation of streptozotocin (NSC 85998) in mice, dogs and monkeys. *Drug Chem Toxicol* 1980;3:201–212.
73. Mansford KRL, Opie L: Comparison of metabolic abnormalites in diabetes mellitus induced by streptozotocin or by alloxan. *Lancet* 1968;1:670–671.

74. Palmano KP, Whiting PH, Hawthorne JN: Free and lipid myo-inositol in tissues from rats with acute and less severe streptozotocin-induced diabetes. *Biochem J* 1977;167:229–235.
75. Miethke H, Wittig B, Nath A, Jungermann K: Gluconeogenic-glycolytic capacities and metabolic zonation in liver of rats with streptozotocin, non-ketotic as compared to alloxan, ketotic diabetes. *Histochemistry* 1986;85:483–489.
76. Carter WJ, Younathan ES: Studies on protection against the diabetogenic effect of alloxan by glucose. *Proc Soc Exp Biol Med* 1962;109:611–612.
77. Scheynius A, Taljedal IB: On the mechanism of glucose protection against alloxan toxicity. *Diabetologia* 1971;7:252–255.
78. Zawalich WS, Beidler LM: Glucose and alloxan interactions in the pancreatic islets. *Am J Physiol* 1973;224:963–966.
79. Ganda OP, Rossini AA, Like AM: Studies on streptozotocin diabetes. *Diabetes* 1976;25:595–603.
80. Rossini AA, Cahill GJ Jr, Jeanloz DA, Jeanloz RW: Anomeric specificity of a 3-O-methyl-D-glucopyranose against alloxan diabetes. *Science* 1975;188:70–71.
81. Brown MR, Dyck PJ, McClearn GE, et al: Central and peripheral nervous system complications. *Diabetes* 1982;31(suppl 1):65–70.
82. Engerman RL, Kern TS: Experimental galactosemia produces diabetic-like retinopathy. *Diabetes* 1984;33:97–100.
83. Kern TS, Engerman RL: Kidney morphology in experimental hyperglycemia. *Diabetes* 1987:36:244–249.
84. Williams CA, MacDonald I: Metabolic effects of dietary galactose. *Wld Rev Nutr Diet* 1982;39:23–52, and references cited.
85. Cori CF: The fate of sugar in the animal body. I. The rate of absorption of hexoses and pentoses from the intestinal tract. *J Biol Chem* 1925;66:691–715.
86. Riklis E, Quastel JH: Effects of cations on sugar absorption by isolated surviving guinea pig intestine. *Can J Biochem Physiol* 1959;36:347–362.
87. Csaky TZ, Thale M: Effect of ionic environment on the intestinal sugar transport. *J Physiol* 1960;151:59–65.
88. Crane RK: Intestinal absorption of sugars. *Physiol Rev* 1960;40:789–825.
89. Harding LJ, Grant GA, Glaister D: Metabolism of galactose. II. The behavior of rat towards moderate amounts of galactose. *Biochem J* 1934;28:257–264.
90. Newstead GC: Serum carbohydrate levels following galactose and galactose plus glucose given to rats. *Proc Nutr Soc* 1979;38:38A.
91. Mitchell HS, Merriam OA, Cook GM: The relation of ingested carbohydrate to the type and amount of blood urine sugar and to the incidence of cataract in rats. *J Nutr* 1937;13:501–511.
92. Poiffait A, David C, Adrian J: L'absorption intestinale du glucose, et du galactose chez le rat, mesuree par les hexosemies. *Intl J Vit Nutr Res* 1982:52:90–95.
93. Dvornik D, Millen J, Hicks D, Cayen M, Sredy J: The pharmacokinetics of aldose reductase inhibitors. Presented at the Intl Symposium on polyol pathway and its role in diabetic complications, Oct 1980, Kashikojima, Japan.
94. Day PL: Blood sugar in rats rendered cataractous by dietary procedures. *J Nutr* 1936;12:395–404.
95. Millen J, et al: Unpublished results from the Ayerst Research Laboratories.
96. Goresky CA, Bach GC, Nadeau BE: On the uptake of materials by the intact liver. The transport and net removal of galactose. *J Clin Invest* 1973;52:991–1009.
97. Henderson JM, Hanna SS: Effective liver blood flow: Determination by galactose clearance. *Can J Surg* 1983;26:129–132.

98. Keiding S: Galactose elimination capacity in the rat. *Scand J Clin Lab Invest* 1973;31:319–325.
99. Cryer A, Bartley W: Adaptation of rats to a diet high in galactose. *Int J Biochem* 1973;4:385–392.
100. Locatto ME, Fernandez MC, Puche RC: The hyperglycemia of experimental galactosemia. *Medicina* 1975;35:499–504.
101. Poiffait A, David C, Adrian J: Repercussions chez le rat d'une consommation prolongée de lactose ou de lactose hydrolysé. 2. Digestibilité, rétention et utilisation des constituants du lactose. *Intl J Vit Nutr Res* 1982;52:96–101.
102. Mangeot M, Djabal A, Myara I, Cherruau B, Lemonnier A: Surcharge expérimentale en galactose: études métaboliques in vivo chez le rat adulte. *Diab Métab* 1986;12:115–116.
103. Robison WG, Kador PF, Akagi Y, et al: Prevention of basement membrane thickening in retinal capillaries by a novel inhibitor of aldose reductase, tolrestat. *Diabetes* 1986;35:295–299.
104. Stewart MA, Sherman WR, Kurien MM, Moonsammy GI, Wisgerhof M: Polyol accumulations in nervous tissue of rats with experimental diabetes and galactosemia. *J Neurochem* 1967;14:1057–1066.
105. Giroix MH, Mallaisse-Lagae F, Sener A, Malaisse WJ: Hexose metabolism in pancreatic islets. Galactose transport phosphorylation and oxidation. *Mol Cell Biochem* 1985;66:61–64.
106. McCaleb, M, et al: Unpublished results from the Ayerst Research Laboratories.
107. Gjedde A: Blood-brain transfer of galactose in experimental galactosemia, with special reference to the competitive interaction between galactose and glucose. *J Neurochem* 1984;43:1654–1662.
108. Daniel PM, Love ER, Pratt OE: Inhibition of glucose transport into the brains of suckling rats by raising the level of galactose in the blood. *J Physiol* 1980; 305:44P–45P.
109. Leloir LF: The enzymatic transformation of uridine diphosphate glucose into a galactose derivative. *Arch Biochem Biophys* 1951;33:186–190.
110. Van Heyningen R: Formation of polyols by the lens in the rat with "sugar" cataracts. *Nature* 1959;184:194–195.
111. Wells WW, Pittman TA, Egan TJ: The isolation and identification of galactitol from the urine of patients with galactosemia. *J Biol Chem* 1964;239:3192–3195.
112. Egan TJ, Wells WW: Alternate metabolic pathway in galactosemia. *Am J Dis Child* 1966;111:400–405.
113. Pirie A, Van Heyningen R: The effect of diabetes on the content of sorbitol, glucose, fructose and inositol in the human lens. *Exp Eye Res* 1964;3:124–131.
114. Williamson JR, Chang K, Jeffrey JR, et al: Sex steroid modulation of diabetes-induced increases in lens polyol content. *Invest Ophthalmol Vis Sci* 1986;27(suppl):136.
115. Quan-Ma R, Wells WW: The distribution of galactitol in tissues of rats fed galactose. *Biochem Biophys Res Comm* 1965;20:486–490.
116. Wells WW, Chin T, Weber B: Quantitative analysis of serum and urine sugars by gas chromatography. *Clin Chim Acta* 1964;10:352–359.
117. Lefevre PG, Davies RI: Active transport into the human erythrocyte: Evidence from comparative kinetics and competition among monosaccharides. *J Gen Physiol* 1951;34:515–524.
118. Wick AN, Drury DR: Action of insulin on the permeability of cells to sorbitol. *Am J Physiol* 1951;166:421–423.
119. Stewart MA, Kurien MM, Sherman WR, Cotlier EU: Inositol changes in nerve and lens of galactose fed rats. *J Neurochem* 1968;15:941–946.

120. Stewart MA, Sherman WR, Kurien MM, Moonsammy GI, Wisgerhof M: Polyol accumulations in nervous tissue of rats with experimental diabetes and galactosemia. *J Neurochem* 1967;14:1057–1066.
121. Sigal H, Berry G, Yandrasitz J, Segal S: Absence of hepatic myo-inositol depletion in galactosemic rats. *Clin Res* 1986;34:554.
122. Mellinkoff S, Roth B, MacLaggan J: Galactosemia with hepatic damage. *J Pediatr* 1945;27:338–342.
123. Bruck E, Rapoport S: Galactosemia in an infant with cataracts. Clinical observations and carbohydrate studies. *Am J Dis Child* 1945;70:267–276.
124. Beutler E: Wyngaarden JB, Smith LH Jr (eds): *Textbook of Medicine,* ed 17. W B Saunders Co, 1985, vol 1, p 1104.
125. Simonelli F, DeRosa G, Rinaldi E, Auricchio L: Possible role of galactose-1-P-uridyl transferase activity deficiency in red blood cells in the development of the presenile and senile cataract. *Ophthalmol Res* 1986;18:309–312.
126. Van Heyningen R: Galactose cataract: A review. *Exp Eye Res* 1971;11:415–428.
127. Beutler E, Matsumoto F, Kuhl W, et al: Galactokinase deficiency as a cause of cataracts. *N Engl J Med* 1973;288:1203–1206.
128. Cohn RM, Segal S: Galactose metabolism and its regulation. *Metabolism* 1973;22:627–642.
129. Cori CF, Cori GT: Carbohydrate metabolism. *Ann Rev Biochem* 1934;3:151–174.
130. Tygstrup N, Schmidt A, Thieden HID: The galactose utilization rate in liver slices from man and rat and its relation to the lactate/pyruvate ratio of the medium. *Scand J Clin Lab Invest* 1971;28:27–31.
131. Wells WW, Pittman TA, Wells HJ, Egan TJ: The isolation of galactitol from the brains of galactosemia patients. *J Biol Chem* 1965;240:1002–1004.
132. Quan-Ma R, Wells HJ, Wells WW, Sherman FE, Egan TJ: Galactitol in the tissues of a galactosemic child. *Am J Dis Child* 1966;112:477–478.
133. Gitzelmann R, Curtius H, Schneller I: Galactitol and galactose-1-phosphate in the lens of a galactosemic infant. *Exp Eye Res* 1967;6:1–3.
134. Kalckar HM, Kinoshita JH, Donnell GN: Galactosemia: Biochemistry, genetics, pathophysiology, and developmental aspects. *Biol Brain Dysfunction* 1973;1:31–88.
135. Gray GM, Ingelfinger FJ: Intestinal absorption of sucrose in man: Interrelation of hydrolysis and monosaccharide product absorption. *J Clin Invest* 1966;45:388–398.
136. Craig JW, Drucker WR, Miller M, et al: Metabolism of fructose by the liver of diabetic and non-diabetic subjects. *Proc Soc Exp Biol Med* 1951;78:698–702.
137. Cahill GF Jr, Ashmore J, Earle AS, Zottu S: Glucose penetration into liver. *Am J Physiol* 1958;192:491–496.
138. Adelman RC, Ballard FJ, Weinhouse S: Purification and properties of rat liver fructokinase. *J Biol Chem* 1967;242:3360–3365.
139. Koivisto VA: Fructose as a dietary sweetener in diabetes mellitus. *Diabetes Care* 1978;1:241–246 and references cited.
140. Froesch ER: Disorders of fructose metabolism. *Clin Endocrinol Metab* 1976;5:599–611.
141. Froesch ER: Fructose metabolism in adipose tissue. *Acta Med Scand* 1972;542(suppl):37–46.
142. Cohen AM, Teitelbaum A: Effect of dietary sucrose and starch on oral glucose tolerance and insulin-like activity. *Am J Physiol* 1964;206:105–108.
143. Cohen AM, Teitelbaum A: Effect of different levels of protein in "sucrose" and "starch" diets on the glucose tolerance and growth. *Metabolism* 1966;15:1034–1038.
144. Cohen AM, Rosenmann E: Diffuse intercapillary glomerulosclerosis in sucrose-fed rats. *Diabetologia* 1971;7:25–28.

145. Rosenmann E, Teitelbaum A, Cohen AM: Nephropathy in sucrose-fed rats. Electron and light microscopic studies. *Diabetes* 1971;20:802–810.
146. Taylor SA, Price RG, Kang SS, Yudkin J: Modification of the glomerular basement membrane in sucrose-fed and streptozotocin-diabetic rats. *Diabetologia* 1980;19: 364–372.
147. Kang SS, Price RG, Bruckdorfer KR, Worcester NA, Yudkin J: Dietary induced renal damage in the rat. *Proc Nutr Soc* 1976;36:27A.
148. Rosenmann E, Cohen AM: Nephropathy in Cohen's diabetic rat, in Shafrir E, Renold AE (eds): *Lessons from animal diabetes.* London, Libbey, 1984, pp 398–401.
149. Rosenmann E, Yanko L, Cohen AM: Female sex hormone and nephropathy in Cohen diabetic rat (genetically selected fructose-fed). *Horm Metab Res* 1984;16:11–16.
150. Cohen AM, Rosenmann E: Effect of the estrogen antagonist, tamoxifen, on development of glomerulosclerosis in the Cohen diabetic rat. *Diabetes* 1985;34:634–638.
151. Cohen AM, Teitelbaum A, Saliternik R: Genetics and diet as factors in development of diabetes mellitus. *Metabolism* 1972;21:235–240.
152. Rosenmann E, Yanko L, Cohen AM: Comparative study of the pathology of sucrose-induced diabetes in the rat and adult-on set diabetes in man. *Isr J Med Sci* 1975;11:753–761.
153. Yanko L, Rosenmann E, Cohen AM: A correlative study on the occurrence of retinopathy and nephropathy in sucrose-fed diabetic rats. *Acta Diabet Lat* 1975;12: 52–65.
154. Papachristodoulou D, Heath H, Kang SS: The development of retinopathy in sucrose-fed and streptozotocin-diabetic rats. *Diabetologia* 1976;12:367–374.
155. Heath H, Hamlett YC: The sorbitol pathway: Effect of streptozotocin induced diabetes and the feeding of a sucrose-rich diet on glucose, sorbitol and fructose in the retina, blood and liver of rats. *Diabetologia* 1976;12:43–46.
156. Ludvigson MA, Sorenson RL: Immunohistochemical localization of aldose reductase. II. Rat and kidney. *Diabetes* 1980;29:450–459.
157. Hutton JC, Schofield PJ, Williams JF, Hollows FC: Sorbitol metabolism in the retina: Accumulation of pathway intermediates in streptozotocin-induced diabetes in the rat. *Austr J Exp Biol Med Sci* 1974;52(pt 2):361–373.
158. Pocknee RC, Kohner EM, Dollery CT: The effect of hyperglycemia on glucose and sorbitol concentration in normal and diabetic rat retina. *Eur J Clin Invest* 1977;7:244.
159. Papachristodoulou D, Heath H: Ultrastructural alterations during the development of retinopathy in sucrose-fed and streptozotocin-diabetic rats. *Exp Eye Res* 1977; 25:371–384.
160. Yanko L, Cohen AM: Retinal vascular changes in Cohen diabetic rats, in Sharfir E, Renold AE (eds): *Lessons from animal diabetes.* London, Libbey, 1984, pp 508–512.
161. Kojima K, Suzuki M, Harada T, et al: Experimentally induced diabetic microangiopathy and the polyol pathway. 1st Report: Influence of fructose on the development of microangiopathy. *Folia Ophthalmol Jpn* 1984;35:749–759.
162. Boot-Handford R, Heath H: Identification of fructose as the retinopathic agent associated with the ingestion of sucrose-rich diets in the rat. *Metabolism* 1980;29:1247–1252.
163. Boot-Handford RP, Heath H: The effect of dietary fructose and diabetes on the rat kidney. *Br J Exp Path* 1981;62:398–406.
164. Bellomo G, Comstock JP, Adamo ML, Wen X, Hazelwood RL: Effects of fructose feeding on the polyol pathway in the rat kidney. *Diabetologia* 1986;29:516A.
165. Engerman R, Finkelstein D, Aguirre G, et al: Ocular complications. *Diabetes* 1982;31(suppl 1):82–88.

166. Fukushi S, Merola LO, Tanaka M, Datiles M, Kinoshita JH: Re-epithelialization of denuded corneas in diabetic rats. *Exp Eye Res* 1980;31:611–621.
167. Datiles MB, Kador PF, Fukui HN, Hu TS, Kinoshita JH: Corneal re-epithelialization in galactosemic rats. *Invest Ophthalmol Vis Sci* 1983;24:563–569.
168. Kinoshita JH, Fukushi S, Kador P, Merola LO: Aldose reductase in diabetic complications of the eye. *Metabolism* 1979;28(suppl 1):462–469.
169. Cobo M: Aldose reductase and diabetic keratopathy, pp 87–99 in Cogan DG, moderator: Aldose reductase and complications of diabetes. *Ann Intern Med* 1984;101:82–91.
170. Friend J, Kiorpes T, Thoft RA: Metabolic effects of diabetes mellitus on rabbit corneal epithelium. *Invest Ophthalmol Vis Sci* 1980;19(suppl):75.
171. Schultz RO, Matsuda M, Yee RW, Edelhauser HF, Schultz KJ: Corneal endothelial changes in type I and type II diabetes mellitus. *Am J Ophthalmol* 1984;98:401-410.
172. Yee RW, Matsuda M, Kern TS, Engerman RL, Edelhauser HF: Corneal changes in diabetic dogs. *Curr Eye Res* 1985;4:759–766.
173. Kinoshita JH, Kador P, Datiles M: Aldose reductase in diabetic cataracts. *JAMA* 1981;246:257–261.
174. Mitchell HS, Dodge WM: Cataract in rats fed on high lactose rations. *J Nutr* 1935;9:37–49.
175. Mitchell HS, Dodge WM: Nutritional cataract in rats. *J Biol Chem* 1934;105:61–62.
176. Mitchell HS: Cataract in rats fed on galactose. *Proc Soc* 1935;32:971–973.
177. Yudkin AM, Arnold CH: Cataract formation in rats fed on a diet containing galactose. *Proc Soc Exp Biol Med* 1935;32:836–837.
178. Sasaki T: Untersuchungen der Linse, des Blutes und des Kammerwassers von Ratten bei Galaktoseverfutterung. I. Klinische Beobachtungen bei Galaktosekatarakt. *Graefe's Arch Ophthalmol* 1938;138:351–364.
179. Mitchell HS, Cook GM: Galactose cataract in rats. *Arch Ophthalmol* 1938;19:22–33.
180. Patterson JW: Effects of galactosemia. *Anat Record* 1960;138:395–398.
181. Patterson JW, Patterson ME, Kinsey VE, Reddy DVN: Lens assays on diabetic and galactosemic rats receiving diets that modify cataract development. *Invest Ophthalmol* 1965;4:98–103.
182. Patterson JW: Effect of blood supply on the development of cataracts. *Am J Physiol* 1955;180:495–497.
183. Lerman S: The lens in human and experimental galactosemia. *NY State J Med* 1962;62:785.
184. Kinoshita JH: Cataracts in galactosemia. *Invest Ophthalmol* 1965;4:786–799.
185. Lerman S: Carbohydrate metabolism in the rat lens as related to the age of the animal. *Arch Ophthalmol* 1961;65:181–183.
186. Patterson JW: Hyperglycemia and galactose cataracts. *Am J Physiol* 1954;177:541–543.
187. Keiding S, Mellemgaard L: Dose dependence of galactose cataract in the rat. *Acta Ophthalmol* 1972;50:174–182.
188. Tygstrup N, Lundquist F: The effect of ethanol on galactose elimination in man. *J Lab Clin Med* 1962;59:102–109.
189. Ribaya-Mercado JD, Gershoff SN: Effects of magnesium on galactose-induced cataract formation and lens aldose reductase activity in rats. *Nutr Res* 1986;6:699–708.
190. Simard-Duquesne N, Greselin E, Gonzalez R, Dvornik D: Prevention of cataract development in severely galactosemic rats by the aldose reductase inhibitor, tolrestat. *Proc Soc Exp Biol Med* 1985;178:599–605.
191. Simard-Duquesne N, Dvornik D: Galactitol accumulation and irreversible lens opacities in galactosemic rats. *Invest Ophthalmol* 1973;12:82–83.

192. Cotlier E: Hypophysectomy effect on lens epithelium and galactose cataract development in rats. *Arch Ophthalmol* 1962;67:476–482.
193. Sippel TO: Change in the water, protein, and glutathion contents in the lens in the course of galactose cataract development in rats. *Invest Ophthalmol* 1966;5:568–575.
194. Kinoshita JH, Merola LO, Satoh K, Dikmak E: Osmotic changes caused by the accumulation of dulcitol in the lenses of rats fed with galactose. *Nature* 1962;194: 1085–1087.
195. Kinoshita JH, Merola LO, Dikmak E: Osmotic changes in experimental galactose cataracts. *Exp Eye Res* 1962;1:405–410.
196. Reddy VN, Schwass D, Chakrapani B, Lim CP: Biochemical changes associated with development and reversal of galactose cataracts. *Exp Eye Res* 1976;23:483–493.
197. Hu T, Datiles M, Kinoshita JH: Reversal of galactose cataract with sorbinil in rats. *Invest Ophthalmol Vis Sci* 1983;34:640–644.
198. Beyer-Mears A, Cruz E, Varagiannis E: Reversal of Stage I sugar cataract by sorbinil, an aldose reductase inhibitor. *Pharmacology* 1985;31:88–96.
199. Okuda J, Yashima K, Inagaki K, Miwa I: Effects of an aldose reductase inhibitor, 1-[(p-bromophenyl)-sulfonyl]hydantoin, on cataract formation and tissue polyol levels in galactosemic rats. *Chem Pharm Bull* 1985;33:2990–2995.
200. Kinoshita JH, Merola LO: Hydration of the lens during the development of galactose cataract. *Invest Ophthalmol* 1964;3:577–584.
201. Patterson JW, Bunting KW: Changes associated with the appearance of mature sugar cataracts. *Invest Ophthalmol* 1965;4:167–173.
202. Kinoshita JH, Futterman S, Satoh K, Merola LO: Factors affecting the formation of sugar alcohols in ocular lens. *Biochim Biophys Acta* 1963;74:340–350.
203. Smith MG: Polyol dehydrogenases. 4. Crystallization of the L-iditol dehydrogenase of sheep liver. *Biochem J* 1962;83:135–144.
204. Eklund H, Horjales E, Jornvall H, Branden CI, Jeffery J: Molecular aspects of functional differences between alcohol and sorbitol dehydrogenases. *Biochemistry* 1985;24:8005–8012.
205. Sasaki T: Untersuchungen der Linse, des Blutes und des Kammerwassers von Ratten bei Galaktoseverfütterung. II. Mitt Uber die Linsenkapselpermeabilität und über den Zuckergehalt von Blut, Kammerwasser und Linse bei der Galaktose-Katarakt. *Graefe's Arch Ophthalmol* 1938;138:365–379.
206. Patterson JW, Bunting KW: Lens cell permeability and cataract formation. *Proc Soc Exp Biol Med* 1964;115: 1156–1158.
207. Fournier DJ, Patterson JW: Lens regeneration after mature galactose cataract formation. *Proc Soc Exp Biol Med* 1970;135:377–379.
208. Parmar NS, Ghosh MN: Effect of gossypin, a flavonoid, on the formation of galactose-induced cataracts in rats. *Exp Eye Res* 1979;29:229–232.
209. Hu T, Merola LO, Kuwabara T, Kinoshita JH: Prevention and reversal of galactose cataract in rats with topical sorbinil. *Invest Ophthalmol Vis Sci* 1984;25:603–605.
210. Beyer-Mears A, Cruz E, Nicolas-Alexandre J: Sorbinil effect on sugar cataract progression and recovery. An initial study. *Invest Ophthalmol Vis Sci* 1982;21:154.
211. Bakker A: Zur Pathogenese der Galaktosekatarakt. *Graefe's Arch Ophthalmol* 1939;140:531–542.
212. Willoughby Cashell GT, Kon SK: Diseases of the lens. 1. Studies in lactose and galactose cataracts in rats. *Trans Ophthalmol* Soc 1939;59:199–218.
213. Patterson JW, Patterson ME: Point of irreversibility of galactose cataracts in the rat. *Proc Soc Exp Biol Med* 1965;118:324–326.
214. Unakar NJ, Genyea C, Reddan JR, Reddy VN: Ultra-structural changes during the development and reversal of galactose cataracts. *Exp Eye Res* 1978;26:123–133.

215. Gifford SR, Bellows J: Histologic changes in the lens produced by galactose. *Arch Ophthalmol* 1979;21:346–358.
216. Unakar NJ, Tsui J: Sodium-potassium-dependent ATP-ase. II. Cytochemical localization during the reversal of galactose cataract in rats. *Invest Ophthalmol Vis Sci* 1980;9:378–385.
217. Beyer-Mears A, Farnsworth PN: Regional analyses of the opaque galactose cataract and the reversal process. *Metab Pediatr Ophthalmol* 1980;4:9–14.
218. Unakar NJ, Price G, Tsui J: Acid phosphatase I. Cyto-chemical localization in lenses of normal and galactose-fed rats. *Ophthalmol Res* 1982;14:83–97.
219. Price G, Tsui J, Unakar NJ: Arylsulfatase in normal and cataractous lens. *Micron* 1982;13:471–472.
220. Gorthy W: Cataracts in the aging rat lens. Morphological and acid phosphatase histochemistry of incipient forms. *Exp Eye Res* 1978;27:301–322.
221. Harries W, Tsui J, Unakar NJ: Ultrastructural cyto-chemistry: Effect of sorbinil on arylsulfatases in cataractous lenses. *Curr Eye Res* 1985;4:657–666.
222. Chaikoff IL, Lachman GS: Occurrence of cataract in experimental pancreatic diabetes. *Proc Soc Exp Biol Med* 1933;31:237–241.
223. Dohan FC, Fish CA, Lukens FDW: Induction and course of permanent diabetes produced by anterior pituitary extract. *Endocrinology* 1941;28:341–357.
224. Foglia VG, Cramer FK: Experimental production of diabetic cataract in the rat. *Proc Soc Exp Biol Med* 1944;55:218–219.
225. Bailey CC, Bailey OT, Leech RS: Alloxan diabetes with diabetic complications. *N Engl J Med* 1944;230:533–536.
226. Charalampous FC, Hegsted DM: Effect of age and diet on development of cataracts in the diabetic rat. *Am J Physiol* 1950;161:540–544.
227. Patterson JW: Course of diabetes and development of cataracts after injecting dehydroascorbic acid and related substances. *Am J Physiol* 1951;165:61.
228. Patterson JW: Development of diabetic cataracts. *Am J Ophthalmol* 1952;35:68–72.
229. Siegel EG, Trapp VE, Wollheim CB, Renold AE, Schmidt FX: Beneficial effects of low-carbohydrate—high-protein diets in long-term diabetic rats. *Metabolism* 1980;29: 421–428.
230. Rodriguez RR, Krehl WA: The influence of diet and insulin on the incidence of cataracts in diabetic rats. *Yale J Biol Med* 1951;24:103–108.
231. Verheyden MC: Cataracte experimentale provoquee par la streptozotocine (NSC-37,917). *Bull Soc Belge Ophthalmol* 1967;147:479–485.
232. Von Sallmann L, Grimes P: Eye changes in streptozotocin diabetes in rats. *Am J Ophthalmol* 1971;71:312–319.
233. Gonzalez AM, Sochor M, McLean P: The effect of an aldose reductase inhibitor (sorbinil) on the level of metabolites in lenses of diabetic rats. *Diabetes* 1983; 32:482–485.
234. Malone JI, Leavengood H, Peterson MJ, et al: Red blood cell sorbitol as an indicator of polyol pathway activity. *Diabetes* 1984;33:45–49.
235. Fukushi S, Merola LO, Kinoshita JH: Altering the course of cataracts in diabetic rats. *Invest Ophthalmol Vis Sci* 1980;19:313–315.
236. Simard-Duquesne N, Greselin E, Dubuc J, Dvornik D: The effect of a new aldose reductase inhibitor (tolrestat) in galactosemic and diabetic rats. *Metabolism* 1985;34: 885–892.
237. Poulsom R, Heath H: Inhibition of aldose reductase in five tissues of the streptozotocin-diabetic rat. *Biochem Pharmacol* 1983;32:1495–1499.

238. Peterson MJ, Sarges R, Aldinger CE, MacDonald DP: CP-45,634: A novel aldose reductase inhibitor that inhibits polyol pathway activity in diabetic and galactosemic rats. *Metabolism* 1979;28(suppl 1):456–470.
239. Beyer-Mears A, Cruz E: Reversal of diabetic cataract by sorbinil, an aldose reductase inhibitor. *Diabetes* 1985;34:15–21.
240. Schmidt FH, Siegel E, Trapp V, Schreiber M: Effects of low-carbohydrate diets in long-term diabetic rats in Shafrir E, Renold AE (eds): *Lessons from animal diabetes.* London, Libbey, 1984, pp 631–636.
241. Lee SM, Schade SZ, Doughty CC: Aldose reductase NADPH and $NADP^+$ in normal galactose-fed and diabetic rat lens. *Biochim Biophys Acta* 1985;841:247–253.
242. Sasaki K, Kuriyama H, Yeh LI, Fukuda M: Studies on diabetic cataract in rats induced by streptozotocin. *Ophthalm Res* 1983;15:185–190.
243. Kuriyama H, Sasaki K, Fukuda M: Studies on diabetic cataract in rats induced by streptozotocin. II. Biochemical examinations of rat lenses in relation to cataract stages. *Ophthalm Res* 1983;15:191–197.
244. Engerman RL: Animal models of diabetic retinopathy. *Trans Am Acad Ophthalmol Otolaryngol* 1976;81:710–715.
245. Musacchio I, Palermo N, Rodriguez R: Microaneurisms in the retina of diabetic rats. *Lancet* 1964;1:146.
246. Toussaint D: Lesions retiniennes au cours de diabete alloxanique chez le rat. *Bull Soc Belge Ophthalmol* 1966;143:648–654.
247. Kojima K: Electron microscopic studies on the retina and choroid in alloxan diabetic rats. *Acta Soc Ophthalmol,* Japan 1971;75:1598–1709.
248. Orloff M, Lee S, Charters A, et al: Long term studies of pancreas transplantation in experimental diabetes mellitus. *Ann Surg* 1975;182:198–205.
249. Heath H, Rutter AC: Retinal angiography in the iminodipropionitrile-treated alloxan diabetic rat. *Br J Exp Pathol* 1966;47:116–120.
250. Leuenberger P, Cameron D, Stauffacher W, Renold A, Babel J: Ocular lesions in rats rendered chronically diabetic with streptozotocin. *Ophthalmol Res* 1971;2:189–204.
251. Leuenberger P, Beachemin ML, Babel J: Experimental diabetic retinopathy. *Arch Ophthalmol,* Paris 1974;34:289–302.
252. Sosula L, Beaumont P, Hollows F, Jonson K: Dilatation and endothelial proliferation of retinal capillaries in streptozotocin-diabetic rats. *Diabetologia* 1972;11:926–935.
253. Hori S, Mukai N: Ultrastructural lesions of retinal pericapillary Müller cells in streptozotocin-induced diabetic rats. *Graefe's Arch Klin Exp Ophthalmol* 1980; 213:1–9.
254. Robison WG, Kador PF, Kinoshita JH: Retinal capillaries: Basement membrane thickening by galactosemia prevented with aldose reductase inhibitor. *Science* 1983;221:1177–1179.
255. Frank RN, Keirn RJ, Kennedy A, Frank KW: Galactose-induced retinal capillary basement membrane thickening: Prevention by sorbinil. *Invest Ophthalmol Vis Sci* 1983;24:1519–1529.
256. Robison WG, Kador PF, Akagi Y, Kinoshita JH: Basement membrane thickening in ocular vessels of galactosemic rats prevented with aldose reductase inhibitors. *Invest Ophthalmol Vis Sci* 1984;25(suppl):66.
257. Patz A, Maumenee AE: Studies on diabetic retinopathy. I. Retinopathy in a dog with spontaneous diabetes mellitus. *Am J Ophthalmol* 1962;54:532–541.
258. Patz A, Berkow J, Maumenee A, Cox J: Studies on diabetic retinopathy. II. Retinopathy and nephropathy in spontaneous canine diabetes. *Diabetes* 1965;14:700–708.
259. Sibay R, Hausler E: Eye findings in two spontaneously diabetic related dogs. *Am J Ophthalmol* 1967;63:289–294.

260. Gepts W, Toussaint D: Spontaneous diabetes in dogs and cats. *Diabetologia* 1967;3:249–265.
261. Engerman R, Bloodworth J: Experimental diabetic retinopathy in dogs. *Arch Ophthalmol* 1965;73:205–210.
262. Hausler H, Sibay T, Campbell J: Retinopathy in a dog following diabetes induced by growth hormone. *Diabetes* 1964;13:122–126.
263. Engerman RL, Davis MD, Bloodworth MB: Retinopathy in experimental diabetes: Its relevance to diabetic retinopathy in man, in Rodriquez R, Vallance-Owen J (eds): *Diabetes.* Amsterdam, Excerpta Medica, 1971, pp 261–267.
264. Engerman R, Bloodworth JM, Nelson S: Relationship of microvascular disease in diabetes to metabolic control. *Diabetes* 1977;26:760–769.
265. Gibbs G, Wilson R, Ho CK: Experimental diabetes in the monkey. *Proc 2nd Intl Congr* Primates. Karger, New York, 1969, vol 3, pp 169–173.
266. Bresnick GH, Engerman R, Davis MD, DeVenecia G, Myers FL: Patterns of ischemia in diabetic retinopathy. *Trans Am Acad Ophthalmol Otolaryngol* 1976;81:694–709.
267. Beaumont P, Schofield PJ, Hollows FC, Williams JF, Steinbeck AW: Growth hormone sorbitol, and diabetic capillary disease. *Lancet* 1971;1:579–581.
268. Gabbay KH, Kinoshita JH: Growth hormone, sorbitol, and diabetic capillary disease. *Lancet* 1971;1:913.
269. Akagi Y, Yajima Y, Kador PF, Kuwabara T, Kinoshita JH: Localization of aldose reductase in the human eye. *Diabetes* 1984;33:562–566.
270. Poulsom R, Heath H: Inhibition of aldose reductase in five tissues of the streptozotocin-diabetic rat. *Biochem Pharmacol* 1983;32:1495–1499.
271. Poulsom R, Mirrlees DJ, Earl DCN, Heath H: The effects of an aldose reductase inhibitor upon the sorbitol pathway, fructose-1-phosphate and lactate in the retina and nerve of streptozotocin-diabetic rats. *Exp Eye Res* 1983;36:751–760.
272. Poulsom R, Boot-Handford RP, Heath H: The effects of long-term treatment of streptozotocin-diabetic rats with an aldose reductase inhibitor. *Exp Eye Res* 1983;37:507–515.
273. Stribling D, Mirrless DJ, Harrison HE, Earl DCN: Properties of ICI 128,436, a novel aldose reductase inhibitor, and its effects on diabetic complications in the rat. *Metabolism* 1985;34:336–344.
274. Engerman RL, Kern TS: Progression of incipient diabetic retinopathy during good glycemic control. *Invest Ophthalmol Vis Sci* 1986;27(suppl):44.
275. Bloodworth JMB Jr, Engerman RL, Powers KL: Experimental diabetic microangiopathy. I. Basement membrane statistics in the dog. *Diabetes* 1969;18:455–458.
276. Engerman RL, Kern TS: Experimental galactosemia produces diabetic-like retinopathy. *Diabetes* 1982;31 (suppl 2):26A.
277. Shanks E, D'Amico DJ, Gragoudas ES: Experimental model of diabetic retinopathy in the rat: Effects of dietary galactose and sorbinil on retinal basement membranes. *Invest Ophthalmol Vis Sci* 1985;26(suppl):28.
278. Dvornik D, Millen J, Kemper C: Prevention by tolrestat of the biochemical and morphological changes in galactose-fed rats. *Diabetes* 1986;35(suppl 1):215A.
279. Robison WG Jr, Kinoshita JH, Kador PF: The polyol pathway in retinal microangiopathy. *Drugs* 1986;32(suppl 2):19–22.
280. MacGregor LC, Matschinsky FM: Treatment with aldose reductase inhibitor or with myo-inositol arrests deterioration of the electroretinogram of diabetic rats. *J Clin Invest* 1985;76:887–889.

281. Vinores SA, Campochiaro PA, May E, Blaydes S, Williams ER: Hyperglycemia associated ultrastructural damage and induction of aldose reductase expression in retinal pigment epithelial (RPG) cells. *Invest Ophthalmol Vis Sci* 1986;27(suppl):144.
282. Brown MR, Dyck PJ, McClearn GE, et al: Central and peripheral nervous system complications. *Diabetes* 1982;31(suppl 1):65–70 and references cited.
283. Ward JD: Diabetic neuropathy, in Alberti KGMM, Krall LP (eds): *The Diabetes Annual I.* Elsevier Science Publishers, 1985, pp 288–308 and references cited.
284. Brown MJ, Asbury AK: Diabetic neuropathy. *Ann Neurol* 1984;15:2.
285. Gabbay KH, Merola LO, Field RA: Sorbitol pathway: Presence in nerve and cord with substrate accumulation in diabetes. *Science* 1966;151:209–210.
286. Ludvigson MA, Sorenson RL: Immunohistochemical localization of aldose reductase. I. Enzyme purification and antibody preparation—localization in peripheral nerve, artery, and testes. *Diabetes* 1980;29:438–449.
287. Gabbay KH: The polyol pathway and the complications of diabetes. *N Engl J Med* 1973;288:831–836.
288. Christiansen JEJ, Varnek L, Gregersen G: The effect of an aldose reductase inhibitor (Sorbinil®) on diabetic neuropathy and neural function of the retina: A double-blind study. *Acta Neurol Scand* 1985;71:164–167.
289. Jakobsen J: Peripheral nerves in early experimental diabetes. *Diabetologia* 1978;14:113–199.
290. Myers RR, Costello ML, Powell HC: Increased endoneurial fluid pressure in galactose neuropathy. *Muscle Nerve* 1979;2:299–303.
291. Powell HC, Costello ML, Myers RR: Endoneurial fluid pressure in experimental models of diabetic neuropathy. *J Neuropath Exp Neurol* 1981;40:613–624.
292. Powell HC, Costello ML, Myers, RR: Galactose neuropathy. Permeability studies, mechanism of edema, and mast cell abnormalities. *Acta Neuropath* 1981;55:89–95.
293. Powell HC, Myers RR: Schwann cell changes and demyelination in chronic galactose neuropathy. *Muscle Nerve* 1983;6:218–227.
294. Eliasson SG: Nerve conduction changes in experimental diabetes. *J Clin Invest* 1964;43:2352–2358.
295. Preston GM: Peripheral neuropathy in the alloxan-diabetic rat. *J Physiol* 1967;189:49P–50P.
296. Hilderbrand JA, Joffroy A, Graff G, Coers C: Neuromuscular changes with alloxan hyperglycemia. Electrophysiological, biochemical and histological study in rats. *Arch Neurol* 1968;18:633–641.
297. Miyoshi T, Goto I: Serial in vivo determinations of nerve conduction velocity in rat tails. Physiological and pathological changes. *Electroenceph Clin Neurophysiol* 1973;35:125–131.
298. Sharma AK, Thomas PK: Peripheral nerve structure and function in experimental diabetes. *J Neurol Sci* 1974;23:1–15.
299. Goto I, Peters HA: Serial in vivo determination of motor conduction velocity in tails of alloxanized non-diabetic and diabetic rats. *J Neurol Sci* 1974;22:177–182.
300. Moore SA, Peterson RG, Felten DL, O'Connor BL: A quantitative comparison of motor and sensory conduction velocities in short- and long-term streptozocin- and alloxan-diabetic rats. *J Neurol Sci* 1980;48:133–152.
301. Yagihashi S, Nishihira M, Baba M: Morphometrical analysis of the peripheral nerve lesions in experimental diabetes rats. *Toku J Exp Med* 1979;129:139–149.
302. Sugimura K, Windebank AJ, Natarajan V, et al: Interstitial hyperosmolarity may cause axis cylinder shrinkage in streptozocin diabetic nerve. *J Neuropath Exp Neurol* 1980;39:710–721.

303. Brismar T, Sima AAF: Changes in nodal function in nerve fibers of the spontaneously diabetic BB-Wistar rat: Potential clamp analysis. *Acta Physiol Scand* 1981;113: 499–506.
304. Jakobsen J, Lundbaek K: Neuropathy in experimental diabetes: An animal model. *Br Med J* 1976;2:278–279.
305. Jakobsen J: Axonal dwindling in early experimental diabetes. IA. Study of cross sectioned nerves. *Diabetologia* 1978;12:539–546.
306. Sharma AK, Thomas PK, De Molina AP: Peripheral nerve fiber size in experimental diabetes. *Diabetes* 1977;26:689–692.
307. Jakobsen J: Early and preventable changes of peripheral nerve structure and function in insulin-deficient diabetic rats. *J Neurol Neurosurg Psychiatry* 1979;42:509–518.
308. Nukada H: Increased susceptibility to ischemic damage in streptozocin-diabetic nerve. *Diabetes* 1986;35:1058–1061.
309. Dahlin LB, Meiri KF, MacLean WG, Rydevik B, Sjostrand J: Effects of nerve compression on fast axonal transport in streptozotocin-induced diabetes mellitus. *Diabetologia* 1986;29:181–185.
310. Greene DA, De Jesus PV Jr, Winegrad AI: Effects of insulin and dietary myoinositol on impaired nerve conduction velocity in acute streptozocin diabetes. *J Clin Invest* 1975;5:1326–1336.
311. Longo FM, Powell HC, Lebeau J, et al: Delayed nerve regeneration in streptozotocin diabetic rats. *Muscle & Nerve* 1986;9:385–393.
312. Tomlinson DR, Mayer HJ: Defects of axonal transport in diabetes mellitus—a possible contribution to the aetiology of diabetic neuropathy. *J Auton Pharmac* 1984;4:59–72 and references cited.
313. Sidenius P, Jakobsen J: Axonal transport in experimental diabetes. *Clin Physiol* 1985;5(suppl 5):14–18.
314. Powell H, Knox D, Lee S, et al: Alloxan diabetic neuropathy: Electron microscopic studies. *Neurology* 1977;27:60–66.
315. Powell HC, Myers RR: Axonopathy and microangiopathy in chronic alloxan diabetes. *Acta Neuropathol* 1984;65:128–137.
316. Jakobsen J, Sidenius P: Nerve morphology in experimental diabetes. *Clin Physiol* 1985;5(suppl 5):9–13.
317. McCallum KNC, Sharma AK, Blanchard DS, et al: The effect of continuous subcutaneous insulin therapy on morphological and biochemical abnormalities of peripheral nerves in experimental diabetes. *J Neurol Sci* 1986;74:55–67.
318. Ivor LP, Wolf PL, Costello ML, Powell HC: Elevated hemoglobin A in streptozocin diabetes and with sucrose and galactose diets. *Clin Chem* 1979;25:1076.
319. Yue DK, Hanwell MA, Satchell PM, Handelsman DJ, Turtle JR: The effects of aldose reductase inhibition on nerve sorbitol and myoinositiol concentrations in diabetic and galactosemic rats. *Metabolism* 1984;33:1119–1122.
320. Mizisin AP, Myers RR, Powell HC: Endoneurial sodium accumulation in galactosemic rat nerves. *Muscle Nerve* 1986;9:440–444.
321. Sharma AK, Thomas PK, Baker RWR: Peripheral nerve abnormalities related to galactose administration in rats. *J Neurol Neurosurg Psychiatry* 1976;39:794–802.
322. Myers RR, Powell HC: Galactose neuropathy: Impact of chronic endoneurial edema on nerve blood flow. *Ann Neurol* 1984;16:587–594.
323. Tuck RR, Schmelzer JD, Low PA: Endoneurial blood flow and oxygen tension in the sciatic nerve of rats with experimental diabetic neuropathy. *Brain* 1984;107:935–950.
324. Gabbay KH, Snider JJ: Nerve conduction defect in galactose-fed rats. *Diabetes* 1972;21:295–300.

325. Simmons DA, Winegrad AI, Martin DB: Significance of tissue myo-inositol concentrations in metabolic regulation in nerve. *Science* 1982;217:848–851.
326. Simmons DA, Winegrad AI, Martin DB: Significance of myo-inositol concentrations in metabolic regulation. *Trans Assoc Am Phys* 1982;95:292–298.
327. Mayer JH, Tomlinson DR: The influence of aldose reductase inhibition and nerve myo-inositol on axonal transport and nerve conduction velocity in rats with experimental diabetes. *J Physiol* 1983;340:25P–26P.
328. Tomlinson DR, Moriarty RJ, Mayer JH: Prevention and reversal of defective axonal transport and motor nerve conduction velocity in rats with experimental diabetes by treatment with the aldose reductase inhibitor sorbinil. *Diabetes* 1984;33:470–476.
329. Freeten P, Tomlinson DR, Townsend J: Prevention of axonal transport defects, in vagus and sciatic nerves of diabetic rats, by aldose reductase inhibition. *Br J Pharmacol* 1984;82:265P.
330. Mayer JH, Tomlinson DR, McLean GW: Slow orthograde axonal transport of radiolabelled protein in sciatic motoneurons of rats with short-term experimental diabetes: Effect of treatment with an aldose reductase inhibitor or myo-inositol. *J Neurochem* 1984;43:1265–1270.
331. Greene DA, Lattimer SA: Impaired rat sciatic nerve sodium-potassium adenosine triphosphatase in acute streptozocin diabetes and its correction by dietary myo-inositol supplementation. *J Clin Invest* 1983;72:1058–1063.
332. Greene DA, Lattimer SA: Impaired energy utilization and Na,K-ATPase in diabetic peripheral nerve. *Am J Physiol* 1984;246:E311–E318.
333. Greene DA, Yagihashi S, Lattimer SA, Sima AAF: Nerve Na^+,K^+-ATPase, conduction, and myo-inositol in the insulin-deficient BB rat. *Am J Physiol* 1984;247:E534–E539.
334. Brismar T: Neuropathy-functional abnormalities in the BB rat. *Metabolism* 1983;32(suppl 1):112–117.
335. Greene DA: Metabolic abnormalities in diabetic peripheral nerve: Relation to impaired function. *Metabolism* 1983;32(suppl 1):118–123.
336. Sima AAF: Can the BB-rat help to unravel diabetic neuropathy? *Neuropath Appl Neurobiol* 1985;11:253–264 and references cited.
337. Brismar T, Sima AAF: Changes in nodal function in nerve fibers of the spontaneously diabetic BB-Wistar rat. Potential clamp analysis. *Acta Physiol Scand* 1981;113: 499–506.
338. Sima AAF, Lattimer SA, Yagihashi S, Greene DA: Axoglyal dysjunction. A novel structural lesion that accounts for poorly reversible slowing of nerve conduction in the spontaneously diabetic Bio-Breeding rat. *J. Clin Invest* 1986;77:474–484.
339. Greene DA, Lattimer SA, Sima AAF: Acute paranodal nerve fiber swelling and conduction slowing in the insulin-deficient BB rat reflects myo-inositol depletion and Na/K-ATPase deficiency rather than sorbitol accumulation. *Clin Res* 1986;34:683.
340. Gillon KRW, Hawthorne JN: Sorbitol, inositol and nerve conduction in diabetes. *Life Sci* 1983;32:1943–1947.
341. Meyer JH, Tomlinson DR: Prevention of defects of axonal transport and nerve conduction velocity by oral administration of myo-inositol or an aldose reductase inhibitor in streptozocin-diabetic rats. *Diabetologia* 1983;25:433–438.
342. Kemper C, Dvornik D: Prevention of neural myoinositol depletion in diabetic rats by aldose reductase inhibition with tolrestat. *Proc Soc Exp Biol Med* 1986;82:505–510.
343. Yue DK, Hanwell MA, Satchell PM, Turtle JR: The effect of aldose reductase inhibition on nerve conduction velocity in diabetic rats. *Diabetes* 1982;31:789–794.
344. Hotta N, Kakuta H, Fukasawa H, et al: Effects of a fructose-rich diet and the aldose reductase inhibitor, ONO-2235, on the development of diabetic neuropathy in streptozocin-treated rats. *Diabetologia* 1985;28:176–180.

345. Greene DA, Lattimer SA: Relationship of polyol (sorbitol) pathway inhibition to a myo-inositol-mediated defect in sodium-potassium ATPase activity. *Diabetes* 1984;33:712–716.
346. Carroll PB, Thornton BM, Greene DA: Glutathione redox state is not the link between polyol pathway activity and myoinositol-related Na^{+}-K^{+}-ATPase defect in experimental diabetic neuropathy. *Diabetes* 1986;35:1282–1285.
347. Cameron NE, Leonard MB, Ross IE, Whiting PH: The effects of sorbinil on peripheral nerve conduction velocity, polyol concentrations and morphology in the streptozotocin-diabetic rat. *Diabetologia* 1986;29:168–174.
348. Dvornik D, Sredy J, Hicks D, Sawicki D, Ackerman D: Polyol pathway and myoinositol content in peripheral nerve of long–term streptozocin (STZ)-diabetic rats. *Diabetes* 1987;36(suppl 1):185A.
349. Inserra JJ, Fossile A, Notvest RR, Keim K: Auditory-evoked brainstem response (ABR) as a measure of nerve transmission time in rats. *Fed Proc* 1986;45:463.
350. Fedele D, Martini A, Cardone C, et al: Impaired auditory brain-stem evoked responses in insulin-dependent diabetic subjects. *Diabetes* 1984;33:1085–1089.
351. Notvest RO, Inserra JJ: Tolrestat, an aldose reductase inhibitor, prevents nerve dysfunction in conscious diabetic rats. *Diabetes* 1987;36:500–504.
352. Kolta MG, Wallace LJ, Gerald MC: Streptozocin-induced diabetes affects rat urinary bladder response to autonomic agents. *Diabetes* 1985;34:917–921.
353. Kudlacz EM, Wallace LJ, Gerald MC: In vitro and in vivo analysis of diabetic rat urinary bladder function. *Pharmacologist* 1986;28:227.
354. Yagihashi S, Sima AAF: Diabetic autonomic neuropathy in BB rat. Ultrastructural and morphometric changes in parasympathetic nerves. *Diabetes* 1986;35:733–743.
355. Yagihashi S, Sima AAF: Diabetic autonomic neuropathy in the BB rat. Ultrastructural and morphometric changes in sympathetic nerves. *Diabetes* 1985;34:558–564.
356. Mauer SM, Steffes MW, Goetz FC, Sutherland DER, Brown DM: Diabetic nephropathy. A perspective. *Diabetes* 1983:32(suppl 2):52–55.
357. Steffes MW, Ellis EN, Mauer SM: Complications of diabetes mellitus and factors affecting their progression. *Clin Chem* 1986;32:B54–B61 and references cited.
358. Ellis EN, Mauer SM: Diabetic nephropathy, in Alberti KGMM, Krall LP (eds): *The Diabetes Annual*. Elsevier Science Publishers, 1985, pp 309–322.
359. Mogensen CE, Andersen MJF: Increased kidney size and glomerular filtration rate in early juvenile diabetes. *Diabetes* 1973;22:706–712.
360. Mogensen CE, Andersen MJF: Increased kidney size and glomerular filtration rate in untreated juvenile diabetes: Normalization by insulin treatment. *Diabetologia* 1975:11:221–224.
361. Christiansen JS, Gammelgaard J, Tronier B, Svendsen PA, Parving HH: Kidney function and size in diabetics before and during initial insulin treatment. *Kidney Int* 1982;683–688.
362. Puig JG, Anton FM, Grande C, et al: Relation of kidney size to kidney function in early insulin-dependent diabetes. *Diabetologia* 1981;21:363–367.
363. Christiansen JS, Gammelgaard J, Frandsen M, Parving HH: Increased kidney size, glomerular filtration rate and renal plasma flow in short-term insulin-dependent diabetes. *Diabetologia* 1981;20:451–456.
364. Wiseman M, Viberti GC: Kidney size and glomerular filtration rate in Type I (insulin-dependent) diabetes mellitus revisited. *Diabetologia* 1983;25:530 (letter).
365. Ellis EN, Steffes MW, Goetz FC, Sutherland DER, Mauer SM: Relationship of renal size to nephropathy in Type I (insulin-dependent) diabetes. *Diabetologia* 1985;28:12–15.
366. Ross J, Goldman JK: Effect of streptozotocin-induced diabetes on kidney weight and compensatory hypertrophy in the rat. *Endocrinology* 1971;88:1079–1082.

367. Seyer-Hansen K: Renal hypertrophy in streptozotocin-diabetic rats. *Clin Sci Mol Med* 1976;51:551–555.
368. Seyer-Hansen K: Renal hypertrophy in experimental diabetes: Relation to severity of diabetes. *Diabetologia* 1977;13:141–143.
369. Seyer-Hansen K, Hansen J, Gundersen JHG: Renal hypertrophy in experimental diabetes. *Diabetologia* 1983;18:501–505.
370. Seyer-Hansen K: Renal hypertrophy in experimental diabetes mellitus. *Kidney Int* 1983;23:643–646.
371. Kroustrup JP, Gundersen HJG, Østerby R: Glomerular size and structure in diabetes mellitus. III. Early enlargement of the capillary surface. *Diabetologia* 1977; 13:207–210.
372. Mogensen CE, Østerby R, Gundersen HJG: Early functional and morphologic vascular renal consequences of the diabetic state. *Diabetologia* 1979;17:71–76.
373. Rasch R, Rytter-Norgaard JO: Renal enlargement: Comparative autoradiographic studies on ^{3}H-thymidine uptake in diabetic and uninephrectomized rats. *Diabetologia* 1983;25:280–287.
374. Sochor M, Baquer NZ, McLean P: Glucose over-utilization in diabetes: Evidence from studies on the changes in hexokinase, the pentose phosphate pathway and glucuronate-xylulose pathway in rat kidney cortex in diabetes. *Biochem Biophys Res Comm* 1979; 86:32–39.
375. Steer KA, Sochor M, Gonzalez AM, McLean P: Regulation of pathways of glucose metabolism in the kidney. Specific linking of pentose phosphate pathway activity with kidney growth in experimental diabetes and unilateral nephrectomy. *FEBS Lett* 1982;150:494–498.
376. Steer KA, Sochor M, McLean P: Renal hypertrophy in experimental diabetes. Changes in pentose phosphate pathway activity. *Diabetes* 1985;34:485–490.
377. Del Val M, Beyer-Mears A, Regan T: Proteinuria and renal hypertrophy in experimental and spontaneously diabetic dogs. *Diabetes* 1986;35(suppl 1):203A.
378. Sochor M, Kunjara S, Greenbaum AL, McLean P: Renal hypertrophy in experimental diabetes. Effect of diabetes on the pathways of glucose metabolism: Differential response in adult and immature rats. *Biochem J* 1986;234:573–577.
379. Wald H, Scherzer P, Popovtzer MM: Enhanced renal tubular Na,K-ATPase in streptozotocin-induced diabetes mellitus: Possible role in electrolyte homeostasis. *Kidney Int* 1986;29:410.
380. Cohen MP, Dasmahapatra A, Shapiro E: Reduced glomerular sodium/potassium adenosine triphosphatase activity in acute streptozotocin diabetes. *Diabetes* 1985;34:1071–1074.
381. Martino G, Botte L, Guala L, Covello C: Metabolic and ultrastructural aspects of diabetic glomerulopathy. *J Endocrinol Invest* 1986:9:87–95.
382. Romen W, Takahashi A: Autoradiographic studies on the proliferation of glomerular and tubular cells of the rat kidney in early diabetes. *Virchow's Arch* 1982; 40:339–345.
383. Broulik PD, Schreiber J: Effect of alloxan diabetes on kidney grown in intact and castrated mice. *Acta Endocrinol* 1982;99:109–111.
384. Rasch R, Norgaard OR: Experimental diabetic nephropathy, in Shafrir E, Renold AE (eds): *Lessons from animal diabetes.* London, Libbey, 1984, pp 392–397.
385. Del Castillo E, Fuenzalida R, Uranga J: Increased glomerular filtration rate and glomerulopressin activity in diabetic dogs. *Horm Metab Res* 1977;9:46–53.
386. Michels LD, Keane WF, Davidman M: Glomerular function in alloxan diabetes and the effect of insulin. *Clin Res* 1980;28:455A.

387. Hostetter TH, Troy JL, Brenner BM: Glomerular hemodynamics in experimental diabetes. *Kidney Int* 1981;19:410–415.
388. Koch-Jensen P, Christiansen JS, Steven K, Parving HH: Renal function in diabetic rats. *Acta Endocrinol* 1981;97(suppl 242):25.
389. Gartner K: Glomerular hyperfiltration during the onset of diabetes mellitus in two strains of diabetic mice. *Diabetologia* 1978;15:59–63.
390. Brown DM, Andres GA, Hostetter TH, et al: Kidney complications. *Diabetes* 1982;31(suppl 1):71–81.
391. Zatz R, Meyer TW, Rennke HG, Brenner BM: Predominance of hemodynamic rather than metabolic factors in the pathogenesis of diabetic glomerulopathy. *Proc Natl Acad Sci* 1985;82:5963–5967.
392. Zatz R, Dunn BR, Meyer TW, et al: Prevention of diabetic glomerulopathy by pharmacological amelioration of glomerular capillary hypertension. *J Clin Invest* 1986;77:1925–1930.
393. Zatz R, Brenner BM: Pathogenesis of diabetic microangiopathy. The hemodynamic view. *Am J Med* 1986;80:443–453.
394. Mogensen CE, Steffes MW, Deckert T, Christiansen JS: Functional and morphological renal manifestations in diabetes mellitus. *Diabetologia* 1981;21:89–93.
395. Viberti GC: Early functional and morphological changes in diabetic nephropathy. *Clin Nephrol* 1979;12:47–53.
396. Mogensen CE, Christensen CK: Predicting diabetic nephropathy in insulin-dependent patients. *N Engl J Med* 1984;311:89–93.
397. Keen H, Chlouverakis C, Fuller J, Jarrett RJ: The concomitants of raised blood sugar: Studies in newly detected hyperglycemics. II. Urinary albumin excretion, blood sugar levels. *Guy's Hosp Rep* 1969;118:247–252.
398. Viberti GC, Keen H: The patterns of proteinuria in diabetes mellitus. *Diabetes* 1984;33:686–692.
399. Viberti GC, Mackintosh D, Keen H: Determinants of the penetration of protein through the glomerular barrier in insulin-dependent diabetes mellitus. *Diabetes* 1983; 32(suppl 2):92–95.
400. Wiseman MJ, Viberti GC: Genesis and evolution of proteinuria in diabetes mellitus. *Ric Clin Lab* 1985:15:9–16.
401. Rasch R, Mogensen CE: Urinary excretion of albumin and total protein in normal and streptozotocin diabetic rats. *Acta Endocrinol* 1980;95:376–381.
402. Mauer SM, Brown DM, Matas AJ, Steffe MW: Effects of pancreatic islet transplantation on the increased urinary albumin excretion rates in intact and uninephrectomized rats with diabetes mellitus. *Diabetes* 1978;27:959–964.
403. Cooper ME, Allen TJ, Jerums G, Doyle AE: Accelerated progression of diabetic nephropathy in the spontaneously hypertensive streptozotocin diabetic rat. *Clin Exp Pharmacol Physiol* 1986;13:655–662.
404. Mogensen CE: Renal function changes in diabetes. *Diabetes* 1976;25:872–879.
405. Viberti GC, Pickup JC, Jarrett RJ, Keen H: Effect of control of blood glucose on urinary excretion of albumin and B_2-microglobulin in insulin-dependent diabetics. *N Engl J Med* 1979;300:638–641.
406. Feldt-Rasmussen B, Mathiesen ER, Hegedus L, Deckert T: Kidney function during 12 months of strict metabolic control in insulin-dependent diabetic patients with incipient nephropathy. *N Engl J Med* 1986;314:665–670.
407. KROC Collaborative Study Group: Blood glucose control and the evolution of diabetic retinopathy and albuminuria: A preliminary multicenter trial. *N Engl J Med* 1984;311:365–372.

408. Deckert T, Lauritzen T, Parving HH, Christiansen JS, Steno Study Group: Effect of two years of strict metabolic control on kidney function in long term insulin dependent diabetes. *Diabet Nephropath* 1984;3:6–10.
409. Bending, JJ, Viberti, GC, Watkins, PJ, Keen, H: Intermittent clinical proteinuria and renal function in diabetes: Evolution and the effect of glycemic control. *Br Med J* 292:83-86 (1986).
410. Rasch R: Prevention of diabetic glomerulopathy in streptozotocin diabetic rats by insulin treatment. Albumin excretion. *Diabetologia* 1980;18:413–416.
411. Pennell JP, Meinking TL: Pattern of urinary proteins in experimental diabetes. *Kidney Int* 1982;21:709–713.
412. Steffes MW, Brown DM, Basgen JM, Matas AJ, Mauer SM: Glomerular basement membrane thickness following islet transplantation in the diabetic rat. *Lab Invest* 1979;41:116–118.
413. Østerby R: Early phases in the development of diabetic glomerulopathy. *Acta Med Scand* 1975;541(suppl):1–80.
414. Stout LC, Folse DS, Meier J, et al: Quantitative glomerular morphology of the normal and diabetic baboon kidney. *Diabetologia* 1986;29:734–740.
415. Rohrbach R: Reduced content and abnormal distribution of anionic sites (acid proteoglycans) in the diabetic glomerular basement membrane. *Virchows Arch* 1986;51:127-135.
416. Brenner BM, Hostetter TH, Humes HD: Molecular basis of proteinuria of glomerular origin. *N Engl J Med* 1978;298:826–833.
417. Cortes P, Dumler F, Sastry KSS, Verghese CP, Levin NW: Effects of early diabetes on uridine diphosphosugar synthesis in the rat renal cortex. *Kidney Int* 1979; 21:676–682.
418. Brownlee M, Spiro RG: Glomerular basement membrane metabolism in the diabetic rat. In vivo studies. *Diabetes* 1979;28:121–125.
419. Spiro RG, Spiro MJ: Effect of diabetes on the biosynthesis of the renal glomerular basement membrane. Studies on glucosyltransferase. *Diabetes* 1971;20:641–648.
420. Romen W, Lange HW, Hempel K, Heck TH: Studies on the collagen metabolism in rats. II. Turnover and amino acid composition of the collagen of the glomerular basement membrane in diabetes mellitus. *Virchow's Arch* 1981;36:313–320.
421. Sternberg M, Andre J, Peyroux J: Inhibition of the alpha-glucosidase specific for collagen disaccharide units in diabetic rat kidney by in vivo glucose levels: Possible contribution to basement membrane thickening. *Diabetologia* 1983;24:286–289.
422. Falk RJ, Scheinman JI, Mauer SM, Michael AF: Polyantigenic expansion of basement membrane constituents in diabetic nephropathy. *Diabetes* 1983;32:34–39.
423. Kefalides NA: Basement membrane research in diabetes mellitus. *Collagen Rel Res* 1981:1:295–299.
424. Mauer SM, Steffes MW, Ellis EN, et al: Structural-functional relationships in diabetic nephropathy. *J Clin Invest* 1984;74:1143–1155.
425. Gellman DD, Pirani CL, Soothill JF, et al: Structure and function in diabetic nephropathy. The importance of diffuse glomerulosclerosis. *Diabetes* 1959;8:251–256.
426. Hostetter TH, Olson JL, Rennke HG, Venkatachalam MA, Brenner BM: Hyperfiltration in remnant nephrons: A potentially adverse response to renal ablation. *Am J Physiol* 1981;24:F85–F93.
427. Carrie BJ, Myers BD: Proteinuria and functional characteristics of the glomerular barrier in diabetic nephropathy. *Kidney Int* 1980;17:667–676.
428. Winetz JA, Golbertz HB, Spencer RJ, Lee JA, Myers BD: Glomerular function in advanced human diabetic nephropathy. *Kidney Int* 1982;21:750–756.

429. Steffes MW, Brown DM, Mauer SM: Diabetic glomerulopathy following unilateral nephrectomy in the rat. *Diabetes* 1978;27:35–41.
430. Steffes MW, Vernier RL, Brown DM, Basgen JM, Mauer SM: Diabetic glomerulopathy in the uninephrectomized rat resists amelioration following islet transplantation. *Diabetologia* 1982;23:347–353.
431. Steffes MW, Brown DM, Basgen JM, Mauer SM: Amelioration of mesangial volume and surface alterations following islet transplantation in diabetic rats. *Diabetes* 1980; 29:509–515.
432. Brown DM, Steffes MW, Thibert P, Azar S, Mauer SM: Glomerular manifestations of diabetes in the BB rat. *Metabolism* 1983;32(suppl 1):131–135.
433. Federlin K, Bretzel RG: Reversibility of diabetic glomerulopathy by islet transplantation in experimental animals. *Pediatr Adolesc Endocrinol* 1981;9:326–332.
434. Fine LG, Bradley T: Adaptation of proximal tubular structure and function: Insights into compensatory renal hypertrophy. *Fed Proc* 1985;44:2727–2733.
435. Fine LG, Badie-Dezfooly B, Lowe AG, et al: Stimulation of Na^+/H^+ antiport is an early event in hypertrophy of renal proximal tubular cells. *Proc Natl Acad Sci* 1985; 82:1736–1740.
436. Viberti GC, Mackintosh D, Bilous RW, Pickup JC, Keen H: Proteinuria in diabetes mellitus: Role of spontaneous and experimental variation in glycemia. *Kidney Int* 1982;21:714–720.
437. Gabbay KH, O'Sullivan JB: The sorbitol pathway in diabetes and galactosemia: Enzyme and substrate localization and changes in kidney. *Diabetes* 1968;17:300.
438. Gabbay KH, Cathcart ES: Purification and immunologic identification of aldose reductases. *Diabetes* 1974;23:460–468.
439. Hutton JC, William JF, Schofield PJ, Hollows FC: Polyol metabolism in monkey-kidney epithelial-cell cultures. Sorbitol synthesis. *Eur J Biochem* 1974;49:347–353.
440. Kinoshita JH, Dvornik D, Kraml M, Gabbay KH: The effect of an aldose reductase inhibitor on the galactose-exposed rabbit lens. *Biochim Biophys Acta* 1968;158: 472–475.
441. Boot-Handford R, Heath H: The effects of aldose reductase inhibitors on the metabolism of cultured monkey kidney epithelial cells. *Biochem Pharmacol* 1981;30:3065–3069.
442. Hutton JC, Schofield PJ, Williams JF, Hollows FC: The localization of sorbitol pathway activity in the rat renal cortex and its relationship to the pathogenesis of the renal complications of diabetes mellitus. *Austr J Exp Biol Med Sci* 1975;53:49–57.
443. Corder CN, Collins JG, Brannan TS, Sharma J: Aldose reductase and sorbitol dehydrogenase distribution in rat kidney. *J Histochem Cytochem* 1977;25:1–8.
444. Kikkawa R, Umemura K, Haneda M, et al: Evidence for existence of polyol pathway in cultured rat mesangial cells. *Diabetes* 1987;36:240–243.
445. Kern TS, Engerman RL: Immunohistochemical distribution of aldose reductase. *Histochem J* 1982;14:507–515.
446. Corder CN, Braughler JM, Culp PA: Quantitative histo-chemistry of the sorbitol pathway in glomeruli and small arteries of human diabetic kidney. *Folia Histochem Cytochem* 1979;17:137–146.
447. Ono H, Shibata M: Sorbitol in the kidney of NSY mice with congenital hyperglycemia. *J Japan Diab Soc* 1982;25:243–245.
448. Bauman JW Jr, Farnsworth PN: Effect of aldose reductase inhibition on natriuresis and proteinuria in diabetic rats. *Kidney Int* 1986;29:391.
449. Sochor M, Kunjara S, McLean P: Sorbinil reduces kidney sorbitol and fructose concentrations in experimental diabetes. *Diabetologia* 1984;27:333A.

450. Beyer-Mears A, Nicholas-Alexandre J, Cruz E: Sorbinil inhibition of renal aldose reductase. *Fed Proc* 1982;41:858.
451. Beyer-Mears A, Ku L, Cohen MP: Glomerular polyol accumulation in diabetes and its prevention by oral sorbinil. *Diabetes* 1984;33:604–607.
452. Kikkawa R, Kitamura E, Fujuwara Y, et al: Impaired contractile responsiveness of diabetic glomeruli to angiotensia II. A possible indication of mesangial dysfunction in diabetes mellitus. *Biochem Biophys Res Comm* 1986;136:1185–1190.
453. Troyer DA, Schwertz DW, Kreisberg JI, Venkatachalam MA: Inositol phospholipid metabolism in the kidney. *Ann Rev Physiol* 1986;48:51–71.
454. Bauman JW Jr: Proteinuria in long term streptozotocin diabetes in rats. *Life Sci* 1980;27:2121–2124.
455. Beyer-Mears A, Varagiannis E, Cruz E: Effect of sorbinil on reversal of proteinuria. *Diabetes* 1985;34(suppl 1):109A.
456. Bauman JW Jr, Robinson D, Farnsworth PN: Physiologic and structural changes related to glomerular proteinuria in diabetic rats treated with aldose reductase inhibitor. *Diab Res Clin Pract* 1985;(suppl 1):S35–S36.
457. Palmano KP, Whiting PH, Hawthorne JN: Free and lipid myo-inositol in tissues from rats with acute and less severe streptozotocin-induced diabetes. *Biochem J* 1977; 167:229–235.
458. Beyer-Mears A, Cruz E, Dillon P, Tanis D, Roche M: Diabetic renal hypertrophy diminished by aldose reductase inhibition. *Fed Proc* 1983;44:505.

Chapter 4
Aldose Reductase Inhibitors

by Dushan Dvornik, D.Sc.

Synopsis

More than 60 years after the discovery of insulin, there is as yet no scientific proof that good blood glucose control in man prevents or retards the development of diabetic complications. This is not surprising since, until recently, it has been practically impossible to maintain blood glucose in insulin-dependent diabetic subjects over long periods of time at levels approaching normoglycemia. Conventional therapy for diabetic hyperglycemia has, therefore, not prevented the development of microvascular complications involving the peripheral nerves, eye, and kidney.

Under physiological conditions, glucose is one of the most tightly regulated metabolic substrates: while counter-regulatory mechanisms maintain normal brain function by protecting against hypoglycemia, the upper limit of blood glucose is kept in balance (mainly by insulin secretion) with the limited capacity of glycolysis, hexose phosphate shunt and glycogen formation, i.e., the primary pathways of glucose utilization. Experimental evidence generated in the past 20 years strongly suggests that once the primary pathways are saturated, as in diabetes, in virtually all of the examined tissues the excess glucose is metabolized via the polyol pathway (aldose reductase and polyol dehydrogenase). As the intracellular glucose concentrations increase, the aldose reductase-catalyzed sorbitol formation also increases and saturates the capacity of the polyol dehydrogenase to oxidize sorbitol to fructose. Sorbitol does not readily pass through cell membranes; hence it accumulates. It is now well established that intracellular sorbitol accumulation and the resulting osmotic stress initiate the progression of biochemical and functional changes that cause cataract. In the peripheral nerves of acutely diabetic animals, sorbitol accumulation is closely related to myoinositol depletion and suppression of Na/K-ATPase, and it is assumed that this is the primary abnormality leading to dysfunction and damage of the diabetic nerve. Abnormalities of the polyol and myoinositol pathways and Na/K-ATPase function have also been shown to occur in the retina and in the kidney.

The pivotal role of aldose reductase (AR) in these pathways has been demonstrated by the use of AR inhibitors; this has inspired the concept that AR inhibition could offer a pharmacological approach to the prevention, arrest, and possibly reversal of specific diabetic complications. This chapter summarizes the results obtained with AR inhibitors, both in vitro and in vivo, and reviews the clinical evidence for the efficacy of several AR inhibitors in diabetic patients.

As indicated in the following chart, in animal models of diabetic complications, AR inhibitors have been shown to prevent a series of biochemical, functional, and morphological changes induced by elevated sugar concentrations.

HYPERGLYCEMIA-INDUCED CHANGES IN ANIMAL MODELS OF DIABETES AND THEIR PREVENTION BY AR INHIBITORS

Type of change	Hyperglycemia-induced alterations prevented by AR inhibitors
Biochemical	Polyol accumulation Myoinositol depletion Na/K-dependent ATPase impairment Endoneurial Na accumulation
Functional	MNCV decrease Axonal transport decrease (RBC deformability, filterability, viscosity) Glomerular filtration Vascular permeability Corneal re-epithelization
Structural	Cataract BM thickening

While reversal of such changes by AR inhibitors was demonstrated in early cataract development and in deficient axonal transport and conduction velocity in peripheral nerves, the results are as yet scanty and reflect the general lack of information on factors rendering the progression of functional and morphological changes in a diabetic tissue irreversible.

Since the first clinical study on the effect of alrestatin on diabetic neuropathy, conducted in four diabetic subjects, several thousands of diabetic patients have been and are currently being treated with second generation AR inhibitors to determine their effect on neuropathy, retinopathy, and nephropathy. At present, the problems of study design, variables to be evaluated, and, particularly, of patients to be selected are the same whether we examine the effect of improved glycemic control or an AR inhibitor on any of these diabetic complications. In both approaches, the outcome will depend on the extent of tissue damage at the time of intervention and the duration of intervening treatment, whether it be aldose reductase inhibition or improved glycemic control. The positive results obtained in a multicenter, double-blind study in diabetic patients with chronic painful/paresthetic neuropathy and treated with tolrestat for one year support the view that clinical benefit from AR inhibitor therapy for an established complication can be expected upon prolonged treatment.

In other clinical studies in diabetic patients, beneficial effects of the AR inhibitor sorbinil in diabetic patients were reported in a case of keratopathy and in several cases of limited joint mobility.

Contents

CONCEPT OF ALDOSE REDUCTASE INHIBITION

The introduction into medical practice of insulin in 1922 has markedly reduced death due to ketoacidosis and increased the life expectancy of the diabetic patient. As a cause of death, however, diabetic coma has been more than supplanted by the composite category of cardiorenal disease, which accounts for about 80% of all deaths in patients with diabetes mellitus.[1] The effects of chronic diabetes have thus been unmasked,[2] and since 1950, it has been evident that while prolonging life, conventional insulin treatment does not prevent the appearance of such disabling complications of long-term diabetes mellitus[3] as neuropathy, nephropathy, retinopathy, corneal epitheliopathy, cataract, accelerated arteriosclerosis and increased susceptibility to infection.

Four points can be made about the complications of chronic diabetes:

1. In spite of the accepted concept that "appropriate therapy should include a serious effort to achieve levels of blood glucose as close to those in the nondiabetic state as feasible,"[4] conventional contemporary therapy is only partly effective at best[5] and does not prevent the development of diabetic retinopathy, nephropathy, or polyneuropathy.[6] Even very meticulous glycemic control by continuous subcutaneous insulin infusion resulted in controversial findings ranging from no effect[7,8] and some regression[9] to significantly less progression of retinopathy.[10]
2. The onset, rate of progression, and clinical expression of many diabetic complications depend mainly on the duration and severity of diabetic hyperglycemia.[11]
3. The target organs of many diabetic complications do not require insulin for their uptake of glucose. The lens, nerve, kidney, retina and capillaries are thus directly exposed to systemic glucose concentrations occurring in subjects with diabetes mellitus.[12] Systemic hyperglycemia is thus translated into tissular hyperglycemia.
4. Experimental evidence obtained during the last two decades indicates that in diabetes mellitus, the metabolic disposition of excess glucose appears to proceed via the polyol pathway in virtually all of the affected tissues.

The polyol pathway consists of two enzymes, aldose reductase (alditol: $NADP^+$ 1-oxidoreductase, EC 1.1.1.21) and the polyol dehydrogenase (L-iditol: NAD^+ 5-oxidoreductase, EC 1.1.1.14). Because of the low affinity of aldose reductase for glucose, the activity of the polyol pathway is very low at physiological glucose concentrations. Because of this low activity, the physiological role of the polyol pathway remains unknown.[13–15] The currently available experimental evidence indicates, however, that aldose reductase activity is increased[16] and the flux through the polyol pathway enhanced[17] when sugar concentrations are elevated because of diabetes or galactosemia.

The involvement of aldose reductase in the development of diabetic complications was first suggested by the elucidation of its role in the pathogenesis of sugar cataracts. As discussed in Chapter 2, the process of cataract development is initiated by an increase in osmotic pressure[18] due to the intracellular accumulation of polyols[19] formed from the excess sugar by the action of aldose reductase.* Unless the excess sugar is lowered, the mounting osmotic pressure results in progressive loss of functional and structural integrity of the lens. Kinoshita's postulate that aldose reductase is pivotal in the pathogenesis of sugar cataract[18,22–25] was substantiated by the demonstration that cataract formation can be prevented by agents inhibiting aldose reductase. The effect was first demonstrated in vitro by Kinoshita et al[26] with tetramethyleneglutaric acid (TMG) (AY-20,037), the first non-cytotoxic inhibitor of aldose reductase, discovered in 1967 at Ayerst Research Laboratories. TMG was not absorbed when given orally,[27,28] but was later found to be active when administered topically to the rat conjunctival sac.[29,30]

The first observation of aldose reductase (AR) inhibition in vivo was made by Kinoshita[25] in rabbits given the AR inhibitor AY-20,263 by intraocular injection. This was followed by the discovery of the first orally effective inhibitor, AY-22,284 (alrestatin), synthesized in 1969.

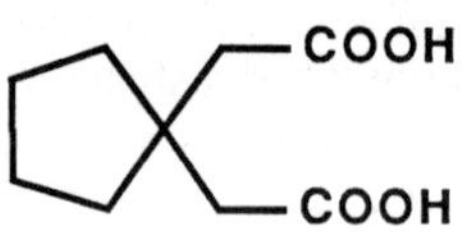

AY-20,037 (TMG)

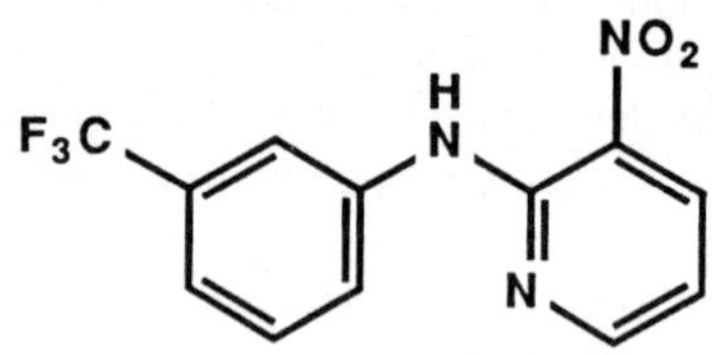

AY-20,263

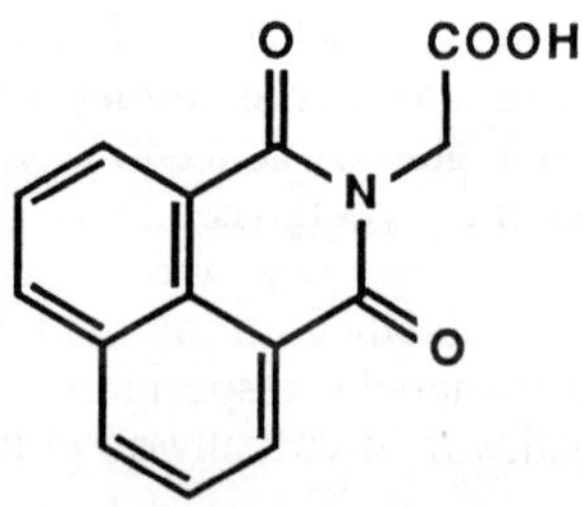

AY-22,284 (Alrestatin)

*Pertinently, addition of sorbitol to the diet had no effect on lens and kidney sorbitol levels in normal and diabetic rats[20] or on plasma and erythrocyte sorbitol levels in normal and diabetic human subjects.[21] Thus, the regulation of endogenous sorbitol production appears unaffected by the sorbitol content of the diet.[21]

The demonstration that administration of alrestatin decreased polyol accumulation in the lens and the sciatic nerve of diabetic and galactosemic rats[27] has provided the basis for a pharmacological approach to the control of diabetic complications.[31] The concept of AR inhibition has attracted many investigators, and within 15 years of the discovery of alrestatin, many hundreds of compounds were synthesized and tested for their inhibitory effect on aldose reductase. Several hundred of them were found to inhibit the enzyme in vitro, a few dozen were active in vivo, and about half a dozen are at present being tested in man. The chemical types of compounds synthesized and the relationship of their chemical structure and AR inhibition in vivo are reviewed in Chapter 5.

Work on the role of aldose reductase in the development of diabetic complications has progressed from initial studies of cataractogenesis to current studies of virtually all tissues that display diabetic pathology.[32,33] Thus far, inhibitors of aldose reductase have been reported to delay or prevent the onset of sugar cataracts in diabetic and galactosemic rats,[34] to reverse delayed re-epithelialization of denuded corneas in diabetic rats and humans,[35] to reverse decreased axonal transport and improve nerve conduction velocity in diabetic rats[36] and humans,[37–39] to symptomatically improve painful diabetic neuropathy,[37,38] to prevent retinal capillary basement membrane thickening in galactosemic[40–44] and diabetic fructose-fed rats,[45] to ameliorate limited joint mobility in diabetic patients,[46] and to prevent increased vascular permeability in diabetic and galactosemic rats.[33]

Before describing the experimental procedures developed to demonstrate AR inhibition in vitro and in vivo, we will review the distribution of the enzyme aldose reductase in the mammalian organism.

DISTRIBUTION OF ALDOSE REDUCTASE IN THE MAMMALIAN ORGANISM

Aldose reductase belongs to a larger family of aldehyde reductases that are monomeric, NADPH-dependent oxidoreductases. Since the catalyzed reduction of aldehydes is largely in favor of alcohol formation, with the reverse reaction occurring only to a very limited extent, the name "reductase" rather than "oxidoreductase" is used.[47,48] Because of their wide distribution in mammalian tissues, their relatively broad and low substrate specificity, and uncertainty about their physiological role,[13–15,49] the nomenclature used in the identification of aldehyde reductases[47,48,50,51] is confusing, despite attempts to make it uniform.[51,52] Representative examples of differences in nomenclature are shown in Table 1.

Mammalian tissues contain two major aldehyde reductases. The predominant enzyme in many tissues, particularly in the liver, brain, and kidney, is an enzyme variously designated by such names as "high Km-form," ARI, AR2, etc. (Table 1), which we will refer to as L-hexonate dehydrogenase. The other major enzyme, previously designated as "low Km-form," AR2, and so forth (Table 1), is aldose reductase, first described by Hers[73] in sheep seminal vesicles and then isolated and characterized in calf lenses by Hayman and Kinoshita.[74] Aldose reductase activity has been demonstrated in a variety of tissues (Table 2). The enzyme is localized in the cytoplasm of the cell.[66]

Table 1. Nomenclatures used for aldehyde reductases.

EC	Names appearing in the literature
1.1.1.2	L-Hexonate dehydrogenase[53,54]
	High Km reductase[55]
	Glucuronate reductase (EC 1.1.1.19)[56]
	L-Gulonate:NADP$^+$ oxidoreductase[56]
	L-Gulonate dehydrogenase[56]
	Daunorubicin pH 8.5 reductase[57]
	Lactaldehyde reductase (EC 1.1.1.55)[56]
	1,2-Propanediol:NADP$^+$ oxidoreductase[56]
	Aldehyde reductase II[51]
	AR1[58,59]
	AR3[60]
	Pig kidney aldehyde reductase[61]
	Pig liver aldehyde reductase[58]
	Human liver aldehyde reductase[62]
	Mevaldate reductase (EC 1.1.1.33)[56,57]
	Mevalonate:NADP$^+$ oxidoreductase[56]
	H4:3 Aldehyde reductase[63,64]
	AR-A[50]
	ALR-1[32]
1.1.1.21	Aldose reductase[65]
	Low Km reductase[55]
	L-Alditol:NADP$^+$ 1-oxidoreductase (EC 1.1.1.21)[66]
	AR2[60]
	Aldehyde reductase I[51]
	Pig muscle aldehyde reductase[67]
	Pig brain aldose reductase[68]
	Prostaglandin E 9-ketoreductase[69]
	L-Glycol dehydrogenase[70]
	Glyceraldehyde reductase[71]
	AR II[59]
	H4:2 Aldehyde reductase[63,64]
	AR-B[50]
	ALR-2[32]
Not classified	Carbonyl reductase[72]
	ARI
	Daunorubicin pH 6.0 reductase[57]
	AR-C[50]
	ALR-3[32]

The major difference between aldose reductase and hexonate dehydrogenase is their capacity to accept as substrate some biologically occurring carbohydrate derivatives, such as D-glucose or D-xylose, as compared with D-glucuronic acid. As

Table 2. Tissues in which aldose reductase activity has been demonstrated.

Tissue	Species
Lens	Bovine,[75,76] rat,[77–79] human,[78] rabbit[80,81]
Retina	Bovine,[82] BB rat[77]
Sciatic nerve	Rabbit,[59] BB rat[83]
Brain	Ox,[54,59,84,85] bovine,[82] human,[51,64,66,86] pig[15,68]
Liver	Calf,[87] human[88]
Kidney	Bovine[89,90]
Renal papilla	Bovine[82]
Pancreas	Bovine,[82] rat[91]
Muscle	Human,[51,92] pig,[67] chicken breast[93,94]
Aorta	Human[51]
Seminal vesicle	Ruminants,[95] sheep[96]
Erythrocyte	Human[51,76,97,98]
Placenta	Sheep,[96] bovine,[99] human,[100–103] ruminants[95]
Testis	BB rat[83]
Embryo	Rat[104,105]
Umbilical cord	Human (endothelial cells)[106]
Yeast	Rhodotorula[107]

illustrated in Table 3, the affinity of aldose reductase (expressed as the Km*) for the aldo-hexoses is somewhat greater than for D-glucuronate, while hexonate dehydrogenase has a much higher affinity for D-glucuronate.

Despite their apparent enzymatic and physicochemical likeness, aldose reductase, hexonate dehydrogenase, and carbonyl reductase, isolated from human tissues, have no common antigenic determinants.[108] The absence of im-

Table 3. Comparison of the substrate affinities (Km) of aldose reductase (AR) and hexonate dehydrogenase (HD). Expressed in mmol/L.

	Ox brain[a]		Human brain		Pig[d]		Human RBC[e]	
Substrate	AR*	HD	AR	HD[b]	AR Muscle	HD Kidney	AR	HD
D-Glucose	37	175	90[b,c]	390	51	**	155	ND
D-Galactose	12	159	110[c]				142	ND
D-Xylose	15.7	192	16[b,c]	260	8.4	2300		
D-Glucuronate	17.5	1.7	33[b];4[c]	4.6	10	5.8	1.2	2.5

*For calf brain AR, the Km values were 70 for D-glucose, 5 for D-xylose, 20 for D-galactose, and 4 for D-glucuronate.[74]
**Activity detectable at 600 mM.
ND = Not detectable
[a]Moonsammy and Stewart[54]
[b]O'Brien and Schofield[64]
[c]Wermuth and Von Wartburg[66]
[d]Flynn and Cromlish[67]
[e]Das and Srivastava[97]

*Km, the Michaelis-Menten constant, represents the substrate concentration at which the enzymatic reaction attains half-maximal velocity. Km is the inverse of the dissociation constant for the enzyme/substrate complex.

munochemical cross-reactivity between the three enzymes enables the determination of aldose reductase by immunochemical methods, e.g., by enzyme immunoassay without interference from the other reductases.

As shown by Hayman and Kinoshita,[74] the affinity of aldose reductase for aldo-hexoses depends on the 0.02% fraction of the sugar present in free aldehyde form.[109] That the aldehyde form of D-glucose is the substrate for aldose reductase (isolated from bovine lens) with a calculated Km of 0.66 μM was confirmed by Inagaki et al.[110] Actually, Grimshaw[111] has used aldose reductase to measure the ring-opening rate of α-glucopyranose and has shown that the enzyme was not catalyzing the ring-opening reaction. The presence of an α-anomer of glucose-specific aldose reductase in rat pancreatic islet was suggested by Dufrane et al[91,112] based on the finding that the reaction velocity of the enzyme was decreased by two structurally distinct AR inhibitors, TMG and sorbinil. However, the immediate, D-glucose-induced insulin secretion by isolated rat pancreatic islets was not affected by the AR inhibitors sorbinil or statil.[113]

Aldose reductase and hexonate dehydrogenase occur in a variety of mammalian tissues; however, as shown by Clements et al,[114] the lens[83] and sciatic nerve of the rat and rabbit contain only aldose reductase. According to Das and Srivastava,[115] human aorta and muscle also contain only aldose reductase. Aldose reductase appears to be absent from the liver.[66]

Considerable progress has been made in the immunohistochemical localization of aldose reductase in tissues known to be affected by long-term diabetes. The presently available data are shown in Table 4. Two points emerge from these studies. First, as indicated by Ludvigson and Sörenson,[118] knowledge of the cellular localization of aldose reductase also exposes the foci of polyol accumulation, such as the cytoplasm of the Schwann cell, the epithelial lining of the lens, cornea, ciliary body, aorta, and muscular arteries, the Müller cells of the retina, and so forth, thus allowing their evaluation as sites of diabetic lesions. Second, as pointed out by several investigators,[12,119] aldose reductase appears to be associated with cells providing a supportive or nutritional role, such as the Schwann cells of the peripheral nerve, the Sertoli cells of the testis, and the glial (Müller) cells of the retina. It is conceivable that the biochemical and functional deficits caused by the increased flux of glucose through the polyol pathway and polyol accumulation concentrated at foci of aldose reductase progressively lead to functional impairments and morphological changes.

Despite attempts to attribute a physiological role to aldehyde reductases in general and to aldose reductase in particular,[47,50,67,125,126] the conclusion of the 1982 Workshop on the Enzymology of Aldehyde Dehydrogenase and Aldo/Keto Reductase was that "... no vital physiological role can be assigned to any member of the aldehyde-ketone reductase family as yet."[126] Similar conclusions were made at the 1984 Workshop.[14] While stating that the primary role of any of the aldehyde reductases is not known and that the reasons for their distribution are even less clear, Cromlish and Flynn[15,49] wondered whether aldose reductase may be involved in the metabolism of biogenic aldehydes in the brain[127,128] and, perhaps, of predominantly hepatic isocorticosteroid metabolism[129] via the "long-loop side-chain" pathway.[130] Interestingly, the isocorticosteroids are 10 to 1,000 times better

Table 4. Immunohistochemical localization of aldose reductase in animal and human tissues.

Source of aldose reductase	Antiserum raised in	Aldose reductase localized in	Ref.
Bovine kidney	Rabbit	Calf retina	116
Bovine kidney papilla	Rabbit	Rat: lens; retina; optic nerve; pancreas; brain	82
Human placenta	Rabbit	Rhesus: mural cells (cultured)	117
Rat seminal vesicle	Rabbit	Rat: seminal vesicle (epithelial lining); testis (Sertoli cells); sciatic nerve (Schwann cell cytoplasm); aorta and muscular arteries (epithelial lining); lens (epithelial lining and cortical fibers); cornea (epithelial lining); ciliary body (inner layer of epithelium); retina (Müller cells); optic nerve; kidney (inner medulla; loop of Henle; collecting tubules; pelvic space epithelium)	118, 119
Dog kidney	Rabbit	Dog: cornea (endothelium and epithelium); lens (epithelium); ciliary processes (non-pigmented epithelium); retina (inner layers); optic nerve;	120
		aorta (endothelium and smooth muscle); peripheral nerves (Schwann cells); kidney (interstitial cells; loop of Henle; collecting tubules)	121
Dog lens	Goat	Dog: retinal mural cells	122
Human placenta	Rabbit, goat	Human retinal mural cells (cytoplasm)	123
Human placenta	Rabbit, goat	Human eye: cornea (endothelium and epithelium); conjunctiva (basal cell layers); lens (epithelium and superficial fibers); retina (Müller cells); optic nerve (axon)	124
Human brain	Rabbit	Human tissues: liver (hepatocytes, Kupffer cells, bile ducts); kidney (medulla, tubular system, absent in glomerulus); adrenals (cortex); retina (ganglion, nerve fiber and inner nuclear layer); etc.	14

substrates for the hexonate dehydrogenase and aldose reductase than the carbohydrates.[131] The only experimentally documented role of aldose reductase is to catalyze the disposition of excessive amounts of glucose appearing in diabetic tissues that do not require insulin for glucose uptake, and hence become targets of diabetic complications. Aldose reductase, therefore, appears to play an important role in the pathophysiology of the tissue damage found in diabetes and experimental galactosemia. As discussed more extensively in the following sections of this chapter, the role of aldose reductase under such conditions and its involvement in the development of complications of long-term diabetes has been greatly aided by the discovery of agents inhibiting aldose reductase.

PHARMACOLOGICAL EFFECTS OF AGENTS INHIBITING ALDOSE REDUCTASE

Testing in vitro

Inhibition of aldose reductase can be demonstrated either by measuring the activity of the enzyme isolated from a suitable mammalian tissue in the presence of the compound tested or by measuring the effect of the test compound on polyol accumulation in an isolated tissue containing aldose reductase and incubated in the presence of high sugar concentrations.

Inhibition of aldose reductase activity

Aldose reductase is assayed spectrophotometrically by measuring the decrease in the absorbance of NADPH at 340 nm, based on the following equation:

$$\text{R-CHO} + \text{NADPH} + \text{H}^{+} \rightarrow \text{R-CH}_2\text{OH} + \text{NADP}^{+}$$

The procedure preferred by most investigators is based on the use of an enzyme isolated from a tissue known to contain only aldose reductase. Usually this is the bovine lens,[74] although on occasion rat,[77] rabbit,[80] and dog[132] lenses, and human placenta[102] are also used. Virtually all procedures are based on that described originally by Hayman and Kinoshita,[74] using partially purified aldose reductase isolated from calf lenses, and a spectrophotometric method. The susceptibility of an aldose reductase preparation to inhibition may change with further purification, and highly purified enzyme was reported to be less susceptible to inhibition.[133] Detailed descriptions of the assay method and purification of the enzyme have been provided for calf kidney,[89] seminal vesicle, and placenta of ruminants,[95] and human brain.[66]

A more sensitive fluorometric assay method has been described by Dufrane et al.[112] The method is rapid and useful for the assay of small tissue samples. Walker-Griffin and McNatt[134] have increased the sensitivity of the fluorometric method further by measuring the rat lens aldose reductase-catalyzed oxidation of benzyl alcohol by the 3-acetylpyridine analog of $NADP^+$.

An alternative method of measuring polyol pathway activity[17,135] and aldose reductase inhibition[136,137] is based on the use of [^{13}C] nuclear magnetic resonance (NMR). NMR spectroscopy may also be suitable for non-invasive monitoring of the polyol pathway in the lens.[137] [^{19}F]NMR spectroscopy was used to monitor polyol pathway activity in rat brain.[138]

In the interpretation of results obtained in vitro with agents inhibiting aldose reductase, several questions may arise. First, does a given compound produce similar inhibition with enzyme preparations isolated from different tissues in the same animal species? Second, what inhibition data are obtained with enzyme preparations isolated from the same tissue but in different animal species? Third, will the agent be active when tested in vivo?

Available literature data cannot answer the first question, since with one exception, such comparative studies have not been carried out in the same laboratory with enzyme preparations isolated from tissues in the same species. It is likely that the variations in the reported values (examples shown in Table 5) reflect between-laboratory differences, such as variations in the isolation and handling of the enzyme, rather than tissue-specific differences in susceptibility of aldose reductase to inhibition by the same agent. Only Kador et al[147] have compared the effects of several structurally different inhibitors on aldose reductase isolated from human lens and human placenta. As shown in Table 6, in general, the enzyme obtained from the human placenta was 3.5 to 36.5 times less sensitive to inhibition than that isolated from human lens.

The second question has been addressed in the laboratories of the National Eye Institute (NEI)[147] and Ayerst.[148] Both groups have used structurally different AR inhibitors and have compared their effects on aldose reductase isolated from the lenses of two different species: rat and human, at the NEI, and rat and bovine, at Ayerst. The results reported by Kador et al[147] (Table 7) though variable, indicate that of the compounds tested more displayed greater inhibitory activity with the human lens enzyme. At the Ayerst Laboratories, based on results obtained with a series of flavonoids, aldose reductase isolated from rat lens was more sensitive to inhibition than that prepared from bovine lenses (Table 8). The differences between the inhibitory values obtained with some other compounds in the two lens enzyme

Table 5. In vitro inhibitory activity of various agents on aldose reductase from various human tissues.

Compound	IC_{50}		
	Lens	**Brain**	**Placenta**
Tetramethyleneglutarate (TMG)	73% at 1×10^{-3}M[a]	53% at 1×10^{-4}M[b]	1.9×10^{-6}M[c] 2.5×10^{-5}M[d] 56% at 2×10^{-4}M[e]
Alrestatin	6×10^{-6}M[f] 41% at 1×10^{-5}M[g] 100% at 1×10^{-4}M[a]	57% at 1×10^{-5}M[g]	6.5×10^{-5}M[d] 1×10^{-6}M[h]
Quercetin	5×10^{-6}M[f]	55% at 1×10^{-5}M[b]	
Sorbinil	2×10^{-7}M[f] 42% at 1×10^{-5}M[g] 93% at 1×10^{-4}M[a]	59% at 1×10^{-5}M[g]	0.7×10^{-6}M[i]
Tolrestat	3×10^{-9}M[j]		1.4×10^{-7}M[j]
Epalrestat	—	—	2.6×10^{-8}M[k]
Statil	—	—	1.5×10^{-7}M[l]

[a]Petrash and Srivastava[88]
[b]Hoffman et al[60]
[c]Terashima et al[139]
[d]Kador et al[102]
[e]Clements and Winegrad[101]
[f]Chaudhry et al[140]
[g]Srivastava et al[141]
[h]Maragoudakis et al[142]
[i]Kinoshita et al[143]
[j]Kador et al[144]
[k]Terashima et al[145]
[l]Stribling et al[146]

Table 6. In vitro inhibitory activity of various compounds on aldose reductase isolated from human tissues and placenta. (Modified from Kador et al[147])

Compound		$IC_{50} \times 10^{-6}M$		
		Placenta (P)	Lens (L)	P/L
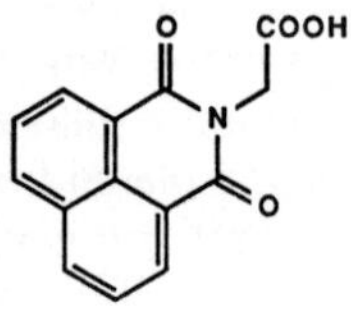		6.5	1.7	3.8
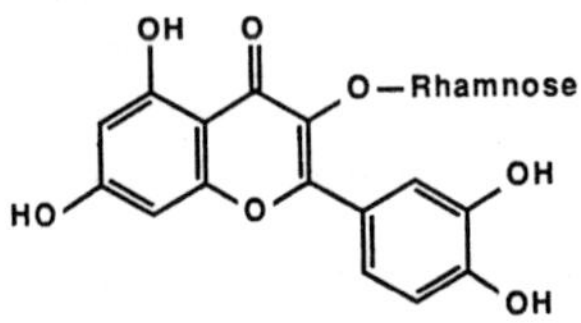		7.1	0.6	11.8
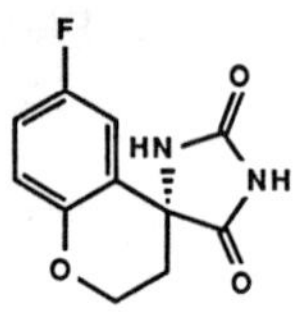		0.7	0.2	3.5
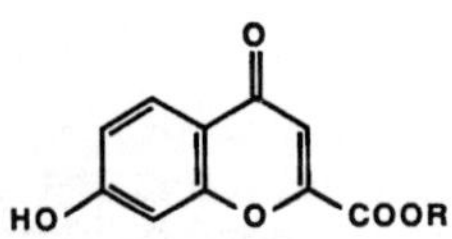	R=H	1.8	0.5	3.6
	R=Et	5.0	0.5	10.0
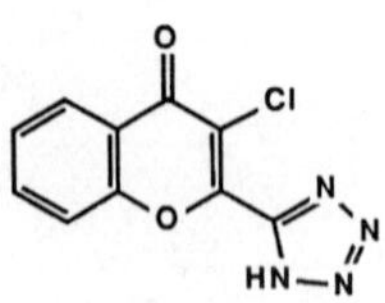		41	1.4	29.3

Table 6. (cont.)

Compound	$IC_{50} \times 10^{-6}M$		
	Placenta (P)	Lens (L)	P/L
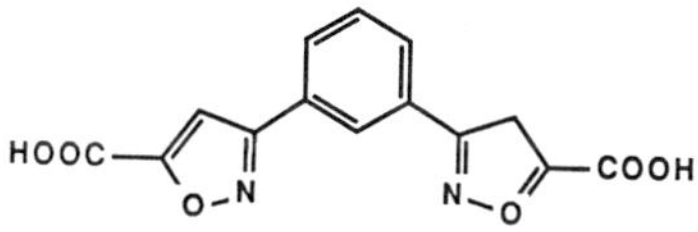	9.2	2.3	4.0
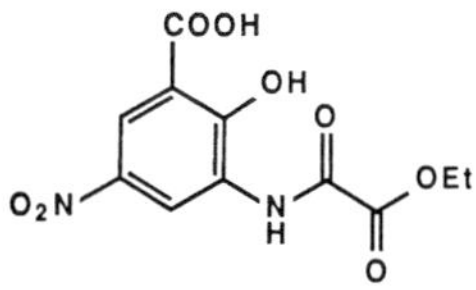	7.3	0.2	36.5
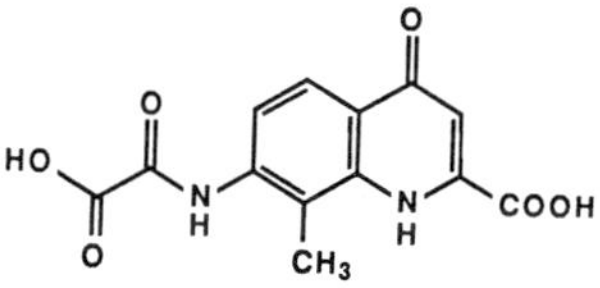	8.3	0.3	27.7
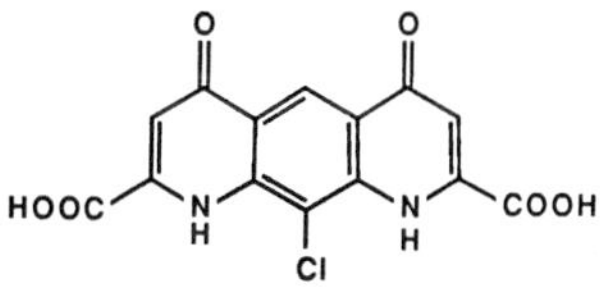	3.6	1.0	3.6
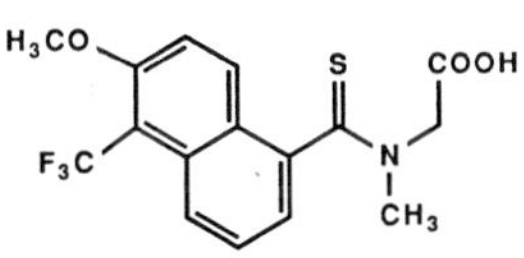	0.1	0.003	33.3

Table 7. In vitro inhibitory activity of various compounds on aldose reductase isolated from rat and human lenses. (Modified from Kador et al[147])

Compound		$IC_{50} \times 10^{-6}M$		
		Human (H)	Rat (R)	H/R
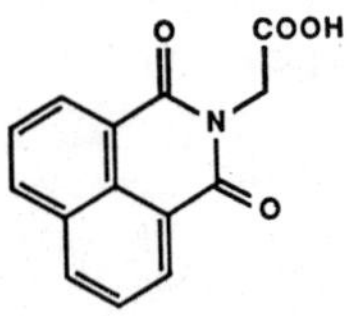		1.7	1.5	1.1
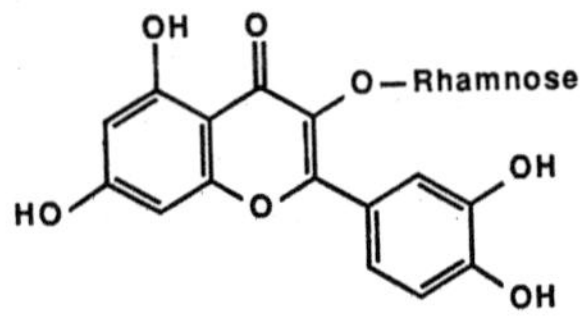		0.6	0.6	1.0
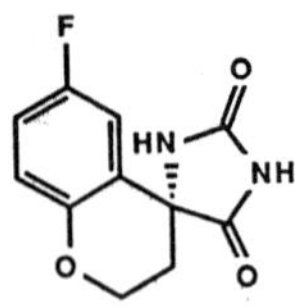		0.2	0.07	2.9
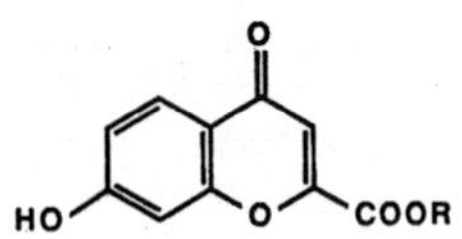	R=H	0.5	2.2	0.2
	R=Et	0.5	2.3	0.2
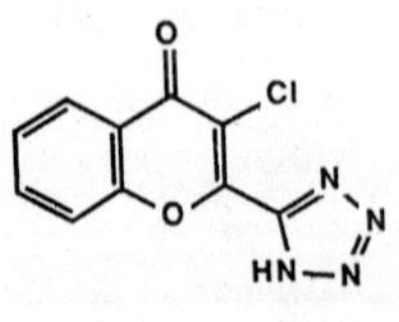		1.4	2.5	0.6

Compound	$IC_{50} \times 10^{-6}M$		
	Human (H)	Rat (R)	H/R
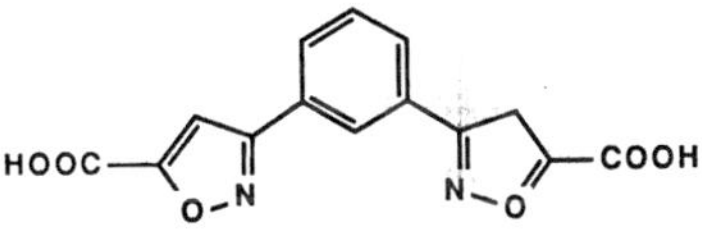	2.3	5.0	0.5
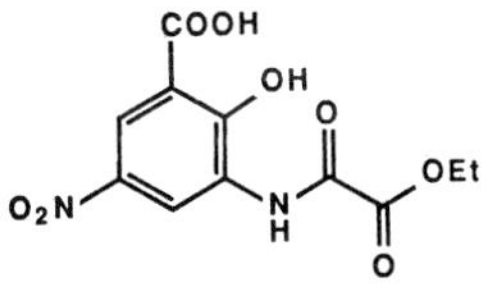	0.2	0.1	2.0
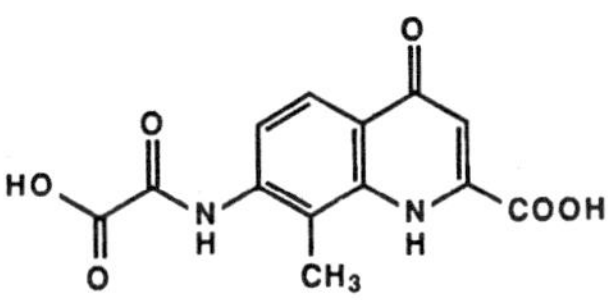	0.3	0.5	0.6
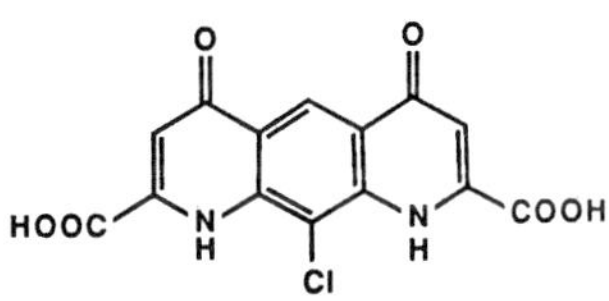	1.0	1.6	0.6
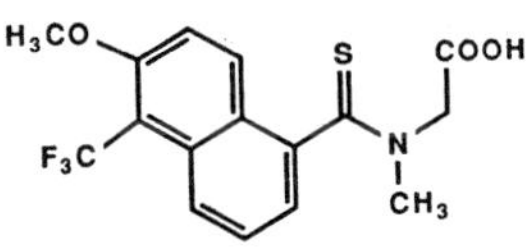	0.003	0.01	0.3

Table 8. In vitro inhibitory activity of various flavonoids on aldose reductase isolated from rat and bovine lenses.[148]

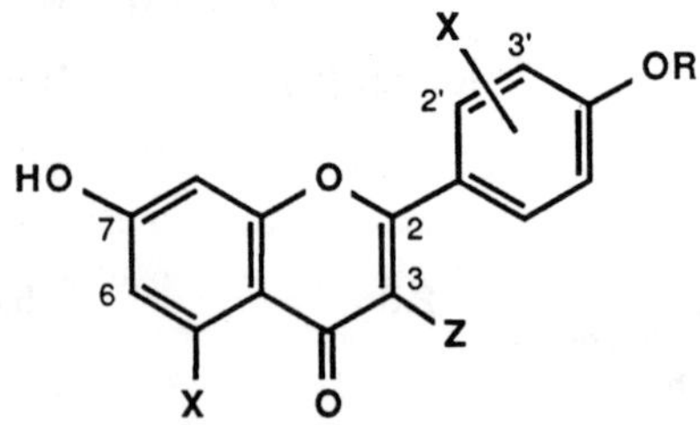

Compound	X	Y	Z	R	$IC_{50} \times 10^{-5}$M		
					Bovine (B)	Rat (R)	B/R
AY-22,950[a]	OH	3′-OH	H	H	4.5	0.5	9.0
Rutin	OH	3′-OH	OR[b]	H	5.0	1.2	4.2
Quercetin	OH	3′-OH	OH	H	5.0	1.5	3.3
Morin	OH	2′-OH	OH	H	2.5	1.3	1.9
Toxifolin	OH	3′-OH	OH[c]	H	4.0	3.0	1.3
Hesperetin	OH	3′-OH	H[c]	CH_3	4.0	3.0	1.3
Kemferol	OH	H	OH	H	4.5	4.5	1.0
Fisetin	H	3′-OH	OH	H	2.5	0.4	6.3

[a]6-CH_3,7-0-glucose
[b]R = Rutinose = rhamnosyl-glucose
[c]2,3-Dihydro-

preparations, however, were not as clear cut (Table 9). On the other hand, Müller et al[149] found no substantial differences in the IC_{50} values for the AR inhibitors sorbinil, AL-1567, and AL-1576 with aldose reductase isolated from rat and bovine lenses. These results are in accordance with those of Conrad and Doughty,[78] who have demonstrated similarity in physical, chemical and kinetic properties of the aldose reductase isolated from bovine, rat, and human lenses. Some kinetic differences between rabbit and rat lens aldose reductase were, however, mentioned by Tanimoto et al.[150]

Comparison of the IC_{50} values for a series of compounds obtained with rat lens aldose reductase in the laboratories of the NEI and Ayerst illustrates the variation that can occur between different laboratories (Table 10). In spite of the variation in IC_{50} values, an appreciation of the relative differences in intrinsic inhibitory activity can be obtained by expressing the IC_{50} values in relation to an AR inhibitor used as reference standard, e.g., alrestatin. A reliable assessment of the relative intrinsic inhibitory activity of structurally distinct AR inhibitors can be made by using results generated under similar experimental conditions, preferably in the same laboratory. The point is illustrated by the IC_{50} values for several known AR inhibitors as reported in the literature (Table 11) and as obtained in Ayerst Laboratories[155] (Table 12). Pertinently, the same relative order is obtained with

Table 9. In vitro inhibitory activity of various agents on aldose reductase from rat and bovine lenses.[148]

Compound	$IC_{50} \times 10^{-6}M$		
	Bovine (B)	Rat (R)	B/R
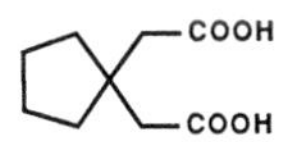	7.0	4.5	1.6
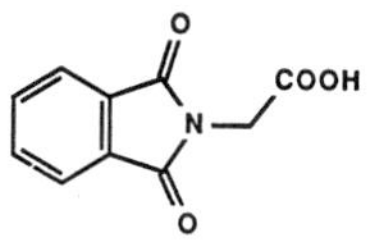	2.5	4.0	0.6
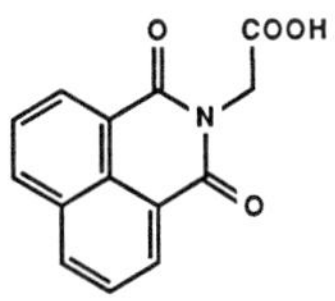	3.5	3.7	0.9
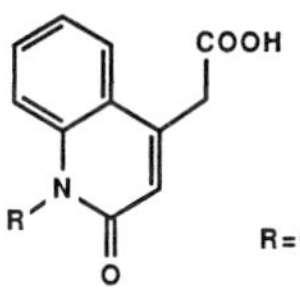 $R{=}CH_2C_6H_4Cl(p)$	0.2	0.04	5.0
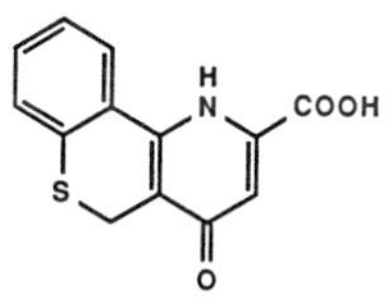	15	25	0.6
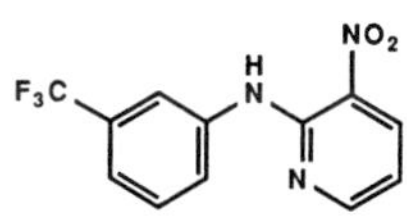	17	21	0.8

bovine and rat lens aldose reductase, though the bovine preparation was uniformly less sensitive to inhibition, with a mean "bovine/rat" ratio of 3.2 ± 1.3 (SD).

Based on their results Kador et al[147] suggested that "the evaluation of AR inhibitors for potential clinical use may require the use of human aldose reductase from the appropriate target tissue." Albeit tentative, this conclusion was interpreted

Table 10. Data from the National Eye Institute (NEI) and Ayerst Laboratories (AY)* on the in vitro inhibitory effect of various agents on aldose reductase isolated from rat lens.

Compound	$IC_{50} \times 10^{-6}M$		IC_{50} relative to alrestatin	
	NEI	AY	NEI	AY
Tetramethyleneglutarate (TMG)	2	4.5	1.0	1.1
Alrestatin	2	4	1.0	1.0
Rutin	2.5	12	1.2	3.0
Quercetin	0.6	15	0.3	3.7
Morin	5	13	2.5	3.2
Toxifolin	5	30	2.5	7.5
Hesperetin	7	30	3.5	7.5
Kemferol	6	45	3.0	11.2
Fisetin	1	4	0.5	1.0

*Based on data from Varma and Kinoshita[151] and unpublished results from the Ayerst Laboratories.[148]

Table 11. In vitro inhibitory activities reported for orally effective AR inhibitors.

AR inhibitor	$IC_{50} \times 10^{-8}M$					
	Bovine lens	Rat lens	Dog lens	Human lens	Human placenta	Human erythrocytes
Tolrestat	3.5[a]	1.1[b]	2.0[b]	0.3[b]	14[b]	3[a]
Statil[c]	2.6	6.6	—	2.0	15	470
Epalrestat[d]	—	1.0	—	—	2.6	150
Sorbinil	50[e];41[g]	25[g];7.0[f]	33[b]	22[b]	68[f]	—
AL-1567	15.6[g]	3.2[g];4.3[h]	—	—	24[h]	—
AL-1576	1.4[g]	0.7[g];2.4[h]	—	—	9[h]	—

[a]Simard-Duquesne et al[152]
[b]Kador et al[144]
[c]Stribling et al[146]
[d]Terashima et al[139]
[e]Peterson et al[153]
[f]Kador et al[147]
[g]Müller et al[149]
[h]Griffin et al[154]

by Flynn[48] to be "related to small differences in the primary structures of the enzymes from various species." As a consequence, since the orally effective AR inhibitors used to date are of the non-competitive type, Flynn concluded that they "will of necessity have different effects because the different primary structures of these enzymes will have different binding properties." We consider both conclusions[48,147] to be overextended. First, in a given laboratory only minor relative differences in inhibitory activity of a series of AR inhibitors are usually observed with aldose reductase from different animal species (see, for example, Tables 7, 9, and 12). Second, since the inhibitory values are usually obtained with partially purified enzyme preparations, it is unlikely that the observed variation reflects differences in the primary structure(s) of aldose reductases from different sources.

Table 12. In vitro comparison of the intrinsic inhibitory acitivity of orally effective AR inhibitors on rat and bovine lens aldose reductase.[155]

AR inhibitor	$IC_{50} \times 10^{-8}$M		
	Bovine (B)	Rat (R)	B/R
Tolrestat	3.5	0.6	5.8
Statil	3.7	1.3	2.8
Epalrestat	4.6	1.4	3.3
AL-1576	5.1	1.6	3.2
AL-1567	16.6	10.6	1.6
Sulindac	53.8	16.2	3.3
Sorbinil	112.0	40.0	2.8

Third, at least five of the widely used AR inhibitors, i.e., TMG,[26] alrestatin,[27] sorbinil,[153] tolrestat,[152] and statil,[146] were discovered through their effect in vitro on partially purified enzyme isolated from calf lenses, applying the procedure of Hayman and Kinoshita.[74] Fourth, except for TMG, all of these AR inhibitors have been found to be effective upon oral administration in both laboratory animals and man. This does not connote, however, that the capacity of a substance to inhibit aldose reductase in vitro implies inhibition (upon oral administration) in vivo. In vivo, the effectiveness of an AR inhibitor depends on the amount of inhibitor available in a given tissue to interact with aldose reductase without diffusional barriers intervening. An effective AR inhibitor must, therefore, attain adequate concentrations at the sites of aldose reductase in any tissue prone to develop diabetic complications due to the aldose reductase-catalyzed disposition of excess glucose. In any such tissue the pharmacodynamics of an AR inhibitor correspond to its intrinsic inhibitory activity and to its concentration at the site of aldose reductase. Such concentrations are determined by the pharmacokinetics of the AR inhibitor, i.e., by the processes determining its absorption, distribution, metabolism and elimination. These processes may vary between tissues in the same species (Table 13) or between species, and in addition, they may depend on any variable that can affect the pharmacokinetics of the AR inhibitor.[157]

Effect of aldose reductase inhibitors on hexonate dehydrogenase

In view of the apparent physico-chemical resemblance between aldose reductase and hexonate dehydrogenase and their overlapping substrate specificity,[47,48,50,57] several investigators have examined, in vitro, the effect of known AR inhibitors on hexonate dehydrogenase [7,15,67,97,158–160] (Tables 14 and 15). Despite the variation in the reported values, particularly for the hexonate dehydrogenase, the results indicate that, at high concentrations, all of the AR inhibitors tested can also inhibit hexonate dehydrogenase, albeit to a different degree. The results shown in Table 15 indicate that tolrestat and statil are more aldose reductase-specific than sorbinil since considerably higher concentrations are required to inhibit hexonate dehydrogenase to the same degree as aldose reductase: 8 to 29 times for sorbinil, 10 to 217 times for tolrestat, and 20 to 323 times higher for statil, respectively. It is,

Table 13. In vitro comparison of the intrinsic inhibitory activity of orally effective AR inhibitors in rat lens, and of the effects on polyol synthesis in rat erythrocyte, sciatic nerve, and lens, incubated in hexose-rich medium.[156]

	$IC_{50} \times 10^{-8}M$			
AR Inhibitor	**Lens AR**	**Polyol synthesis, in vitro**		
		Erythrocytes[a]	**Sciatic nerve[a]**	**Lens[b]**
Tolrestat	0.6	1.2	54	100
Statil	1.3	11	140	180
Epalrestat	1.4	130	280	310
Sorbinil	40	74	220	1200

[a]Incubated in 25 to 50 mM glucose
[b]Incubated in 30 mM galactose

Table 14. In vitro inhibition of aldose reductase and hexonate dehydrogenase reported for tetramethyleneglutarate, alrestatin, and sorbinil.

AR inhibitor	**Conc. (mM)**	**Percent inhibition of**					
		Aldose reductase			**Hexonate dehydrogenase**		
		a	**b**	**c**	**a**	**b**	**c**
Tetramethyleneglutarate	0.2			77			27
(TMG)	0.5			86			41
Alrestatin	0.1	73	42		40	51	
	0.01	54	26		8	11	
	0.05			70			15
Sorbinil	0.1	74	64		83	94	
	0.01	55	36	48	54	80	68
	0.05			95			85

[a]Pig muscle AR, pig kidney HDH (Flynn and Cromlish[67])
[b]Pig brain AR and HDH (Cromlish and Flynn[15])
[c]Human erythrocyte AR and HDH (Das and Srivastava[97])

therefore, not very likely that doses required to produce a clinically effective degree of aldose reductase inhibition would also affect hexonate dehydrogenase.

Since the physiological role of hexonate dehydrogenase is unknown,[14,126] the consequence(s) of its inhibition under physiological conditions cannot be considered with any degree of confidence. In diabetes, on the other hand, in tissues containing both aldose reductase and hexonate dehydrogenase, hexonate dehydrogenase, in view of its lower affinity for glucose, may not be able to compete with aldose reductase for the available glucose. In tissues containing only hexonate dehydrogenase, to the extent that hexonate dehydrogenase converts glucose to sorbitol,[54] its inhibition by a non-specific AR inhibitor would, in fact, be desirable.

Table 15. Comparative inhibition in vitro of aldose reductase and hexonate dehydrogenase by tolrestat, statil, and sorbinil.

AR inhibitor	$IC_{50} \times 10^{-8}$								
	Aldose reductase (AR)			Hexonate dehydrogenase (HDH)			HDH/AR		
	a	b	c	a	b	c	a	b	c
Tolrestat	0.6	1.1	1.8	130	11	136	217	10	76
Statil	1.3	1.6	61	420	190	1190	323	119	20
Sorbinil	40	7.0	35	380	200	295	9.5	29	8.4

[a]Rat lens AR, pig kidney HDH (Millen et al[155])
[b]Rat lens AR, rat kidney HDH (Sato et al[159])
[c]Rat lens AR, rat kidney HDH (Skau et al[160])

Effect on polyol accumulation

Because it cannot compete with hexokinase for the available glucose, the activity of aldose reductase is barely detectable at physiological glucose concentrations. Therefore, for inhibition of aldose reductase to be measured, its activity must be increased by elevating the ambient concentration of glucose (or galactose) beyond the saturation level of hexokinase (or galactokinase). This is accomplished by incubating an aldose reductase-containing tissue in a medium enriched with glucose (or galactose), followed by the measurement of intracellular sorbitol (or galactitol) concentration in the presence and absence of an agent to be tested for its inhibitory effect on aldose reductase. Commonly, the lens, sciatic nerve, and erythrocytes are used.

Being avascular and dependent on the uptake of its nutrient from the aqueous humor, the lens is ideal for such studies, since the in vitro conditions mimic its behavior under physiological conditions.[161,162] In fact, the increased production of polyol by aldose reductase in the presence of high sugar concentrations[163–168] and the inhibition of aldose reductase[26,168] were first demonstrated in the lens. The same technique was used by Gabbay[169,170] to demonstrate aldose reductase activity and its inhibition in sciatic nerve incubated in high-glucose medium.

The lens[82] and sciatic nerve are preferred for such studies because they contain only aldose reductase.[114,170] Thus, the technique of incubating lenses or sciatic nerves in high-sugar medium has been used to demonstrate the activity of AR inhibitors such as TMG,[26,170] sorbinil,[136,153] sulindac,[136] ONO-2235,[139] and tolrestat.[156]

The presence of the polyol pathway in human red blood cells (RBC) and its dependence on ambient glucose concentration was uncovered by Morrison et al.[171] The pathway is active even under physiological conditions, and about 3% of the glucose taken up by the erythrocytes is normally metabolized via the polyol pathway. Therefore, the formation of sorbitol is attributed to aldose reductase rather than L-hexonate dehydrogenase, since the latter has a much lower affinity for glucose.[97] The formation of sorbitol from glucose by partially purified aldose reductase isolated from human erythrocytes was, in fact, demonstrated by Srivastava et al.[98] Because of the poor penetration of cell membranes by polyols,[172,173] the sorbitol concentration in RBCs was found to be about five times higher than in plasma.[171] When erythrocytes are incubated in a high-glucose medium, the intracellular sorbitol and fructose levels are increased in conjuction with the glucose concentrations,[174] reflecting the low affinity of aldose reductase for glucose as compared with that of hexokinase.[175]

The presence of aldose reductase in human erythrocytes was initially questioned,[82,176] and the NADPH-linked reduction of glucose was attributed to the action of L-hexonate dehydrogenase. Later, the presence of aldose reductase in human RBCs was demonstrated by Crabbe and colleagues,[76,177] who found its activity to be higher in diabetic patients with retinopathy and cataract.[71,178] The initial observations of Morrison et al[171] were confirmed by Malone et al[179] and amplified by their finding of significantly higher RBC sorbitol levels in children with diabetes [28.0 $\pm$ 18.9 nmol/g hemoglobin ($\pm$SD)] as compared with a non-diabetic cohort (10.1 $\pm$ 7.2 nmol/g). That the RBC sorbitol levels in subjects with diabetes are indeed about twice as high as those in non-diabetics has been corroborated in a number of studies.[179-187] Of relevance is the finding of Barretto et al[188] that erythrocyte sorbitol dehydrogenase activity was significantly lower in IDDM patients [0.22 $\pm$ 0.08 U/min.g Hb ($\pm$SD)] than in normal subjects 0.34 $\pm$ 0.09 U/min.g Hb]. Recently, Srivastava et al[51] established the presence of aldose reductase and hexonate dehydrogenase in human erythrocytes immunochemically and also by isolating, purifying, and characterizing the enzyme.[97] Wirth and Wermuth,[14] on the other hand, were again unable to detect aldose reductase in human RBC immunohistochemically.

The use of human RBC incubated in a high-glucose medium as a test to demonstrate the activity of an AR inhibitor was introduced by Malone et al[179,180] with TMG and was later used by several investigators[139,146,152,156,189] to measure the polyol-lowering capacity of other AR inhibitors.

We have used the procedure involving incubation of different aldose reductase-containing tissues in sugar-rich medium to develop some perception of the interaction between factors affecting the bioavailability of an AR inhibitor at the sites of aldose reductase.[157] Comparison of the IC_{50} values obtained with the AR inhibitors tolrestat,[156] statil, epalrestat, and sorbinil in rat RBC, sciatic nerve, and lens shows that, for all AR inhibitors tested, the IC_{50} values increased in the same sequence, i.e., RBC, sciatic nerve, lens (Table 13). The observation that different inhibitor concentrations in the incubation medium are required to produce in different tissues the same degree of AR inhibition suggests that the rates of tissular inhibitor uptake are different.

The rate of uptake of a systemically available AR inhibitor by the erythrocyte can also be demonstrated ex vivo, i.e., by collecting the RBC from laboratory animals or human subjects given an AR inhibitor by mouth, then incubating the RBC in hexose-rich medium. This is illustrated below by the results obtained with erythrocytes [incubated in 25 mM (450 mg/dL) glucose] collected from dogs two hours after oral administration of an AR inhibitor.[157]

AR Inhibitor	Dose mg/kg	Inhibition of RBC sorbitol synthesis (%)
Tolrestat	5	66
AL-1576	5	54
(±)Sorbinil	5	36.5
Statil	5	30.5
Epalrestat	20	0

The technique using incubation of erythrocytes with galactose was also selected to demonstrate the presence of an AR inhibitor, statil, in the plasma of human subjects given the drug by mouth. The correlation of plasma AR inhibitor concentrations with the RBC galactitol concentration, i.e., degree of AR inhibition, indicated an IC_{50} of approximately 3.3×10^{-5}M (13 μg/mL) achieved by oral doses of 600 mg to 1000 mg of statil.[190]

Aldose reductase, isolated from human aorta, brain,[115] and RBC[98,191] was reported to be activated by ambient glucose concentrations.[192] The activated form exhibited altered kinetics and was less sensitive to the AR inhibitors alrestatin and sorbinil.

Another tissue capable of synthesizing sorbitol is the human platelet. As demonstrated by Bidot-Lopez et al,[193] in contrast to platelets from non-diabetics, those of diabetic subjects contain sorbitol, with the levels directly corresponding to the plasma glucose concentration. Upon incubation in a glucose-rich medium, the platelets from non-diabetic and diabetic subjects were shown to synthesize sorbitol. The biosynthesis of sorbitol was prevented by adding alrestatin to the medium.[194]

The presence of aldose reductase in monkey-kidney epithelial-cell cultures was suggested by the presence of sorbitol upon incubating the culture in glucose-rich medium and by preventing sorbitol formation with TMG.[195] The finding was corroborated with the structurally distinct AR inhibitors ICI-105,552 and two flavonoids.[196]

Aldose reductase was also localized in the cultured human retinoblastoma cell line Y-79 by Russell et al.[197] Upon incubation in a medium containing 30 mM (540 mg/dL) galactose, considerable accumulation of galactitol occurred. The accumulation was reduced by adding sorbinil to the medium.

Li et al[198] have reported that the sorbitol content of cultured bovine retinal capillary pericytes was increased by high glucose concentration in the culture medium and that the increase was reduced in concentration-dependent fashion by sorbinil. The glucose-induced increase in pericyte collagen synthesis[199] was not, however, affected by sorbinil.[198] The D-glucose transport by cultured bovine retinal capillary pericytes is an insulin-dependent, sodium-independent, stereospecific carrier-mediated transport process, which does not require a direct input of metabolic energy.[200] Holman et al[201] were able to culture canine and human retinal capillary pericytes that continued to express the cytoplasmic aldose reductase. AR activity was demonstrated by production of xylitol by cells grown in medium supplemented with xylose; xylitol production was prevented by the AR inhibitor tolrestat.

Hexitol-producing activity was also demonstrated in microvessels isolated from dog retina and incubated with galactose;[202] the activity was inhibited by sorbinil.

The presence of aldose reductase in rat embryos was suggested by the finding of increased sorbitol concentrations upon incubation of cultured rat embryos[104] or rat conceptuses (embryos, visceral yolk sacs, and ectoplacental cones)[105] in the presence of high glucose concentrations. Supporting evidence was provided by decreasing the amounts of sorbitol formed by adding to the incubation medium either statil[104,105] or sorbinil.[105] At 1×10^{-5}M, sorbinil decreased sorbitol accumulation by 82% and statil, by 70% at 5×10^{-5}M.[105]

Testing in vivo

As mentioned earlier, under physiological ambient sugar concentrations AR activity is so low that intracellular polyol levels are practically undetectable in the majority of tissues containing aldose reductase. To measure AR activity in vivo, the activity must be enhanced by increasing the supply of the sugar serving as substrate. Experimentally, high systemic sugar concentrations are produced by inducing diabetes or by feeding a diet rich in galactose. Under such conditions, the AR activity or its inhibition can be determined either directly or indirectly: directly, by measuring polyol concentrations in tissue(s) known to contain aldose reductase, or indirectly, by measuring in selected tissues the changes initiated by activation of the polyol pathway, the intracellular polyol accumulation, or both. Changes may be functional, such as nerve conduction velocity or axonal transport, or they may be morphological, such as lenticular opacity or capillary basement membrane thickening.

Diabetes is usually induced by a single intravenous or intraperitoneal injection of streptozocin (STZ). Within 48 hours, plasma glucose concentrations reach a level of at least 250 to 300 mg/dL, and they continue to rise over time to about 500 mg/dL. The accumulation of sorbitol is readily detectable several days after induction of diabetes. As shown in Table 16, the relative accumulation of sorbitol in rats is much greater in the lens than in the sciatic nerve. A linear relationship between the concentrations of glucose, sorbitol, and fructose in the nerve of STZ-induced diabetic rats was originally shown by Gabbay et al[204] and confirmed by Ward et al.[205]

Table 16. Sorbitol levels in the sciatic nerve and lens of streptozocin-induced diabetic rats.

Strain (Body wt.)	Dose of streptozocin (mg/kg)	Days of diabetes	Group	Sorbitol (nmol/mg ± SE)		Ref. No.
				Sc. nerve	Lens	
Sprague Dawley			ND	0.07 ± 0.02	0.15 ± 0.03	183
(150-240 g)	85, i.v.	8	D	1.08 ± 0.11	22.5 ± 2.3	
Sprague Dawley			ND	0.08 ± 0.01	0.52 ± 0.05	152
(150 g)	55, i.v.	21	D	1.30 ± 0.11	37.22 ± 2.51	
Wistar			ND	0.15 ± 0.04	0.36 ± 0.05	203
(250 g)	75, i.v.	28	D	1.55 ± 0.07	27.35 ± 2.18	

ND = Non-diabetic; D = Diabetic

As discussed in Chapter 3, orally administered galactose is readily absorbed, distributed, and metabolized in rats via the Leloir pathway (shown in Chapter 3, Fig 1, page 166) to glucose-1-phosphate, which can then enter the glycolytic pathway. Galactose present in excess of the saturation point of galactokinase, the rate-limiting enzyme of the Leloir pathway, is converted by aldose reductase to galactitol, which is readily detectable in tissues of galactosemic rats[19,206,207] and galactosemic human subjects.[208] Since the affinity of aldose reductase for galactose is much greater than that of L-hexonate dehydrogenase,[54] the galactitol found in tissues of galactosemic rats was most likely formed in situ[172] by the action of aldose reductase (Table 4).

In addition, aldose reductase has a greater affinity for D-galactose (Km, 20 mM) than for D-glucose (Km, 70 mM).[74] This is due to the different configuration of carbon atom 4. In contrast to glucose, the 4-hydroxy group of galactose is axial, making the cyclic hemi-acetal form less stable; a higher proportion of galactose is thus in the "open" aldehyde form[109] needed for acceptance as substrate for aldose reductase.[74,110] Furthermore, by being a poor substrate for the polyol dehydrogenase,[23,209] in contrast to sorbitol, galactitol is not further oxidized. The intracellular galactitol concentration thus becomes very elevated. These properties of galactose, coupled with its facile absorption after oral administration, result in very fast attainment of high tissue galactitol levels.

Galactose is administered to laboratory animals either by gastric intubation or admixture with the diet, the latter being preferred in chronic studies. As illustrated in Table 17, similar tissue galactitol levels are produced by either mode of administration. As shown in Chapter 3, Fig 3, page 171, the accumulation of galactitol in the diaphragm, sciatic nerve, and lens in rats is correlated with the amount of galactose ingested. The rate of galactitol accumulation in the sciatic nerve and lens of the galactose-fed rat is distinctly faster than the rate of sorbitol accumulation in the diabetic rat. Similar tissue polyol accumulation was thus achieved after four days of 10% galactose feeding or 21 days of STZ-induced diabetes (Table 18).

Table 17. Galactitol accumulation in rats given galactose by gastric intubation or admixed with the diet.[210]

Mode of galactose administration (for three days)	Galactitol accumulation (nmol/mg ± SE)		
	Diaphragm	Heart	Lens
Gastric intubation, 12 g/kg/day	4.6 ± 0.3	6.2 ± 0.5	16.6 ± 1.1
10% of diet	4.5 ± 0.7	7.9 ± 1.3	14.4 ± 1.4

Another advantage of galactose-fed animal models is that the biochemical, functional, and morphological changes associated with polyol accumulation appear to occur in the presence of insulin. Galactose slightly increases insulin output in the presence of a stimulatory concentration of glucose, but fails to provoke insulin release in the absence of glucose.[211] Therefore, it is useful to demonstrate the effectiveness of an AR inhibitor in both diabetic and galactosemic laboratory animals.

Table 18. Comparison of polyol accumulation in streptozocin-induced diabetic rats and in rats fed galactose with the diet.[210]

Treatment	Duration (days)	Polyol accumulation (nmol/mg ± SE)	
		Sciatic nerve	Lens
Streptozocin (55 mg/kg, i.v.)	21	1.22 ± 0.11[a]	36.70 ± 2.51[a]
10% Galactose in the diet	4	1.59 ± 0.16[b]	29.73 ± 1.21[a]

[a]Sorbitol
[b]Galactitol

Effect of AR inhibitors on tissue polyol accumulation and myoinositol depletion

Polyol accumulation

The effectiveness of an AR inhibitor in vivo is usually expressed as the dose, in mg/kg, that produces a specified decrease in tissue polyol levels. Preferably, dose-dependency is determined, and the ED_{50}, which is the dose causing 50% decrease in polyol accumulation, is calculated. Since tissue polyol accumulation is dependent on the experimental conditions, it is not unusual that for a given AR inhibitor the estimated effective doses vary within and between laboratories.

Alrestatin

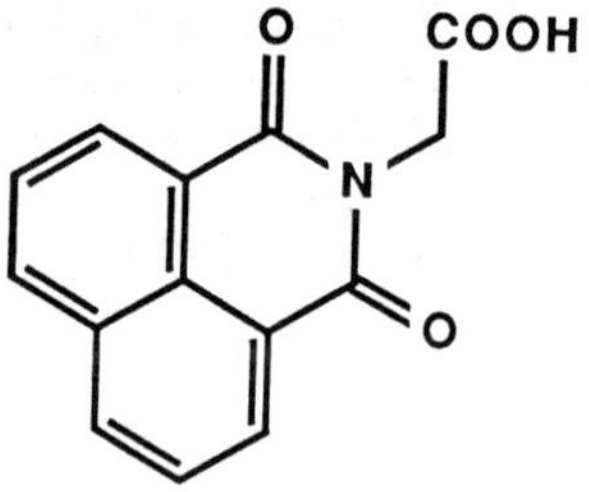

Alrestatin

That aldose reductase can be inhibited in vivo in the lens and sciatic nerve, two tissues known to contain only aldose reductase[114] was demonstrated in 1973 in STZ-induced diabetic rats and in rats fed galactose and treated with alrestatin (AY-22,284).[27] The results, presented in Table 19, illustrate the different experimental conditions used to detect a drug effect on polyol accumulation. The effects of alrestatin on sorbitol and fructose levels in the sciatic nerve of STZ-diabetic rats fed 72% fructose in the diet are summarized in Table 20.

Sorbinil

The effects of the uncompetitive AR inhibitor sorbinil (CP-45,634)[153] on polyol accumulation in the sciatic nerve and lens of diabetic and galactosemic rats obtained under different experimental conditions are presented in Tables 21 and 22. Sorbinil was also shown to decrease polyol accumulation in the kidney[218] and glomeruli[219] of diabetic rats (Table 23), and to decrease the accumulation of galactitol in the renal cortex and medulla of rats fed 50% galactose with the diet.[220]

Table 19. Effect of alrestatin on polyol accumulation in diabetic and galactose-fed rats. (From Dvornik et al[27])

Rat model	Alrestatin (% of diet)	Duration (days)	Group	Polyol accumulation (nmol/mg ± SE)	
				Sciatic nerve	Lens
Streptozocin-induced diabetic (85 mg/kg, i.v.)	0.6	21	Control	2.03 ± 0.11	—
			Treated	1.15 ± 0.16[a]	
10% Galactose-fed	0.7	3	Control	—	14.43 ± 0.77
			Treated	—	7.19 ± 0.49[b]
30% Galactose-fed	0.7	7	Control	3.29 ± 0.82	—
			Treated	0.82 ± 0.16[c]	

[a]Fructose levels were also decreased from 4.55 ± 0.33 to 2.28 ± 0.22 nmol/mg; for both constituents, $p<0.001$.
[b]$p<0.01$
[c]$p<0.02$

Table 20. Effect of aldose reductase inhibitors on sorbitol and fructose accumulation and tail-nerve conduction velocity in streptozocin-induced diabetic rats fed 72% fructose with the diet. (From Hotta et al[212])

Group	Dose of AR inhibitor (mg/kg/day)	nmol/mg ± SE		MNCV (m/sec ± SE)
		Sorbitol	Fructose	
ND + F	—	0.11 ± 0.02	1.07 ± 0.07	36.3 ± 1.0
D + F	—	0.47 ± 0.04[c]	5.96 ± 0.50[c]	28.3 ± 0.6
D + F + Alrestatin	900	0.17 ± 0.03	2.70 ± 0.65[a]	33.1 ± 0.9[a]
D + F + Epalrestat	50	0.25 ± 0.05[a]	3.14 ± 0.69[a]	33.8 ± 1.3
D + F + Insulin	—	0.22 ± 0.03[a]	2.44 ± 0.35[b]	33.6 ± 1.2

Wistar rats (body wt., 200-250 g) were injected with streptozocin (40 mg/kg, i.v.) and, after 16 days, fed for four weeks 72% fructose with the diet. ND = Non-Diabetic; F = Fructose-fed; D = Diabetic.
[a]$p<0.05$
[b]$p<0.01$
[c]$p<0.001$ as compared with D + F group.

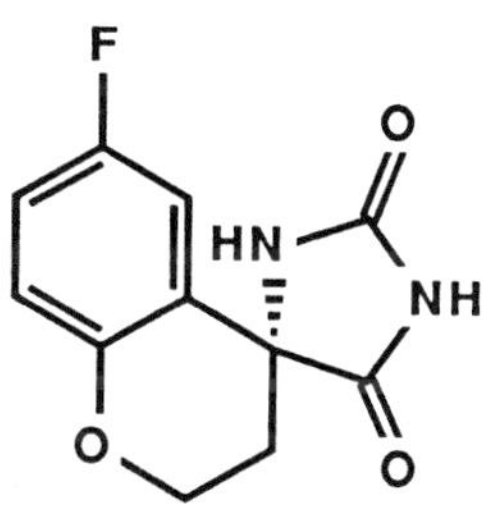

Sorbinil

Partial normalization of RBC sorbitol levels was reported by Yue et al for sorbinil[221] and by Akanuma et al[222] for methosorbinil (M-79,175), the 2-methyl analog of sorbinil.[223]

Table 21. Effect of sorbinil on sorbitol accumulation in diabetic rats.

Strain (Body wt.)	Diabetes induced with (mg/kg)	Sorbinil (mg/kg/day)	Duration	Group	Sorbitol (nmol/mg ± SE)		Ref. No.
					Sciatic nerve	Lens	
Wistar (250 g)	Alloxan (200, s.c.)	40 + 0.05 mg/rat topically	6 d	ND D DT	—	0.33 ± 0.03 12.2 ± 0.52 0.6 ± 0.06	213
Charles River (200-250 g)	STZ (85, i.v.)	5	2 w D + 1 w T	D DT	1.57 ± 0.18 0.13 ± 0.01	25.60 ± 2.37 2.68 ± 0.28	153
Sprague Dawley (150-240 g)	STZ (85, i.v.)	5	2 w D + 1 w T	ND D DT	0.07 ± 0.02 1.08 ± 0.11 0.10 ± 0.02	0.15 ± 0.03 22.5 ± 2.3 4.4 ± 0.8	183
Sprague Dawley (60 g)	STZ (60, i.v.)	20	16 d D + 5 d T	ND D DT	—	0.28 ± 0.05 21.01 ± 1.05 0.43 ± 0.08	214
			30 d	D DT	—	45.31 ± 4.79 1.28 ± 0.20	
Wistar (290-310 g)	STZ (50, i.p.)	25	42 d	ND D DT	0.05 ± 0.01 1.48 ± 0.14 0.09 ± 0.01	—	215
Wistar (270-320 g)	STZ (50, i.p.)	20	10 w	ND D DT	0.25 ± 0.01 2.38 ± 0.17 0.51 ± 0.09	—	216

ND = Non-diabetic; D = Diabetic; DT = Diabetic treated; STZ = Streptozocin; d = day; w = week; T = Treatment.

Table 22. Effect of sorbinil on galactitol accumulation in galactose-fed Sprague Dawley rats.

Body wt.	Galactose (% of diet)	Sorbinil (mg/kg/day)	Duration (days)	Group	Galactitol (nmol/mg ± SE)		Ref. No.
					Sciatic nerve	Lens	
200-250 g	30	11.5	7	G	—	35.24 ± 6.66	153
				GT		1.52 ± 0.02	
50 g	50	1% solution topically to the eye, 3 days pretreatment	5	G	6.6 ± 2.2	74.7 ± 8.0	217
				GT	0.16 ± 0.14	19.0 ± 4.0	

G = Galactose-fed; T = Treated

Table 23. Effect of sorbinil on aldose reductase in the kidney of diabetic rats.

Diabetes induced by	Sorbinil (mg/kg/day)	Duration	Group	Sorbitol		Ref. No.
				Kidney (nmol/mg ± SE)	Glomerulus (nmol/mg protein ± SE)	
Alloxan	10	6 days	ND	0.26 ± 0.01	—	
			D[a]	0.32 ± 0.02		218
			DT	0.25 ± 0.01		
STZ (60 mg/kg, i.v.)	20	6 weeks	ND	—	0.84 ± 0.18	219
			D		6.39 ± 1.74	
			DT		0.48 ± 0.01	
		9 weeks	ND	—	0.43 ± 0.06	
			D		1.31 ± 0.39	
			DT		0.63 ± 0.12	

ND = Non-diabetic; D = Diabetic; DT = Diabetic treated; STZ = Streptozocin
[a]The increase in fructose levels (from 0.17 ± 0.01 to 0.26 ± 0.02) was prevented by sorbinil at a dose of 40 mg/kg/day.

Decreased erythrocyte deformability observed in diabetic rats was prevented by administration of sorbinil at a dose of 20 mg/kg/day.[224] However, in human RBC incubated in 22 mM (396 mg/dL) glucose, 25 μM (9 μg/mL) sorbinil failed to prevent the decrease in deformability in spite of preventing sorbitol accumulation. The finding suggests that the hyperglycemia-induced decrease in erythrocyte deformability may not be linked with AR activity.[225]

Incubation of washed erythrocytes (from normal human subjects) in 50 mM (900 mg/dL) glucose for two hours resulted in a 13% decrease in RBC filterability.[226] This decrease was associated with a marked increase in RBC sorbitol concentration. The fact that both alterations were prevented by the addition of sorbinil (2×10^{-5}M) to the medium implicates aldose reductase in the impairment of RBC filterability. However, in view of the small decrease, sorbitol accumulation may not play an important role in the rheology of erythrocytes from poorly controlled diabetic patients.[226] This view is supported by the finding of Kern et al[227] that, in dogs fed on a 30% galactose diet, despite very high polyol levels [1428 ± 417 nmol/g Hb (±SD)] as compared with poorly controlled diabetic (80 ± 29) or normal dogs (38 ± 13), whole blood filterability was not significantly impaired.

Tolrestat

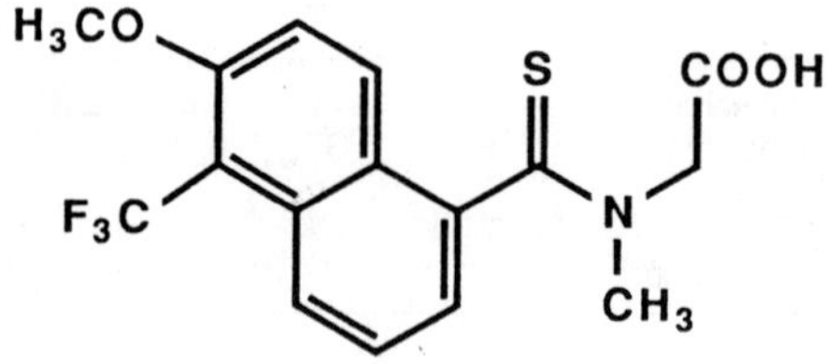

Tolrestat

The dose-dependence of the effect of an AR inhibitor on sorbitol formation in the erythrocytes of diabetic rats may be illustrated by the results obtained with the uncompetitive AR inhibitor tolrestat (AY-27,773; Alredase®).[152] As shown in Table 24, the approximately 2.5 times higher RBC sorbitol levels (attained in 9-day diabetic rats*) decreased in proportion to plasma drug concentrations, without affecting the elevated plasma glucose levels. At a dose of 1.8 mg/kg, tolrestat reduced the RBC sorbitol levels to those found in non-diabetic rats; higher doses caused further lowering. Dose-dependent lowering of RBC sorbitol has also been demonstrated in non-diabetic rats (Table 25); this finding supports the postulate that RBC sorbitol is produced by aldose reductase rather than L-hexonate dehydrogenase.[179]

Table 24. Effect of tolrestat on red blood cell (RBC) sorbitol concentrations in diabetic rats. [From Simard-Duquesne et al[152]]

Tolrestat (mg/kg/day)	Plasma tolrestat (ng/mL ± SE)	Plasma glucose (mg/dL ± SE)		RBC sorbitol (nmol/g Hb ± SE)
		Start	End	
0	0	474 ± 6	416 ± 16	126 ± 6
1.0	<25 ± 2	476 ± 8	444 ± 15	71 ± 4*
1.8	50 ± 7	472 ± 5	422 ± 6	54 ± 3*
3.9	110 ± 9	474 ± 7	439 ± 9	38 ± 3*
7.4	244 ± 24	472 ± 10	432 ± 12	27 ± 2*
ND rats	—	151 ± 3	141 ± 2	49 ± 3

Sprague Dawley rats were used, b.w. 150 g. Diabetes was induced with streptozocin (55 mg/kg, i.v.); ND = Non-diabetic
*p <0.001

In STZ-induced diabetic rats, tolrestat maintained sciatic nerve sorbitol and fructose at levels found in age-matched non-diabetic animals; this was shown in 2-week diabetic rats with a daily dose of 5 mg/kg[228] (Table 26) and in 6-month diabetic rats with a dose of 25 mg/kg/day[230] (Table 27).

*About five times higher RBC sorbitol levels were found in 5-week STZ-diabetic rats.[223]

Table 25. Effect of tolrestat on red blood cell (RBC) sorbitol levels in nondiabetic rats. (From Simard-Duquesne et al[152])

Tolrestat (mg/kg/day for 14 days)	Plasma glucose (mg/dL ± SE)	RBC sorbitol (nmol/g Hb ± SE)
0	145 ± 3	51.0 ± 4.5
1.0	138 ± 3	35.5 ± 3.8
1.9	148 ± 2	33.5 ± 6.2*
3.8	149 ± 3	26.2 ± 4.4**
7.1	149 ± 3	16.5 ± 3.0***

*$p < 0.05$; **$p < 0.01$; ***$p < 0.001$

The effectiveness of an AR inhibitor in animals fed galactose corresponds to the amount of AR inhibitor present at the site of aldose reductase at the time of galactose entry, hence, upon the experimental conditions used. Since large doses of galactose are administered to accumulate galactitol rapidly, particularly in the lens, an orally administered AR inhibitor is being absorbed and transported to the sites of aldose reductase in the presence of large amounts of galactose. For example, the ratio in the diet between an AR inhibitor at a dose of 10 mg/kg and galactose can vary from 1:1400 (with 10% galactose in the diet) to 1:3900 (with 25% galactose in the diet). The differences in tissue galactitol levels found in the absence and presence of an AR inhibitor reflect, therefore, not only its effectiveness upon administration with a diet rich in galactose, but also the rate and extent of AR inhibitor transport to the site of aldose reductase as compared with those of galactose. The pharmacodynamics of an AR inhibitor in galactose-fed rats thus depends on the interplay of the pharmacokinetics of both AR substrate and AR inhibitor. This is illustrated in studies conducted by Simard-Duquesne et al with tolrestat and (±)sorbinil.[152]

That the effectiveness of an AR inhibitor depends on the timing of its administration relative to that of galactose is illustrated by the 2.6- to 4.6-fold decrease in the ED_{50} of tolrestat, as contingent on duration of pretreatment before the animals were given access to the galactose-containing diet. The ED_{50} of tolrestat in diabetic rats has also been increased through pretreatment, albeit to a lesser extent than in galactosemic rats (Table 28). Pretreatment was also used to determine the effect of an AR inhibitor on galactitol accumulation in the erythrocytes and sciatic nerve: rats were pretreated with statil for five days, then given a single oral dose of galactose (15 g/kg), followed after one hour by the measurement of galactitol levels.[146] The influence of pretreatment on the effectiveness of an AR inhibitor, 1-[(p-bromophenyl)sulfonyl] hydantoin (p-Br-PSH), was also reported by Okuda et al.[231]

The effectiveness of an AR inhibitor in galactosemic rats also depends on the amount of galactose ingested, i.e., on the acuteness of severe galactosemia. As shown in Table 29, a decrease of galactose intake from 27.3 g/day for 4 days to 13.3 g/day for 12 days increased the ED_{50} of tolrestat in the lens by a factor of 8.5. For (±)sorbinil, the increase was 1.6-fold.[152]

Table 26. Effect of aldose reductase inhibitors on the levels of glucose, sorbitol, fructose, and myoinositol in the sciatic nerve of Wistar rats with short-term streptozocin-induced diabetes.

Aldose reductase inhibitor (mg/kg/day)	Group	nmol/mg ± SE				Ref. No.
		Glucose	Sorbitol	Fructose	Myoinositol	
Statil 25	ND	0.19 ± 0.05 *	0.01 ± 0.00	0.01 ± 0.00	3.31 ± 0.15 **	229
	NDT	0.76 ± 0.27 *	0.01 ± 0.00	0.01 ± 0.00	4.77 ± 0.12 **	
	D	10.25 ± 0.75 ***	2.19 ± 0.13	4.22 ± 0.33 *	2.65 ± 0.16 ***	
	DT	16.33 ± 0.83 ***	0.27 ± 0.07	2.92 ± 0.40 *	3.96 ± 0.20 ***	
Tolrestat[a] 10	ND	2.49 ± 0.18	0.12 ± 0.04	<0.64	3.00 ± 0.18 *	228
	NDT	3.95 ± 0.87	<0.08	<0.64	3.72 ± 0.24 *	
	D	13.52 ± 1.11 * *	1.77 ± 0.20[+]	3.49 ± 0.48[+]	2.26 ± 0.10 *	
5	DT	26.04 ± 1.30 * *	0.13 ± 0.04	<0.64	3.59 ± 0.19	
10	DT	19.51 ± 1.25 *	<0.08	<0.64	3.25 ± 0.15	
20	DT	16.36 ± 0.85	<0.08	<0.64	3.30 ± 0.19	

ND = Non-diabetic; NDT = Non-diabetic treated (either with statil, for 5 weeks, or with tolrestat, for 2 weeks); D = Diabetic (streptozocin, 50 mg/kg, i.p. for statil, and 55 mg/kg, i.v., for tolrestat); DT = Diabetic treated (with statil or tolrestat).

[a]Given for 10 days before induction of diabetes.

*$p<0.05$; **$p<0.01$; ***$p<0.001$; [+]Massive differences were not analyzed.

Table 27. Effect of tolrestat on glucose, sorbitol, fructose, and myoinositol levels in the sciatic nerve of Wistar rats with long-term streptozocin-induced diabetes. (From Dvornik et al[231])

		nmol/mg ± SE			
Diet	**Group**	**Glucose**	**Sorbitol**	**Fructose**	**Myoinositol**
Normal	ND	1.58 ± 0.10	0.04 ± 0.02	0.51 ± 0.04	3.17 ± 0.28
	NDT	1.58 ± 0.13	nd	0.06 ± 0.01	2.83 ± 0.22
	D	14.81 ± 1.95⁺	1.48 ± 0.25	8.36 ± 1.48	2.88 ± 0.41
	DT	13.48 ± 0.83	0.05 ± 0.02	0.36 ± 0.03	2.77 ± 0.31
68% Sucrose	ND	1.99 ± 0.11	0.09 ± 0.01	0.83 ± 0.08	2.82 ± 0.27
	NDT	1.46 ± 0.12	nd	0.11 ± 0.01	2.66 ± 0.37
	D	43.63 ± 3.72]*	3.76 ± 0.43	9.63 ± 0.80	2.09 ± 0.18
	DT	54.99 ± 5.11]*	0.40 ± 0.03	1.44 ± 0.13	2.99 ± 0.39

ND = Non-diabetic; NDT = Non-diabetic treated with tolrestat (25 mg/kg/day, for 6 months);
D = Diabetic (streptozocin, 25 mg/kg, i.v.); DT = Diabetic treated with tolrestat (25 mg/kg/day, for 6 months); ND = none detected;
*$p<0.05$;
⁺Massive differences were not analyzed.

The effect of an AR inhibitor on tissue polyol accumulation can also be demonstrated in galactosemic dogs.[210] The accumulation of galactitol in RBC, kidney cortex and medulla, aorta, retina, and sciatic nerve of dogs fed for four consecutive days on a diet containing 50% galactose was decreased in dose-dependent fashion by treatment with tolrestat (Table 30). The effect varied among the different tissues, reflecting the interplay in a given tissue of the pharmacokinetics of AR substrate and AR inhibitor.

Epalrestat

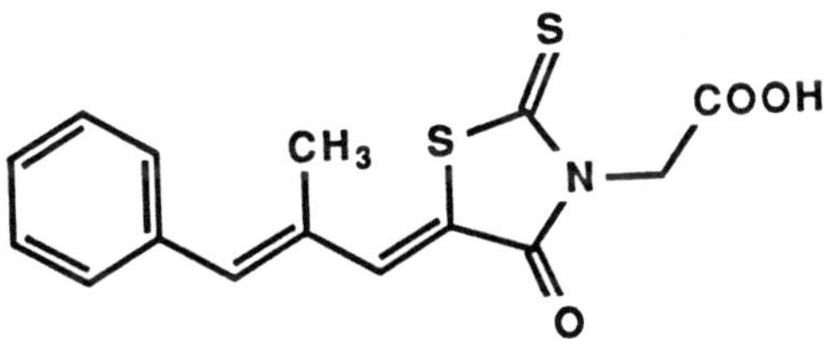

Epalrestat

The effects of the uncompetitive AR inhibitor epalrestat (ONO-2235; Sorbistat)[145] on sorbitol accumulation in the sciatic nerve of STZ-induced diabetic rats are summarized in Table 31. Based on the observation that tissue sorbitol and fructose accumulation in STZ-induced diabetic rats is increased by 30% if 72% fructose is added to their diet,[236] such treatment was used to evaluate the effects of epalrestat and alrestatin on polyol accumulation in the sciatic nerve and on tail-nerve conduction velocity. With the experimental conditions used, neither alrestatin, epalrestat nor insulin decreased the sorbitol and fructose levels by more than 50% to 60% while markedly improving the nerve conduction velocity (Table 20).[212]

Table 28. Effect of tolrestat on polyol accumulation in galactosemic and diabetic rats: Dependence upon the duration of pretreatment. (From Simard-Duquesne et al[152])

Experimental model	Days of pretreatment	ED_{50} (mg/kg/day)	
		Sciatic nerve	Lens
4-Day galactose-fed (20%) rat	0	11.8	128
	3	7.9	91
	6	8.0	45
	9	5.3	35
	12	4.5	28
10-Day STZ-induced diabetic rat	0	9	21
	11	5	12

ED_{50}: Dose decreasing polyol accumulation by 50%.
STZ = Streptozocin (55 mg/kg, i.v.)

Table 29. Effect of tolrestat and (±)sorbinil on galactitol accumulation in the lens of galactose-fed rats: Dependence on the acuteness and severity of galactosemia. (From Simard-Duquesne et al[152])

Experimental model	Galactose intake (g/day)	ED_{50} (mg/kg/day)	
		Tolrestat	(±)Sorbinil
20% Galactose for 4 days	27.3	128	12
15% Galactose for 8 days	20.9	66	11
10% Galactose for 12 days	13.3	15	7.5

Table 30. Effect of tolrestat on galactitol accumulation in dogs fed 50% galactose for 4 days. (From Millen et al[232])

Tolrestat (mg/kg/day)	Galactitol, nmol/mg ± SE*					
	RBC	Aorta	Sciatic nerve	Kidney cortex	Kidney medulla	Retina
0	599 ± 22	8.80 ± 0.44	5.78 ± 0.64	0.65 ± 0.14	3.29 ± 0.46	1.26 ± 0.09
5	99 ± 10	1.33 ± 0.20	2.41 ± 0.47	<0.5	0.27 ± 0.09	0.71 ± 0.17
10	88 ± 6	0.97 ± 0.14	1.57 ± 0.19	<0.5	0.38 ± 0.17	<0.5

Adult male beagle dogs (4 per group), b.w. 8.7 to 15.0 kg, were pretreated for 5 days with placebo or tolrestat.
*For all tolrestat-treated groups, $p<0.01$ as compared to galactose-fed controls.

Table 31. Effect of epalrestat on sorbitol accumulation in the sciatic nerve of diabetic rats.

Strain (Body wt.)	Diabetes induced with	Epalrestat (mg/kg/day)	Duration	Group	Sorbitol (nmol/mg ± SE)	Ref. No.
Sprague Dawley (250 g)	STZ (60, i.v.)	10–40	2 weeks	ND	0.04 ± 0.01	233
				D	0.60 ± 0.15	
				DT (10)	0.19 ± 0.05*	
				DT (20)	0.12 ± 0.01*	
				DT (40)	0.13 ± 0.03*	
Wistar (250 g)	STZ (40, i.v.)	50	2 weeks	ND	0.17	234
				D	0.86	
				DT	0.61*	
Sprague Dawley (230-260)	STZ (60, i.v.)	20, 40	2 weeks	ND	0.23 ± 0.02	235, 236
				D	1.31 ± 0.08	
				DT (20)	0.61 ± 0.26*	
				DT (40)	0.91 ± 0.33*	
Sprague Dawley (220 g)	STZ (65, i.v.)	50	3 weeks	ND	0.08 ± 0.01	237
				D	0.83 ± 0.19	
				DT	0.28 ± 0.14**	

STZ = Streptozocin; ND = Non-diabetic; D = Diabetic; DT = Diabetic treated.
*$p < 0.001$ as compared to D group; **$p < 0.02$ as compared with D group.

The initially reported effect of epalrestat on RBC sorbitol levels was relatively weak and unrelated to dose.[233] The finding was attributed to a difference in the transport rate of epalrestat to erythrocytes and sciatic nerve, since in the latter the compound had decreased sorbitol accumulation.[233] Later, significant decreases in RBC sorbitol levels were reported in STZ-induced diabetic rats given epalrestat orally at a dose of 50 mg/kg/day for eight days (62% decrease),[238] or, given for four weeks to diabetic rats fed on a 72%. sucrose diet (51% decrease).[212]

ICI-105,552

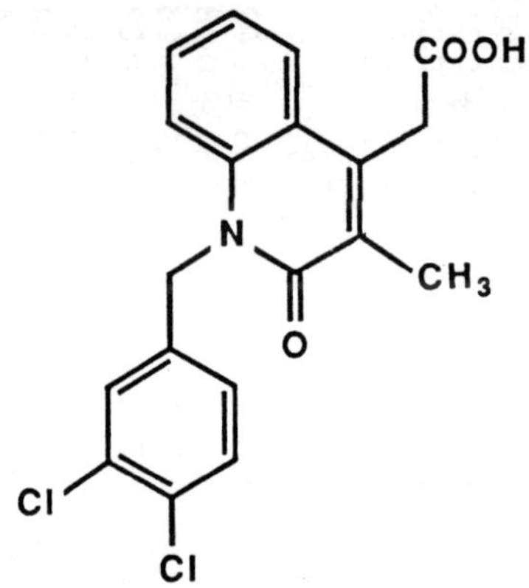

ICI-105,552

The effects of the oxoquinoline AR inhibitor ICI-105,552 on tissue sugar and polyol levels in STZ-induced diabetic rats are shown in Tables 32 and 33.[203,239] The results indicate a drug-induced decrease in sorbitol accumulation in the sciatic nerve, lens, and seminal vesicles, but not in the retina and kidney. Similar results were obtained in diabetic rats treated with ICI-105,552 at a dose of 50 mg/kg/day for 373 days.[240] Tentatively, the authors attributed the dissimilarity in effectiveness to tissue-specific differences in susceptibility of aldose reductase to inhibition. A more likely explanation is that the dissimilarities are due to differences in the tissue pharmacokinetics of an AR inhibitor with moderate intrinsic activity. The argument is supported by reports that renal polyol accumulation in diabetic[218] and galactosemic rats[220] was prevented by the more potent AR inhibitor sorbinil.

Statil

The effective dose of the non-competitive AR inhibitor Statil® (ICI-128,436)[146] varied, depending on the experimental conditions, with an ED_{50} (in mg/kg) in acutely galactosemic rats of 2.2 for erythrocytes and 8.6 for the sciatic nerve (5 in diabetic rats).[146] The results obtained in experiments of longer duration in the renal cortex and retina of STZ-induced diabetic rats are shown in Table 34, and in the sciatic nerve and lens, in Table 35.

Incubation of erythrocytes from IDDM patients or control subjects in 33 mM (560 mg/dL) glucose for three hours resulted in increased RBC viscosity. Addition to the

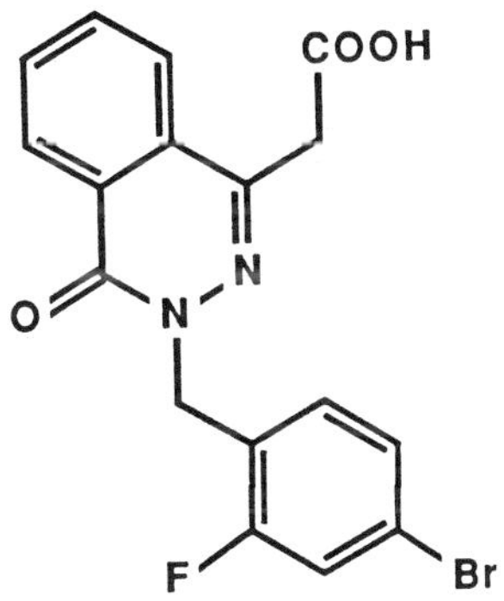

Statil

medium of statil completely inhibited RBC sorbitol synthesis and partially reduced the increase of viscosity in both diabetic and normal subjects.[241]

The greatly increased sorbitol levels found in the growth-retarded embryos of rats with STZ-induced diabetes indicated the presence of a functioning aldose reductase system during organogenesis.[242] Supporting evidence was obtained by preventing sorbitol accumulation (measured on gestational day 11) by giving the mothers statil orally at a dose of 25 mg/kg/day.[243] The results indicate the capacity of statil to penetrate to the site(s) of fetal aldose reductase. Of importance is the finding that the sorbitol accumulation and growth retardation are unrelated events because no change in embryonic or fetal growth was observed in the offsprings of diabetic mothers treated with the AR inhibitor.

Myoinositol depletion

Interest in tissue myoinositol levels was stimulated by the report of Greene et al[244] that the decrease in motor nerve conduction velocity (MNCV) in acute STZ-induced diabetic rats is associated with a decrease in nerve myoinositol, which can be compensated by adding 1% myoinositol to the diet. Addition of 3% myoinositol to the diet of normal rats, however, caused a fall in MNCV. As discussed more extensively in Chapter 2, the finding of Greene et al[244] was corroborated by many investigators in rats with short-term experimentally induced diabetes (Chapter 2, Table 2, page 114) and in rats fed galactose (Chapter 2, Table 3, page 116). However, on occasion, no change was detected.[203] This decrease in nerve myoinositol levels is small, the published values amounting to a median decrease of 22%. However, it was regarded by Simmons et al[245,246] as sufficient to affect the small, rapidly turning over pools of phosphatidylinositol believed to be involved in regulation of nerve metabolism, e.g., of the Na/K-dependent ATPase activity.

It is pertinent that normal myoinositol levels were found in sciatic nerve of rats with experimentally induced diabetes of six months' duration,[230,247] thus suggesting that neural myoinositol depletion could be transient, lasting only until the metabolic derangement attains steady state (see Chapter 2 for a more detailed discussion).

Table 32. Effect of ICI-105,552 on tissue sugar and polyol concentrations in streptozocin-induced diabetic rats. (From Poulsom and Heath[203])

Tissue	Group	Concentration (nmol/mg ± SE) Glucose	Sorbitol	Fructose	Myoinositol
Sc. nerve	ND	1.57 ± 0.12	0.15 ± 0.04	0.63 ± 0.07	2.51 ± 0.11
	NDT	1.56 ± 0.13 **	0.14 ± 0.03 **	0.62 ± 0.06 **	2.39 ± 0.17
	D	10.24 ± 0.37	1.55 ± 0.07	6.43 ± 0.41	2.34 ± 0.10
	DT	9.38 ± 0.72	0.34 ± 0.03 **	2.40 ± 0.25 **	2.15 ± 0.09
Lens	ND	0.31 ± 0.02	0.36 ± 0.05	0.78 ± 0.07	1.31 ± 0.10 **
	NDT	0.31 ± 0.06 **	0.29 ± 0.08 **	1.08 ± 0.24 **	1.05 ± 0.24
	D	5.23 ± 0.67	27.35 ± 2.18	9.64 ± 0.85	0.15 ± 0.01
	DT	5.14 ± 0.27	8.39 ± 1.03 **	7.98 ± 0.54	0.20 ± 0.03
Retina	ND	1.00 ± 0.17	0.29 ± 0.06	0.53 ± 0.13	0.66 ± 0.08
	NDT	0.93 ± 0.18	0.21 ± 0.04 *	0.46 ± 0.16 **	0.67 ± 0.07
	D	7.17 ± 0.77	0.62 ± 0.11	1.13 ± 0.08	0.91 ± 0.14
	DT	8.01 ± 0.72	0.43 ± 0.05	0.90 ± 0.09	0.74 ± 0.08
Kidney	ND	4.78 ± 0.38	0.28 ± 0.06	0.87 ± 0.06	8.09 ± 0.64
	NDT	4.15 ± 0.36 **	0.16 ± 0.02 **	0.83 ± 0.19 **	6.72 ± 0.79
	D	34.00 ± 2.75	0.91 ± 0.08	8.21 ± 1.13	7.54 ± 0.47
	DT	32.20 ± 2.06	0.88 ± 0.09	5.71 ± 0.51	7.63 ± 0.43
Seminal ves. and coag. glands	ND	1.42 ± 0.17	0.30 ± 0.06	2.61 ± 0.45	24.30 ± 2.14
	NDT	1.34 ± 0.17 **	0.22 ± 0.04 *	2.04 ± 0.40 **	30.40 ± 1.43
	D	13.70 ± 3.07	0.59 ± 0.05	5.54 ± 0.31	23.80 ± 2.07
	DT	16.20 ± 6.63	0.43 ± 0.07 *	3.95 ± 0.82	23.00 ± 2.64

ICI-105,552 was administered p.o. at a dose of 50 mg/kg/day for 22 days one week after induction of diabetes with streptozocin (75 mg/kg, i.v.).
ND = Non-diabetic; NDT = Non-diabetic treated; D = Diabetic; DT = Diabetic treated
*$p<0.05$; **$p<0.0001$.

Table 33. Effect of ICI-105,552 on sugar and polyol concentrations in the sciatic nerve and retina of streptozocin-induced diabetic rats. (From Poulsom et al[239])

Tissue	Group	Concentration (nmol/mg ± SE)			
		Glucose	Sorbitol	Fructose	Myoinositol
Sc. nerve	ND	1.94 ± 0.06	0.11 ± 0.01	0.94 ± 0.03	3.61 ± 0.09
	NDT	1.77 ± 0.06	0.08 ± 0.01	0.76 ± 0.05	3.66 ± 0.16
	D	11.47 ± 0.68	1.83 ± 0.11 *	5.73 ± 0.23 *	2.87 ± 0.14 *
	DT	11.43 ± 0.49	0.62 ± 0.06	3.50 ± 0.15	3.07 ± 0.08
Retina	ND	0.81 ± 0.11	0.06 ± 0.01	0.05 ± 0.01	1.07 ± 0.05
	NDT	0.65 ± 0.11	0.04 ± 0.01	0.05 ± 0.01	1.03 ± 0.06
	D	5.78 ± 0.32	0.66 ± 0.04	0.68 ± 0.04	0.93 ± 0.04
	DT	6.97 ± 0.57	0.68 ± 0.06	0.63 ± 0.04	0.90 ± 0.05

ICI-105,552 was administered p.o. at a dose of 50 mg/kg/day for 22 days one week after induction of diabetes with streptozocin (65 mg/kg, i.v.)
ND = Non-diabetic; NDT = Non-diabetic treated; D = Diabetic; DT = Diabetic treated
*$p<0.05$. Massive differences were not analyzed.

Table 34. Effect of statil on polyol accumulation in the renal cortex and retina of diabetic rats. (From Stribling et al[146])

Duration	Statil (mg/kg/day)	Group	Polyol accumulation (nmol/mg ± SE)			
			Renal Cortex		Retina	
			Sorbitol	Fructose	Sorbitol	Fructose
D, 3 to 6 w	20 (kidney)	ND	0.15 ± 0.02	0.33 ± 0.02	0.31 ± 0.10	0.35 ± 0.11
		D	0.64 ± 0.05	0.90 ± 0.05	1.50 ± 0.48	0.41 ± 0.07
T, 5 d	28 (retina)	DT	0.43 ± 0.07*	0.91 ± 0.07	0.53 ± 0.10	0.57 ± 0.14

w = weeks; c = days
ND = Non-diabetic; D = Diabetic; DT = Diabetic treated.
*$p<0.05$

Table 35. Effect of statil on polyol accumulation in the sciatic nerve and lens of diabetic rats. (From Stribling et al[146])

Tissue	Day	Group/Dose (mg/kg/day)	Polyol accumulation (nmol/mg ± SE) Sorbitol	Fructose
Sciatic nerve	74	ND	0.14 ± 0.01	0.68 ± 0.06
		NDT/25	0.10 ± 0.02	0.45 ± 0.04
		D	1.29 ± 0.12	3.77 ± 0.33
		DT/3.125	0.67 ± 0.05	3.16 ± 0.26*
		6.25	0.40 ± 0.05	2.61 ± 0.17
		12.5	0.25 ± 0.01	2.03 ± 0.13
		25.0	0.23 ± 0.05	1.67 ± 0.13
Lens	31	D	46.82 ± 1.99	12.74 ± 0.24
		DT/10	37.45 ± 2.55	13.11 ± 0.34*
		25	12.03 ± 0.94	9.27 ± 0.48
		100	2.15 ± 0.13	2.70 ± 0.16
	74	D	6.78 ± 1.96	6.31 ± 0.29
		DT/10	12.03 ± 0.54	—
		25	16.42 ± 1.29	11.77 ± 0.54
		100	3.10 ± 0.31*	4.40 ± 0.33

Alderly Park rats were used, b.w. 100-120 g for lens, and 290-315 g for sc. nerve.
Diabetes was induced with streptozocin (60 mg/kg, i.v.).
D = Diabetic; DT = Diabetic treated.
*Not significant as compared with D.

A link between aldose reductase and the above-mentioned metabolic abnormalities, as well as the impaired functions induced by diabetes in the peripheral nerve (see below), was demonstrated by the use of AR inhibitors. By preventing the accumulation of sorbitol (and fructose), orally administered AR inhibitors prevented the decrease in nerve myoinositol levels of short-term STZ-induced diabetic rats (Tables 26, 32, 33, 36 and 37).

That neural myoinositol levels are depleted in galactosemia was first observed by Stewart et al.[207,255] In rats fed on a 40% galactose diet, after two weeks, the myoinositol content of the sciatic nerves was decreased by 72%[207]; no further decrease was observed after five months of galactose feeding. We have corroborated the observation in rats fed for 178 days on a 50% galactose diet, which resulted in a 60% decrease in myoinositol levels in the sciatic nerve.[210] This depletion of myoinositol was prevented by the AR inhibitor tolrestat added to the diet at a dose of 7 mg/kg/day, which decreased neural galactitol accumulation by 58%[44] (Table 38). The finding that normal neural myoinositol levels were maintained in the presence of readily detectable galactitol levels suggests that the nerve can tolerate a certain degree of galactitol accumulation without its affecting neural myoinositol metabolism. Interestingly, the typical 25% decrease in myoinositol levels found in the nerves of short-term experimentally diabetic rats is usually associated with lower combined concentrations of sorbitol and fructose (Tables 26, 32, 33, 36 and 37).

Table 36. Effect of AR inhibitors on motor nerve conduction velocity in streptozocin-induced diabetic rats.

Aldose reductase inhibitor (mg/kg/day)	Duration	Group	MNCV (m/sec ± SE)	Sciatic nerve (nmol/mg ± SE)		Ref. No.
				Sorbitol	Myoinositol	
ICI-105,552 (50)	21 days	ND	△: +2.2 ± 1.5	0.08 ± 0.01	2.30 ± 0.10	248
		NDT	+2.1 ± 1.3	<0.05	2.51 ± 0.12	
		D	−6.2 ± 0.7**	1.56 ± 0.22	1.47 ± 0.10**	
		DT	+2.6 ± 1.7	0.08 ± 0.04	2.75 ± 0.20	
Sorbinil (25)	D, 6 weeks T, 9 weeks	ND	43.1 ± 0.5	0.24 ± 0.02	3.92 ± 0.07	249
		D	39.0 ± 0.7**	2.90 ± 0.22**	2.98 ± 0.11**	
		DT	43.3 ± 0.5	0.15 ± 0.01	3.78 ± 0.10	
Sorbinil (20)	14 days	ND	—	0.24 ± 0.01	2.86 ± 0.17	250
		D	—	0.78 ± 0.07**	2.12 ± 0.11*	
		DT	—	0.30 ± 0.06	2.61 ± 0.11	
Sorbinil (25)	42 days	ND	55.9 ± 1.6	0.05 ± 0.01	2.33 ± 0.15	215
		D	43.9 ± 1.2**	1.48 ± 0.14	1.73 ± 0.17*	
		DT	50.5 ± 1.2	0.09 ± 0.01	2.40 ± 0.10	
Epalrestat (10-40)	D, 2 weeks T, 2 weeks	ND	38.8 ± 7.4[a]	0.04 ± 0.01	—	233
		D	23.2 ± 4.7	0.60 ± 0.15		
		DT (10)	28.8 ± 0.5[b]	0.19 ± 0.05[b]		
		DT (20)	30.7 ± 3.2[b]	0.12 ± 0.01[b]		
		DT (40)	30.1 ± 0.7[b]	0.13 ± 0.03[b]		
Epalrestat (50)	2 weeks	ND	33.1[a]	0.17		234
		D	26.2	0.86**		
		DT	31.0	0.61[c]		
Epalrestat (20)	2 weeks	ND	29.4 ± 1.3[a]	0.23 ± 0.02	—	235, 251, 252
		D	24.5 ± 0.4**	1.31 ± 0.08**		
		DT	29.0 ± 1.4[b]	0.61 ± 0.26[c]		

MNCV = Mctor nerve conduction velocity; ND = Non-diabetic; NDT = Non-diabetic treated; D = Diabetic; DT = Diabetic treated
[a]Measured in the tail.
[b]$p<0.01$.
[c]$p<0.001$; as compared with D.
*$p<0.05$.
**$p<0.001$ as compared with ND.

Table 37. Effect of AR inhibitors on orthograde axonal transport, motor nerve conduction velocity, sorbitol and myoinositol levels in the sciatic nerve of 21-day streptozocin-induced diabetic rats.

Aldose reductase inhibitor (mg/kg/day for 21 days)	Group	ChAT accumulation (nmol ACh/hr/nerve ± SE)	MNCV (m/sec ± SE)	nmol/mg ± SE		Ref. No.
				Sorbitol	Myoinositol	
ICI-105,552	ND	5.1 ± 0.4	△: +2.2 ± 1.5	0.08 ± 0.01	2.30 ± 0.10	
(50)	NDT	4.2 ± 0.4	+2.1 ± 1.3	<0.05	2.51 ± 0.12	253
	D	2.8 ± 0.4***	−6.2 ± 0.7***	1.56 ± 0.22+	1.47 ± 0.10*	
	DT	4.7 ± 0.5	+2.6 ± 1.7	0.08 ± 0.01	2.75 ± 0.20	
Sorbinil	ND	5.7 ± 0.5	53.6 ± 1.5	0.08 ± 0.01	2.30 ± 0.10	
(25)	NDT	5.6 ± 0.5	55.6 ± 1.1	0.05 ± 0.01	2.56 ± 0.22	215
	D	2.8 ± 0.4***	43.9 ± 2.0***	1.56 ± 0.22+	1.47 ± 0.10***	
	DT	6.0 ± 0.5	55.0 ± 0.5	0.06 ± 0.03	2.28 ± 0.12	
Statil	ND	4.6 ± 0.5[a]	—	0.17 ± 0.05	3.54 ± 0.22	
(25)	D	3.0 ± 0.3**	—	2.03 ± 0.28+	2.66 ± 0.18**	254
	DT	4.2 ± 0.3	—	0.19 ± 0.04	3.41 ± 0.18	

Wistar rats (b.w. 290-310 g or 350-369 g with statil) were injected with streptozocin (50 mg/kg, i.p.);
ChAT = Choline Acetyl Transferase; MNCV = motor nerve conduction velocity;
ND = Non-diabetic; NDT = Non-diabetic treated; D = Diabetic.
[a]Reversible deficit also found in vagus nerve.
*$p < 0.05$; **$p < 0.01$; ***$p < 0.001$ as compared with ND.
+Massive differences were not analyzed.

Table 38. Effect of tolrestat on galactitol and myoinositol levels in the sciatic nerve of rats fed 50% galactose for 178 days. (From Dvornik et al [44])

Group	Tolrestat[a] (mg/kg/day)	nmol/mg ± SE	
		Galactitol	Myoinositol
Normal diet	0	ND	2.97 ± 0.30
50% Galactose	0	30.0 ± 4.0	1.19 ± 0.10
	7	12.5 ± 0.9*	3.08 ± 0.20*
	20	5.5 ± 1.1*	3.46 ± 0.10*
	40	2.9 ± 0.8*	3.29 ± 0.10*

ND = Not detected.
[a]Rats had access for 14 days to diets containing tolrestat; from Day 15 to 178, 50% galactose was added to the diet.
*$p < 0.05$ as compared with galactosemic control group.

Effect of AR inhibitors on functional changes caused by polyol pathway activation

Effect on nerve conduction velocity

Diabetic polyneuropathy is characterized by the loss of myelinated and unmyelinated axons and by segmental demyelination, which may be secondary to axonal atrophy.[256] The impaired axonal viability is attributed primarily to metabolic derangements in axons caused by hyperglycemia.[235] Physiologically, diabetic neuropathy is characterized by decreased nerve conduction velocity in both sensory and motor nerves. In recently diagnosed subjects with IDDM, motor nerve conduction velocity (MNCV) improved after a few weeks of treatment with insulin and slowed again a few days after withdrawal of the treatment.[257]

Impaired sciatic motor and sensory-nerve conduction velocities in rats made diabetic by pancreatectomy or by administration of alloxan was first reported in 1964 by Eliasson.[258] A definite relationship between a lack of insulin, as manifested by hyperglycemia and the development of impaired sciatic MNCV was demonstrated by Preston[259] in alloxan-induced diabetic rats, and by Gabbay[260] and Greene et al[244] in STZ-induced diabetic rats. The impairment was associated with a decrease in free myoinositol concentrations in the nerve and was abolished by feeding myoinositol.[244]

The results obtained by Hatanaka[251] in STZ-induced diabetic rats suggest that impairment in MNCV became evident after six days of diabetes when the sorbitol content in the sciatic nerve reached a threshold level between 0.81 and 1.27 nmol/mg.

The finding of fructose in the sciatic nerve of rabbits and dogs by Stewart and Passonneau[261] was followed by the demonstration of the presence of the polyol pathway in the sciatic nerve of normal and alloxan-diabetic rats by Gabbay et al[204] and Stewart et al.[262] The elevated levels of sorbitol and fructose found in the diabetic sciatic nerves suggested that as in the pathogenesis of sugar cataracts, aldose reductase localized in the Schwann cells may also play a role in the pathogenesis of diabetic neuropathy.[263] In the meantime, Stewart et al[255] expanded their investigations on the polyol pathway in nervous tissue and reported pronounced galactitol accumulation in the sciatic nerve of rats fed 40% galactose with the diet. Evidence supporting the postulate that polyol accumulation is involved in the development of a defect in MNCV was provided by the demonstration that such a defect was induced in rats fed on a galactose diet, that it was exacerbated by increasing galactose intake, and that it was abolished by galactose withdrawal.[264] Increases in nerve galactitol and water contents closely followed the galactose intake and the MNCV defect. The finding that galactosemia results in decreased MNCV associated with galactitol accumulation and overhydration of the peripheral nerves was later corroborated[265] and amplified by the demonstration of decreased neural myoinositol levels.[207,255]

The involvement of aldose reductase in the initiation of the defect in MNCV was confirmed by Gabbay et al[260] by treating galactose-fed rats with alrestatin, thus preventing both galactitol accumulation[27] and the defect in MNCV. This was the first demonstration that a sugar-induced defect in MNCV can be prevented by administration of an AR inhibitor. This finding was later substantiated by the results obtained in STZ-induced diabetic rats with such structurally different AR inhibitors as ICI-105,552,[248] sorbinil,[215,216,247,249,266] epalrestat,[233-235,237,251,252] and statil[146] (Table 36). The effects of alrestatin and epalrestat on tail-nerve conduction velocity were also investigated in STZ-induced diabetic rats fed 72% fructose with the diet[212] (Table 39). The early metabolic phase of neuropathy in the spontaneously diabetic BB-Wistar rat, including decreased nerve conduction velocity,[268] was prevented by administration of statil.[269]

Three findings in the peripheral nerves are of interest: first, that AR inhibition can reverse motor nerve dysfunction in rats with diabetes of two to nine months' duration (Table 40); second, that AR inhibition can improve the MNCV defect without restoring nerve sorbitol levels to normal,[146,235,251,252,267] thus suggesting that as in the lens, the nerve can withstand some increase in polyol pathway activity without overt damage (Tables 36 and 39); third, that the effect of an AR inhibitor on MNCV, e.g., of statil (Table 41) and epalrestat,[252] may not be dose-dependent.

Table 39. Effect of aldose reductase inhibitors on sorbitol accumulation and motor nerve conduction velocity in 4-month streptozocin-induced diabetic rats. (From Kikkawa et al[267])

Aldose reductase inhibitor (mg/kg/day)	Duration	Group	MNCV (m/sec ± SE)	Sorbitol (nmol/mg ± SE)
Sorbinil		D	33.4 ± 2.2	0.66 ± 0.04
(20)	2 weeks	DT	38.2 ± 3.5*	0.36 ± 0.12*
Epalrestat		D	35.1 ± 2.7	0.57 ± 0.15
(20)	2 weeks	DT	41.1 ± 1.3*	0.30 ± 0.02*

MNCV = Motor nerve conduction velocity; D = Diabetic; DT = Diabetic treated
*$p<0.05$ as compared with D.

Table 40. Effect of sorbinil on motor nerve conduction velocity in streptozocin-induced diabetic rats. (From Yue et al[266])

	Group	Motor nerve conduction velocity (m/sec ± SD) D, 2 months + 4 weeks T	D, 5 months + 4 weeks T	D, 9 months + 4 weeks T
Before	ND	50.1 ± 4.5	52.2 ± 3.3	60.9 ± 4.9
	D	39.8 ± 5.7*	46.1 ± 4.9*	52.8 ± 5.4*
After	NDT	49.7 ± 1.2	57.3 ± 4.9	58.5 ± 4.3
	DT	47.7 ± 6.7**	52.5 ± 3.8**	56.4 ± 2.3**

D = Diabetes; T = Treatment (sorbinil, 5 mg/kg/day);
ND = Non-diabetic treated; DT = Diabetic treated.
$^{*}p<0.01$ $^{**}p<0.001$

Table 41. Effect of statil on motor nerve conduction velocity in streptozocin-induced diabetic rats. (From Stribling et al[146])

Group	Statil (mg/kg/day)	Motor nerve conduction velocity (m/sec ± SE), after 7 days	21 days	42 days	74 days
ND	0	54.66 ± 1.45	58.06 ± 1.45	60.91 ± 1.78	67.46 ± 1.26
NDT	25	55.23 ± 2.11	59.90 ± 1.49	63.31 ± 1.80	67.67 ± 1.70
D	0	48.04 ± 1.81*	55.93 ± 1.48	55.71 ± 2.16	59.01 ± 1.31**
DT	3.125	52.47 ± 0.95	55.97 ± 1.64	61.70 ± 1.05	62.44 ± 1.29*
	6.25	53.05 ± 1.6	58.30 ± 0.81	61.00 ± 1.49	61.89 ± 1.83*

ND = Non-diabetic; NDT = Non-diabetic treated; D = Diabetic; DT = Diabetic treated.
$^{*}p<0.05$; $^{**}p<0.001$ as compared with ND.

The distal nerve transmission time, measured in rats by the auditory-evoked brainstem response, was shown to be prolonged ($p<0.05$) after two weeks of STZ-induced diabetes.[270] The impairment in nerve transmission time was prevented by oral administration of tolrestat at a dose of 20 mg/kg/day.[271]

Effect on sensory function

Stribling et al[272] have reported that STZ-induced diabetic rats develop abnormalities in sensory function, the nature of which depends upon the duration of diabetes. Thus, at nine days' duration, the weight applied to the paw necessary to induce foot withdrawal in diabetic rats was 1.4 times greater than in age-matched non-diabetic rats; the defect was ameliorated by administration of the AR inhibitor statil at a dose of 25 mg/kg/day. After 21 days, however, the diabetic rats became more sensitive to paw pressure, and the effect of statil, more variable. Such decrease in pain threshold was observed in the sand rat, in STZ-induced diabetic rats, and in rats fed on a galactose diet for four weeks.[273]

Effect on sympathetic activity

Yoshida et al[237,238] reported that in 1-week STZ-induced diabetic rats, oral administration of epalrestat, at a dose of 50 mg/kg/day for three weeks, reversed the diabetes-induced decrease in norepinephrine turnover in brown adipose tissue, heart, and pancreas.

Sympathetic activity in patients with diabetic polyneuropathy has been recently reviewed by Fagius.[274]

Effect on axonal transport

The finding that the neuronal synthesis of macromolecules is virtually confined to the nerve cell body[275,276] pointed to the existence of processes capable of transporting these molecules from the nerve cell to the nerve terminals. The existence of intra-axonal translocation was made clear in 1948 by Weiss and Hiscoe.[277] Since then, many investigators have contributed to our understanding of axonal transport and its subdivision into orthograde (anterograde) transport, from the nerve cell body to the periphery, and retrograde transport, from axon terminals and dendrite tips to the cell body. A comprehensive review of this work was prepared recently by Grafstein and Forman.[278]

The structural and functional integrity of the axon depends upon its supply of nutrients via orthograde transport, while retrograde transport is believed to provide feedback to the nerve cell body about the state of the axon terminals. Pertinently, the consequences of experimental impairment of orthograde transport closely resemble the features of neuropathy as seen in chronic diabetes. Axonal transport in diabetes mellitus was recently reviewed by Tomlinson and Mayer[36]; the following points are of relevance to the testing of AR inhibitors.[279]

To date, two methods have been used to study axonal transport. In the first method, the accumulation of an endogenous constituent of axoplasm is measured against a constriction applied to the nerve trunk. The accumulation of the constituent proximal to the constriction is taken as an index of orthograde transport, and accumulation distal to the constriction, as an index of retrograde transport. The second method, known as "pulse labeling," enables the measurement of the rates of transport of different (labeled) axoplasmic constituents. Careful statistical analysis is needed for interpretation of results obtained by pulse labeling. As discussed by Tomlinson and Mayer,[36] the preferred method for the study of orthograde axonal transport uses choline acetyltransferase as marker. The method was first described by Schmidt et al[280] and perfected by Tomlinson and colleagues.[215,281,282]

Pulse labeling has been used to demonstrate that the defect in the orthograde axonal transport of choline transferase, detectable in 3-week STZ-induced diabetic rats, is prevented by daily treatment with AR inhibitors such as ICI-105,552[253,281] sorbinil,[215] and statil.[253] The results in Table 37 demonstrate the relationship between the increased sorbitol levels and the decreases in orthograde axonal transport, MNCV, and myoinositol levels in diabetic rats, and the prevention of all these changes by treatment with an AR inhibitor. Reversal of these changes was effected with sorbinil.[215] Similar results were obtained in a study of axonal transport of ([^{3}H]methyl) choline containing lipids in 3-week STZ-induced diabetic rats.[283]

Mayer and Tomlinson[284] have also used pulse labeling to demonstrate that the diabetes-induced retardation of the slow orthograde axonal transport of [^{3}H]-labeled proline was affected by the AR inhibitor statil. Subsequently, Mayer et al[229] investigated the effect of short-term STZ-induced diabetes on the velocity profile of slow, orthogradely transported proline-labeled proteins in rat sciatic motoneurons. The minor retardation in the faster components of the velocity profile was not modulated by either oral administration of statil (at 25 mg/kg/day) or myoinositol (at 1.5% of diet). It was concluded that first, the major effect of diabetes on axonal transport in cholinergic neurons is to reduce the amount of material in transit without markedly affecting the rate of translocation, and second, that aldose reductase and myoinositol are involved primarily in the mechanism(s) controlling the amount of material transported. Later experiments have confirmed that, in 23-day STZ-diabetic rats, statil (at 25 mg/kg/day) was devoid of any significant effect on the reduced velocity of the slow component-a of axonal transport (of [^{3}H]proline).[285]

With respect to the slow component-b of axonal transport (of [^{3}H]leucine) in rats, both STZ-induced diabetes of 35 days' duration and feeding on a 20% galactose diet for 20 days produced a selective increase in transport velocity. Since it was prevented by either of two AR inhibitors, statil or sorbinil, the increase appears to be related to polyol formation.[286]

The axonal transport of choline acetyltransferase in several cholinergically innervated organs of STZ-induced diabetic rats was decreased after four and eight months by 83% in the iris and 61% in the illeum, but not in the atria or skeletal muscle. Administration of statil at a dose of 25 mg/kg/day prevented depletion at four, but not after eight months of diabetes.[287] In 3-week STZ-induced diabetic rats administration of statil (25 mg/kg) prevented the development of defective axonal transport in cholinergic neurons of the sciatic and vagal nerves.[288] This was associated with prevention of neural sorbitol accumulation and myoinositol depletion, and a 63% reduction in neural fructose levels.

The dependence of both orthograde axonal transport of choline acetyltransferase and nerve conduction velocity on the extent of hyperglycemia, i.e., on the extent of flux of glucose through the polyol pathway, was demonstrated by Mayer et al[289] in spontaneously diabetic BB rats kept moderately hyperglycemic with daily insulin injections.

Effect on Na/K-dependent ATPase activity in nerves and kidney

Acute STZ-induced diabetes in rats is associated with decreased energy utilization and substrate metabolism in the peripheral nerve, despite increased glucose, sorbitol, and fructose levels due to enhanced polyol pathway activity.[290] The findings that the Na/K-dependent ATPase that generates the transmembrane sodium gradient in peripheral nerve consumes the major portion of the tissue's energy flux,[291] and that its activity is reduced in the sciatic nerve of STZ-induced diabetic rats,[292] prompted the suggestion that myoinositol may contribute to the function of Na/K-dependent ATPase.[245,246,290,293] A decrease in the membrane-bound, Na/K-dependent ATPase activity in sciatic nerves of STZ-diabetic rats was indeed prevented by adding 1% myoinositol to their diet.[294] A self-enforcing cycle was postulated to exist between the myoinositol-related activity of the Na/K-dependent ATPase and the sodium-dependent uptake of myoinositol.[295,296] Links between diabetes-induced hyperglycemia, the myoinositol-related Na/K-ATPase defect, and the reversible portion of the slowed nerve conduction velocity were subsequently demonstrated in the insulin-deficient BB rat.[297]

It is of interest that the early metabolic phase of diabetic neuropathy in the BB rat, i.e., decrease in Na/K-dependent ATPase, intra-axonal sodium accumulation, and paranodal swelling as well as slowing of nerve conduction velocity, was also normalized by four-week treatment with an AR inhibitor, statil.[298]

Significantly higher ($p<0.001$) sodium concentrations (295 meq/L) were found in the endoneurial fluid of the sciatic nerve of rats fed for five months on a 40% galactose diet as compared with age-matched controls (152 meq/L).[298] Endoneurial sodium accumulation was associated with edema localized primarily to subperineurial and perivascular areas. Since in galactosemic rats the blood/nerve barrier remains intact,[299] the endoneurial fluid pressure, reported to increase five times above normal,[300] was attributed primarily to the endoneurial accumulation of sodium caused by an "inward sugar concentration gradient."[301] Since the elevated endoneurial sodium concentration, increased water content, and increased interstitial fluid pressure were reversed by treatment with an AR inhibitor, statil, administered orally at a dose of 25 mg/kg/day,[301] it is likely that the phenomena are linked to the aldose reductase-catalyzed conversion of galactose to galactitol rather than to the uptake of galactose per se.

Decrease in Na/K-dependent ATPase activity was also demonstrated by measuring the rate of ouabaine-sensitive [^{86}Rb] uptake by endoneurial preparations of sciatic nerve from STZ-induced diabetic rats.[302] The decrease was significant after six months of diabetes.

Meanwhile, a relationship was shown to exist between the polyol pathway, myoinositol levels, conduction velocity, and orthograde axonal transport in the nerves of diabetic rats. As shown in Table 37, the evidence was obtained by inhibiting aldose reductase. It remained for Greene and Lattimer[303] to demonstrate that the 40% to 45% decrease in nerve Na/K-dependent ATPase activity of STZ-induced diabetic rats is also prevented by inhibiting aldose reductase. As shown in Table 42, treatment with the AR inhibitor sorbinil prevented the 19% decrease in nerve myoinositol levels and the 44% decrease in Na/K-dependent ATPase activity. The finding corroborates the involvement of aldose reductase in the diabetes-induced, myoinositol-mediated Na/K-dependent ATPase activity in the peripheral nerves. In accordance, the Na-dependent amino acid transport, enabled by the transmembrane Na-dependent ATPase, was found to be decreased by over 50% in the peripheral nerve of 2-week alloxan-induced diabetic rabbits.[304] The reduction was prevented by treating the rabbits with either sorbinil (15 mg/kg/day) or myoinositol (100 mg/kg/day).

Table 42. Effect of sorbinil on myoinositol content and ATPase activity in the sciatic nerve of 4-week streptozocin-induced diabetic rats. (From Greene and Lattimer [304])

Group	Plasma glucose (mg/dl ± SE)	Myoinositol (nmol/mg ± SE)	ATPase activity (nmol/mg ± SE)	
			Composite	Ouabain-inhibited
ND	165 ± 5	2.79 ± 0.11	431 ± 10	103.8 ± 3.9
NDT	156 ± 5	2.92 ± 0.13**	455 ± 27***	97.6 ± 6.2***
D	589 ± 28	2.26 ± 0.11	321 ± 12	58.2 ± 2.6
DT	623 ± 25	3.12 ± 0.14	374 ± 18*	95.8 ± 5.0***

ND = Non-diabetic; T = Treated (sorbinil, 20 mg/kg/day, by gavage); D = Diabetic (streptozocin, 60 mg/kg, i.v.); DT = Diabetic treated.
*$p<0.025$; **$p<0.005$; ***$p<0.0001$.

A sorbinil responsive, myoinositol-related Na/K-dependent ATPase defect analogous to that of peripheral nerve was reported to occur in the superior cervical ganglion of 8-week STZ-induced diabetic rats.[305,306] The authors suggested that altered ganglionic myoinositol metabolism in diabetes interferes with autonomic function by diminishing membrane repolarization and muscarinic signal transduction in postsynaptic cells.[306]

Prompted by their finding of sorbitol accumulation and myoinositol depletion in the glomeruli of STZ-induced diabetic rats,[219] Cohen et al[307] have found that as in the peripheral nerve,[294,297,303] the ouabain-inhibited, Na/K-dependent ATPase activity in the glomeruli is also decreased in acutely diabetic rats. The decrease was prevented by the administration of sorbinil at a dose of 20 mg/kg/day. The authors speculated that the effect of sorbinil may be due either to inhibition of aldose reductase or to its specific binding to glomerular membranes,[308] similarly to the binding of the structurally related phenytoin to receptor sites associated with the activation of voltage-sensitive Na-channels in the CNS.[309] However, neither acute STZ-induced diabetes nor sorbinil (at 20 mg/kg/day for 14 to 18 days) produced detectable changes in the glomerular concentration of phosphatidylinositol.[310] The finding does not support the postulate that correspondent changes in myoinositol and phosphatidylinositol contents are contributory to diminished glomerular

Na/K-ATPase activity in diabetes, but are compatible with depletion of glomerular myoinositol in diabetes.

Garner and Spector[311] have found that incubation of bovine renal Na/K-dependent ATPase with glucose-6-phosphate results in glycation, which, in turn, reduces ATP hydrolysis by 40%. Similar substrate inhibition was observed for the renal Na/K-dependent ATPase isolated from patients with NIDDM. Glycation of the bovine renal enzyme in the presence of 30.5 mM glucose or 16.7 mM glucose-6-phosphate was not affected by AR inhibitors, either AL-1567 or sorbinil.[312] However, the kinetics of the glycated Na/K-ATPase tended to be normalized in the presence of AL-1576. The authors have concluded that the AR inhibitors may be acting at the low-affinity ATP-binding site of the Na/K-dependent ATPase, a site also affected by glycation.[312]

According to McCormack et al,[313] sorbinil, at a dose of 20 mg/kg/day, had no effect on insulin clearance and tubular enzymuria in 28-day STZ-induced diabetic rats.

Effect on glomerular filtration

The mechanism(s) by which hyperglycemia induces glomerular hyperfiltration in IDDM patients were investigated by Goldfarb et al[314] in STZ-induced diabetic rats of seven to ten days' duration. Treatment of the diabetic rats for eight days with sorbinil, injected intraperitoneally at a dose of 25 mg/kg, or with myoinositol added to the diet at a 1% level, resulted in a significant amelioration of glomerular hyperfiltration.

Administration of sorbinil (20 mg/kg/day) to STZ-induced diabetic rats prevented the shift of the urinary protein pattern toward higher molecular weights[315,316] and diminished diabetes-induced proteinuria.[317] Sorbinil has also been found to diminish the development of renal hypertrophy.[318]

Effect on vascular permeability

Newly formed subcutaneous tissue in diabetic[319] and galactose-fed rats[320] is characterized by increased vascular permeability. The pathophysiological perturbatious and vascular changes responsible for increased albumin permeation in diabetic rats are readily reversible upon islet transplantation.[321] Increased vascular permeability is associated with increased tissue polyol levels and decreased levels of myoinositol in diabetic[33,322] but not in galactose-fed rats.[320] The involvement of aldose reductase was shown by the finding that the diabetes-induced increases in vascular permeability were preventable either by treatment with sorbinil, at a dose of 25 mg/kg/day[33] or by castration.[322] Treatment of the diabetic or galactose-fed rats with tolrestat or sorbinil also markedly decreased the increased polyol levels in granulation tissue.

Increased permeation of [^{125}I]albumin was also found in the choroid-scleral and anterior uveal, but not retinal vessels of 3-week STZ-induced diabetic mature male rats.[323] The diabetes-induced increase in vascular permeability is an aldose reductase-linked phenomenon, since it was markedly diminished by admixture to the diet of approximately 200 μmol/kg/day of two structurally distinct AR inhibitors tolrestat and sorbinil. The findings also suggest that the earliest diabetes-induced increase in vascular permeability occurs in the uveal vasculature.

According to Lorenzi et al,[324] sorbitol accumulation in cultured human umbilical vein endothelial cells was not affected by adding 1 μmol sorbinil to the incubation medium containing 20 mmol glucose.

Effect on retinal pigmented epithelium

Elevated levels of glucose and sorbitol and decreased myoinositol levels were detected within the choroid, retinal pigmented epithelium (RPE), and all retinal layers of alloxan-induced diabetic rabbits.[325] In addition, the Na/K-dependent ATPase activity in the RPE and the neural retina was reduced.[326] It is of interest that the function of the retinal pigmented epithelium, forming the outer component of the blood-retinal barrier, is impaired after induction of diabetes in pigmented rats, and that the impairment was prevented by treatment with sorbinil, or by myoinositol supplementation.[325] As the major component of the outer blood/retinal barrier, the RPE is pivotal in determining the composition of the retinal extracellular fluid. In 2-week STZ-induced diabetic rats, a progressive decline in c-wave amplitude of the electroretinograms was noted, reflecting impairment of function of the RPE. This decline was arrested by treatment with the AR inhibitor sorbinil (10 mg/kg/day) or by supplementation of myoinositol (650 mg/kg/day).[327]

According to Campochiaro et al,[328] the RPE of non-diabetic rats and humans are immunohistochemically negative for aldose reductase. In contrast, in spontaneously diabetic BB rats, there was an induction of aldose reductase expression in the RPE and a marked increase in the staining intensity of the ciliary body epithelium. While in short-term diabetic human eyes the RPE was negative, in cases of longer duration, aldose reductase was demonstrable in the RPE. The findings suggest a possible association between induction of aldose reductase expression and cellular damage in diabetic RPE.

Effect of AR inhibitors on morphological changes caused by polyol pathway activation

Effect on sugar cataract development

The polyol hypothesis as formulated by Kinoshita[24,25] incriminates aldose reductase in the induction of biochemical changes that in the presence of persisting hyperglycemia, progress to loss of functional and structural integrity of lenticular cells. The most convincing experimental evidence of this hypothesis, and particularly of the pivotal role of aldose reductase, was provided by inhibitors of aldose reductase and their control of sugar-induced cataractogenesis. The cataracts produced in diabetic and galactosemic laboratory animals are now classified as sugar cataracts and are known to be initiated by a common mechanism.[329]

As discussed in greater detail in Chapter 3, experimentally, the process of cataract formation can be reproducibly initiated with high ambient sugar concentrations, both in vitro and in vivo.

The preferred animal model is the galactose-fed rat, since a mature cataract can appear within about four weeks, particularly in young animals, while about three months is required in rats made diabetic. The effectiveness of an AR inhibitor can be determined by investigating its effect either on the initial lenticular changes or on the appearance of the mature cataract. The former are detectable by slit-lamp microscopy, while the latter is visible with the unaided eye. The changes characterizing cataract development in galactosemic rats are differentiated by variations[146,153,330-334] of the classifications of Cotlier[335] and Sippel.[336] For short-term comparative studies, we have developed a model in which rats are exposed for seven days to a diet containing 40% galactose and an AR inhibitor. Based on a four-stage classification,[330] an arbitrary Opacity Index can be calculated.[152] The test is illustrated in Table 43 by results obtained with the AR inhibitors alrestatin and tolrestat.[152]

Table 43. Effect of aldose reductase inhibitors on the initial stages of cataract development in rats fed 40% galactose for seven days. (From Simard-Duquesne et al[337])

Aldose reductase inhibitor	Dose (mg/kg/day)	No. of affected lenses at Stage			Opacity Index
		I	II	III	
Control (10)	—	0	10	10	2.5
Alrestatin (9)	1007	16	2	0	1.1
Tolrestat (10)	28	20	0	0	1.0

Number of rats in parentheses. The lenses were examined by slit-lamp microscopy and graded into four stages.[330] The Opacity Index was calculated by giving no points to Stage 0, one point to Stage I, two points to Stage II, etc., then dividing the sum of the points by the total number of lenses per group.

The first demonstration that mature cataract can be very markedly delayed was made in rats fed a diet containing 30% galactose and 0.7% alrestatin[27] (Fig 1). The sensitivity of the 30-day, 30%-galactose-fed rat model to detect the dose-dependent effect of an AR inhibitor is illustrated with results obtained with tolrestat[337] (Table 44).

Since alrestatin, virtually every orally active AR inhibitor had been tested for its effect on cataract development in galactosemic (Table 45) and/or STZ-induced diabetic rats (Table 46). The results indicate that cataract development can be prevented and, depending upon the extent of lenticular damage, even reversed by inhibiting lens aldose reductase. Of interest is the finding that with Statil[146] prevention of cataract formation was achieved, although the 74-day lenticular sorbitol and fructose levels were higher than those observed in non-diabetic lenses (Table 35). The result suggests that the rat lens can tolerate a certain increase of polyol levels and the associated osmotic pressure without necessarily progressing to cataract development.

Often, AR inhibitors are tested in rats fed on a 50% galactose diet, i.e., in acute galactosemia of such severity that essentially irreversible lenticular damage can occur within five days.[343] The effectiveness of an AR inhibitor in a model of such severity[333] thus depends upon its pharmacokinetics in the presence of huge amounts of galactose, i.e., on the experimental conditions used.[152,337]

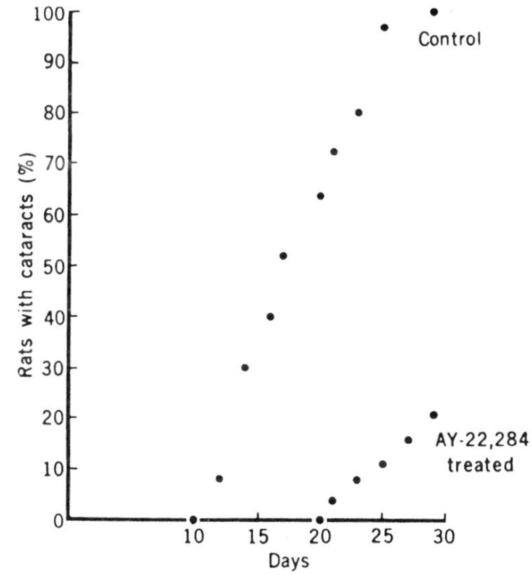

Figure 1. Effect of alrestatin (0.7% of diet) on mature cataract appearance in rats fed 30% galactose for 30 days. (From Dvornik et al[27])

Table 44. Effect of aldose reductase inhibitors on the appearance of mature cataract in rats fed 30% galactose for 31 days. (From Simard-Duquesne et al[337])

	Percentage of lenses with mature cataract				
			Tolrestat (mg/kg/day)		
Day of treatment	**Control**	**Alrestatin, 983 mg/kg/day**	**11**	**16**	**20**
16	0	0	0	0	0
17	0	0	5	0	0
18	0	0	10	0	0
19	5	0	10	0	0
20	10	0	15	5	0
21	25	0	35	5	0
22	40	0	35	5	0
23	45	0	35	5	0
24	45	0	40	10	0
25	65	0	40	15	0
26	70	0	40	15	0
27	70	0	45	15	0
28	70	5	45	15	0
29	80	5	50	15	0
30	85	5	65	15	10
31	90	10	65	15	10

Table 45. Effect of various aldose reductase inhibitors on cataract development in rats fed galactose.

Inhibitor	Dose and mode of admin.	Strain (Body wt.)	Galactose in diet	Duration (days)	Observation	Ref. No.
Alrestatin	0.7% of diet	Sprague Dawley	30%	29	80% Decrease in cataract formation	27
Alrestatin	10% ointment topically to the eye, every 2 hr	Sprague Dawley (60-80 g)	50%	23	Delay in appearance of nuclear cataract	338
Gossypin	15 mg/g diet	Albino (50-60 g)	30%	28	60% Decrease in cataract formation	339
Quercetin	25 mg/g diet	Neonatal	50%	12	Maintaining of lens fiber thickness, density and interdigitations	340
RS-7535	2%, solution topically to the eye or 0.5% of diet	Weanling	35%		Delayed onset of cataract formation	341
Sorbinil	5 and 10 mg/kg with the diet	Charles River (200-250 g)	30%	29	90% Decrease in cataract formation	153
Sorbinil	60 mg/kg with the diet		50%	28	Prevention of lenticular opacification	332
Sorbinil	60 mg/kg, p.o. or 4.25 mg/g diet	Sprague Dawley (50 g)	50%	240	Prevention of cataractous changes	333
Sorbinil	5 mg/g diet	Sprague Dawley (50 g)	50%	40	Prevention of ultrastructural changes	342
Sorbinil	4 mg/kg diet	Sprague Dawley (50 g)	50%	60	Reversal of 5-day old cataractous process (vaculoar stage)	343
Sorbinil	1% solution topically to the eye, 4 times daily	Sprague Dawley (50 g)	50%	21	Prevention and reversal of vacuolar stage (5-day-old) of cataractous process	217
Sorbinil	20 mg/kg	Sprague Dawley (68 ± 12g)	50%	30	Retarded opacification in 10-days old cataractous process	344, 345
Tolrestat	(a) 43 mg/kg (b) 58 mg/kg with the diet	Sprague Dawley (60-80 g)	50%	(a) 207 (b) 277	Prevention of lenticular opacification	337
p-Br-PSH	(a) 25 mg/kg (b) 50 mg/kg	Sprague Dawley (45-60 g)	50%	30	Delayed rate of cataract formation	231

Table 46. Effect of various aldose reductase inhibitors on cataract development in streptozocin-induced diabetic rats.

Aldose reductase inhibitor	Dose (mg/kg)	Animal species (body wt.)	Streptozocin (mg/kg)	Duration of treatment (days)	Observation	Ref. No.
Quercitin	25 mg/g diet + 70 mg/day, p.o.	Octodon degus (90-100 g)	100, i.p. (after 3 days of pretreatm.)	25	Delay in nuclear opacification	346
Sorbinil	60 mg/kg (p.o. for 1 month, then with diet)	Rat, Charles River (∼80 g)	100, i.v.	150	Prevention of lenticular changes	331
Sorbinil	20 mg/kg in the diet	Rat, Sprague Dawley (60 g)	65, i.v.	5 days after 16 days of diab	Arrest of fiber damage	214
				30	Promotion of lenticular changes	
Sorbinil	20 mg/kg, p.o. (30 days after STZ injection	Rat (young)	65, i.v.	7 weeks	Reversal of lenticular changes	347
Statil	50 mg/kg, p.o. (one week after STZ injection)	Rat, Wistar (200 g)	50, i.v.	340 (mean)	Delay of onset and rate of cataract development	334
Statil	10, 20 and 40 mg/kg, p.o.	Rat, Alderly Park (100-120 g)	60, i.v.	80	Delayed cataract development at 10 mg/kg, prevention up to Day 74 with 25 and 100 mg/kg	146

In spite of the severity of the 50% galactose-fed rat model, dose-dependency of the preventive effect of an AR inhibitor on cataract development can be demonstrated by monitoring the progression of lenticular changes with slit-lamp microscopy. The results obtained with various doses of tolrestat listed in Table 47 show that no relevant changes were detected in rats fed on a diet containing 50% galactose and 43 mg (120 μmol)/kg/day of tolrestat for 207 days.[337] Prevention of lenticular changes in 50% galactose-fed rats was previously observed with sorbinil ingested at a dose 60 mg (253 μmol)/kg/day.[333] That cataract development in severely galactosemic rats[333] was completely prevented by treatment with two structurally distinct AR inhibitors strongly supports the postulate that sugar cataract formation, at least in rats, requires the presence of aldose reductase in the lens.[337]

Cataract development in the 50% galactose-fed rat can be reversed by inhibiting

Table 47. Dose-dependence of the preventive effect of tolrestat on cataract development in rats fed 50% galactose for 207 days. (From Simard-Duquesne [337])

Tolrestat (mg/kg/day)	Day	Percentage of lenses at Stage				
		0 + I	*	II	III	IV
9.5	28	0	0	0	10	90
	55	0	0	0	0	100
	28	20	0	5	35	30
	55	30	10	0	0	70
19	109	0	10	0	0	90
	150	0	10	0	0	90
	207	0	10	0	0	90
	28	55	0	15	10	20
	55	20	35	0	0	45
28	109	20	25	0	0	55
	150	15	30	0	0	55
	207	20	25	0	0	55
	28	100	0	0	0	0
	55	70	30	0	0	0
43	109	70	30	0	0	0
	150	70	30	0	0	0
	207	70	30	0	0	0
	28	100	0	0	0	0
	55	89	11	0	0	0
58	109	94	6	0	0	0
	150	100	0	0	0	0
	207	83	17	0	0	0

All rats had for 14 days access to diets containing tolrestat; from Day 15 to 207, 50% galactose was added to the diet. All untreated galactosemic rats used as control had bilateral mature cataract after 28 days of ingesting 50% galactose with the diet.

*Faint lenticular changes detected by slit-lamp microscopy as isolated pin dots or shadows in the center of the lens.

aldose reductase, provided treatment is started within the first five[343] to seven[348] days, i.e., in the early vacuolar stage of cataractogenesis.[217,330] According to Hu et al,[343] in rats fed on 50% galactose, the point of irreversibility seems to be associated with a peak galactitol level of about 75 nmol/mg lens.[23,217] This is similar to the finding of 69 ± 3 nmol/mg lens (±SE) after four-day feeding[337] and of 72 nmol/mg by Beyer-Mears et al[348] after a seven-day feeding period.* These results imply that the lens can tolerate a certain polyol level and the associated osmolality without initiating irreversible lenticular changes. For example, Keiding and Mellemgaard[349] detected no nuclear cataracts in rats fed a 15% galactose diet for 75 days, while after four days such diet was reported to produce 42.2 ± 2.7 nmol (±SE) galactitol per mg lens.[337] A related observation was that in rats fed on a 50% galactose diet and treated topically with sorbinil for five days, no histopathologically detectable changes were found in the lens in the presence of 19.0 ± 4.0 nmol (±SE) galactitol per mg lens.[217] Furthermore, in two separate studies in rats fed for 178 and 207 days on diets containing 50% galactose and 0.03% tolrestat (corresponding to 40[44] to 43 mg/kg/day[152]) we detected no relevant lenticular changes by slit-lamp microscopy, yet the clear lenses contained 35 ± 4 and 30 ± 2 nmol galactitol per mg lens, respectively. A similar observation was reported by Stribling et al[146] in lenses of diabetic rats treated with statil.

Effect on capillary basement membrane thickening

Basement membranes are part of the extracellular matrix that forms a continuous sheet surrounding endothelial and epithelial cells. They act as support for the epithelial cell, as a recognition factor during regeneration, and as a semipermeable barrier to modulate the passage of macromolecules.[350] The glomerular basement membrane consists of at least four different macromolecules: a unique Type IV collagen; laminin, another glycoprotein linked covalently to the collagenous part; a heparan sulfate-like glycosaminoglycan with a peptide core covalently linked to the Type IV collagen; and amyloid P, also covalently linked to the Type IV collagen.[351]

In human diabetes, most tissues, including those affected by diabetic microvascular disease, such as the eye and the kidney, are characterized by a thickening of the capillary basement membrane.[352] Capillary basement membrane thickening represents a characteristic structural lesion of the small blood vessels in diabetic subjects and is regarded as one of the classical ultrastructural findings in diabetic microangiopathy.[350] Despite some disagreement over measurement methodologies,[350] the precise prevalence of the lesion in the capillaries of skeletal muscles[353] and renal glomeruli,[354] and the relation of these lesions to the age of subject or duration of diabetes,[355-357] the presence of thickened basement membranes in skeletal muscle and glomerular capillaries from diabetic patients has been confirmed in many studies.[358]

---

*When the access to a 50% galactose diet was extended to ten days, Beyer-Mears et al[345] found a lenticular galactose level of 96 ± 7 nmol/mg lens and were able to effect partial reversal (of the vacuoles formed) by feeding the animals for ten days on a normal diet supplemented with sorbinil at a dose of 20 mg/kg/day.

In the dog, long-term experimental diabetes also produced thickening of basement membranes in capillaries of the kidney, retina, and muscle similar to that found in humans.[359] The increase in the width of the basement membranes became statistically significant after two to three years of diabetes.[360] Subsequent studies confirmed that by 60 months of diabetes, retinal capillary aneurysms, pericyte ghosts, obliterated vessels, retinal hemorrhage, and other microvascular abnormalities typical of human diabetes were apparent in all of the alloxan-induced diabetic dogs used in the study. Morphologically, these lesions were very similar to those known to occur in human diabetes.[361] The demonstration that the development of retinopathy in the diabetic dog was markedly inhibited by insulin treatment suggested the involvement of hyperglycemia.[361] This conclusion is supported by the finding in galactose-fed dogs of retinal lesions morphologically similar to those of diabetic dogs.[362]

Of particular interest was the demonstration of Efimov et al[363] that the thickening of the capillary basement membranes in the muscle of six- to nine-month alloxan-induced diabetic rats was significantly decreased by the AR inhibitor alrestatin, given intraperitoneally at a dose of 50 mg/kg/day. This was the first indication that aldose reductase may be involved in the diabetes-induced thickening of capillary basement membranes.

The involvement of aldose reductase in the pathogenesis of the retinal changes was supported by the finding of galactitol accumulation in dog retinal microvessels incubated with 30 mM galactose, and by the observation that the accumulation was reduced by the addition of the AR inhibitor sorbinil to the incubating medium.[364]

Current research on aldose reductase has produced a finding of fundamental importance for the understanding of the mechanism(s) controlling capillary membrane thickening. The finding was a precognition based on insight entailing two components. First, by feeding rats on a 50% galactose diet, the basement membrane thickening and membrane compositional differences in retinal capillaries were found to be similar to those in rats with hereditary diabetes (BB Wistar), and in aging rats.[365] The second component was the concept that the development of such changes could be controlled by AR inhibitors. Several independent studies[40-44,366,367] have demonstrated that long-term severely galactosemic rats developed an approximately two-fold thickening of capillary basement membranes in the outer plexiform layer of the retina; the thickening was less pronounced in other tissues, e.g., in the capillaries of the cremaster muscle, Bruch's membrane, and the inner limiting membrane.[367] The time required for the development of readily discernable changes in the width of basement membranes varied, depending on the amount of galactose added to the diet, from 28 weeks with 50% galactose[40] to 84 weeks with 30% galactose in the diet.[41]

Of significance is the finding that retinal capillary basement membrane thickening was prevented by two structurally distinct AR inhibitors, i.e., the spirohydantoin derivative[368] sorbinil,[40-42] and the sarcosine derivative[369] tolrestat,[43,44,366,370] thus amplifying the involvement of aldose reductase.[43] The results obtained in rats fed for 207 days on a diet containing 50% galactose and tolrestat at a dose corresponding to 43 mg (120 μmol)/kg/day are shown in Fig 2.[43] Subsequently, in rats fed on a 50% galactose diet for six months, the basement

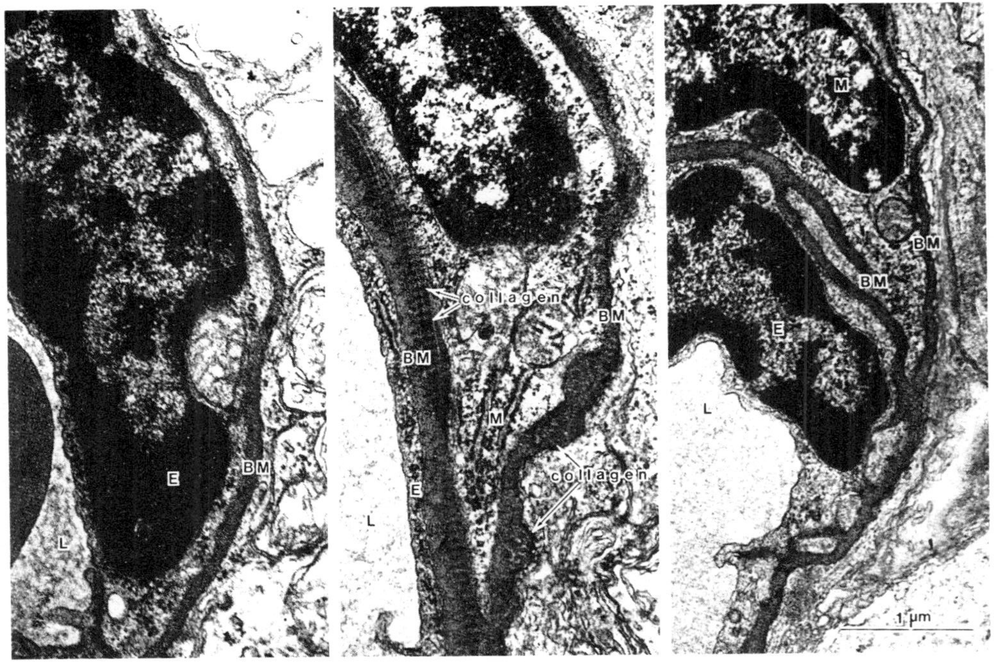

Figure 2. Comparative basement membrane thickness in retinal capillaries of the outer plexiform layer in rats on Purina Laboratory Chow (left), galactose chow (center), and galactose chow supplemented with .03% tolrestat (right) for 207 days. Note the clear banding pattern (640 Å spacing) in the collagen of the thickened basement membrane in the galactose-fed rat. Abbreviations: BM, basement membrane; E, endothelial cell; L, lumen; M, mural cell (x 23,000). (From Robison et al[43])

membrane thickening was prevented by tolrestat at a daily dose of 7 mg (20 μmol)/kg.[44]

In STZ-induced diabetic rats, thickening of retinal and glomerular capillary basement membranes was prevented by administration of the spirohydantoin-type[371] AR inhibitors AL-1567 and AL-1576.[372] According to Stribling et al,[373] the 9.6% increase in retinal capillary basement membrane thickness detected in 6-month STZ-diabetic rats was decreased by treatment with statil, admixed to the diet (0.023% w/w).

A retinopathy resembling the human diabetic disorder was also found in genetically selected rats with low glucose tolerance fed on a diet rich in sucrose.[374-377] The sucrose-induced retinopathy was shown to be due to fructose produced from sucrose.[377,378] Addition of 68% sucrose to the diet of STZ-diabetic rats accelerated the appearance of these retinal changes.[377,379] Treatment with the AR inhibitor epalrestat, at a dose of 50 mg (157 μmol)/kg/day, caused a marked reduction ($p<0.05$) in retinal sorbitol and fructose accumulation[380] and prevented the development of retinal capillary basement membrane thickening.[45,380] These findings suggest a specific role for aldose reductase in capillary basement membrane thickening.

Histochemically, aldose reductase has been localized in all retinal regions displaying diabetic pathology, namely pericytes of retinal capillaries, the Müller cells, and ganglion cells of both rat[119] and man.[123,124]

A 13% increase in renal glomerular basement membrane thickness (2031 ± 122 Å) in STZ-induced diabetic rats fed for 70 days on a 30% galactose diet was reported by Sato et al.[381] The increase was reduced (to 1884 ± 29 Å, as compared with 1796 ± 57 Å found in non-diabetic rats) by daily oral administration of the AR inhibitor methosorbinil. Treatment also reduced polyol accumulation and prevented myoinositol depletion in the glomeruli.

EVIDENCE FOR EFFICACY OF ALDOSE REDUCTASE INHIBITORS IN CLINICAL STUDIES

Neuropathy

Comprehensive reviews were recently written by Boulton and Ward[382] on diabetic neuropathics and pain, and by Gillon et al[383] on the pathology of diabetic neuropathy and the effects of AR inhibitors.

Alrestatin

The first AR inhibitor to be tested clinically in diabetic subjects with polyneuropathy was alrestatin. Initially, Gabbay et al[384] reported remarkable subjective improvement in two diabetic patients with severe neuropathy given alrestatin intravenously at a dose of 50 mg/kg body weight over 24 hours, in four divided doses, for five days. However, no significant changes in sensory or MNCV were observed; nor were there measurable changes in four other diabetic patients with severe neuropathy treated with alrestatin at a dose of 1 g, given four times daily for 30 days. Alrestatin was well tolerated, except that in one patient, fasciculation was observed in the vastus lateralis muscles. After intravenous injection, serum alrestatin concentrations decreased rapidly, corresponding to a half-life of about 50 minutes. The lack of objective evidence of improved nerve function was tentatively attributed to low systemic drug levels, patient selection, and short duration of treatment.

Subsequently, Culebras et al[385] injected alrestatin intravenously, 50 mg/kg/day in four divided doses, for five days, to ten diabetic patients with clinically evident peripheral neuropathy in the lower extremities. A marked increase in sensory conduction velocities was recorded in four of ten patients, a worsened conduction velocity in four, and no change in two patients. Alrestatin produced no side effects. Since the study was not placebo-controlled, the possibility of a placebo effect cannot be excluded.

In another study, Handelsman and Turtle[386] used alrestatin to treat nine diabetic patients with peripheral neuropathy accompanied by severe debilitating pain and an average duration of diabetes of 22 ± 4 years. In a single-blind, placebo-controlled design, the patients received alrestatin orally at an average daily dose of 4.8 ± 0.6 g for eight weeks. No objective benefit from drug treatment was recorded; the subjective benefit noted in most patients was not consistent with a drug effect in all cases. Skin rash was observed in four patients and photosensitivity in two. The authors concluded that further trials may be more rewarding in early diabetic neuropathy, where structural damage is lesser.

Such a study was conducted by Fagius and Jameson[387] in 30 patients with stable diabetes and mean duration of disease of 8.3 years (range, 3 to 44 years), all but three with clinical signs of slight to moderate polyneuropathy evidenced by decreased conduction velocities. Using a double-blind, placebo-controlled design, alrestatin was administered four times daily at a dose of 2 g/day for one week, 4 g/day for five weeks, and 8 g/day for the last six weeks. Subjective improvement of sensation and reduction of symptoms was reported more frequently and was more pronounced among the drug-treated patients. Drug treatment reduced the mean score of sensory impairment and improved the discriminative sensation ($p<0.05$). Vibration thresholds were improved, the degree of significance increasing with duration of treatment. Treatment with alrestatin also improved the conduction velocity of the ulnar nerve ($p<0.01$), but not of the median and tibial nerves. A small improvement of autonomic function was also observed. The authors regarded the results obtained with alrestatin as indicative that "aldose reductase inhibitor treatment may be of value in diabetic polyneuropathy," thus providing "support for the sorbitol pathway hypothesis of diabetic polyneuropathy."

Sorbinil

The clinical program for the study of the therapeutic potential of sorbinil in patients with neuropathy and retinopathy has been presented by Pitts et al.[388]

In a study by Judzewitsch et al,[389] 250 mg of sorbinil was given once daily for nine weeks to patients with chronic diabetes (mean duration from diagnosis, 9.8 years) without clinical symptoms of peripheral neuropathy.[390] A randomized, double-blind, crossover study design was used. Thirty-nine patients completed the study, and five were withdrawn because of development of fever and rash, occurring within six to 14 days of starting sorbinil treatment. The drug caused small increases in nerve conduction velocity in the median motor (+1.19%) and sensory (+2.09%) nerves and in the peroneal motor nerve (+2.00%); these effects were maximal within three weeks and rapidly dissipated when the drug was discontinued. The degree of hyperglycemia remained stable during the study. Interestingly, the increases in nerve conduction velocities observed with nine weeks of sorbinil treatment were of similar magnitude as those observed earlier[391,392] with 12 months of antihyperglycemic therapy.[393] The selective assessment of nerve conduction velocities and the small increases observed prompted several critical comments.[394-396] In their reply,[397] the authors agreed that "current methods of measuring nerve conduction velocity provide only limited information about nerve function..." but felt that "despite the small and variable magnitude of the effect of sorbinil, it would be unwise at this stage to ignore these suggestive findings." (They also corrected the baseline values appearing in Table 1 of the original report.) In an editorial comment on the report, Winegrad et al[390] concluded that the results of Judzewitsch et al "support the view that the polyol pathway plays a part in mediating the effect of hyperglycemia in nerves."

Results obtained in 11 patients with painful diabetic neuropathy and treated with sorbinil were reported by Jaspan et al.[398] The severity of pain made it impossible to have placebo control periods for every patient or to define the length of the placebo period. The study design was thus single-blind and unrandomized. Sorbinil was given once daily at a dose of 250 mg for ten days to five weeks. Eight of the 11 patients noticed substantial relief of pain, generally three to four days after initiation of treatment. Each of the four patients with diabetic amyotrophy reported striking improvement in pain. Autonomic nerve function and nerve conduction velocity improved in six of seven patients tested. Clinical improvement seemed to be related to increase in nerve conduction velocity. Another patient had macular erythematous rash and was withdrawn from the study. The validity of the reported results was questioned by two groups of clinicians,[399,400] mainly because of the study design (single-blind, with subjective or observer-dependent end points), small number of subjects, lack of a reasonable period of double-blind investigation of a placebo group, and because the study measured nerve conduction velocity rather than the amplitude of the action potentials of the sural and common peroneal nerves. (The latter are considered to be the more sensitive electrophysiological indicators of diabetic neuropathy). Abraham et al[400] concluded that "similar placebo-controlled, double-blind investigations are required before sorbinil is credited with a useful role in the treatment of diabetic neuropathy."

Young et al[401] conducted a double-blind, randomized, placebo-controlled crossover study in 15 diabetic subjects with chronic painful neuropathy for longer than one year's duration. Sorbinil was given once daily at a dose of 200 mg for four weeks. The only significant objective changes observed in the trial were improvement in reflex scores, increase in sural nerve sensory potentials, and deterioration in sensory scores in patients receiving sorbinil. However, improvement in pain was reported more frequently ($p<0.02$) by patients taking sorbinil. Four patients

(26.7%) experienced rash with variable leukopenia and lymphadenopathy, which was reversible and resolved within ten days of discontinuing the drug. The authors conclude their report by suggesting that pain of diabetic neuropathy may be mediated by a metabolic disorder rather than structural damage and regard their findings as support for the hypothesis that the polyol pathway is implicated in the pathogenesis of diabetic neuropathy.

The short-term effect of sorbinil, at a dose of 250 mg per day, on severe painful neuropathy was also investigated by Rosenstock et al[402] in a double-blind, placebo-controlled study with 32 patients. Assessment was based on a 20-point subjective neuropathy and pain symptom score. Although sorbinil treatment caused significant improvement of severe pain and overall neuropathy assessment, no difference in these parameters was found after six weeks of therapy. The authors concluded that longer treatment periods are required, preferably in less advanced forms of diabetic neuropathy.

Lehtinen et al[403-406] reported the results from a preliminary study in ambulatory patients with diabetic neuropathy. In a double-blind, crossover, placebo-controlled trial, 43 subjects were given 100 mg sorbinil per day for four weeks; 31[404-406] and 32[403] patients completed the study. There were no statistically significant differences in MNCV and distal latency of the peroneal nerve, F-latency of the median nerve, and sensory nerve conduction velocities during the sorbinil period as compared with the placebo period. The authors attributed the lack of effect to the small dose and short duration of treatment with sorbinil. One patient developed rash, myalgia, and fever, which subsided in two weeks.

The effect of 200 mg sorbinil, given once daily, in 13 patients with symptomatic diabetic neuropathy of mean duration of six years was investigated by Lewin et al[407] in a double-blind, placebo-controlled crossover study. The four-week treatment with sorbinil produced no significant change in motor, sensory, or mixed nerve conduction velocities, in the amplitude of motor or sensory action potentials, or in distal motor latency; the vibration perception thresholds remained unchanged, and there was no significant change in any of the autonomic function tests performed after sorbinil treatment. One patient developed a febrile illness with rash and oral ulceration 21 days after starting sorbinil; this resolved on drug withdrawal. In comparing the results of their study with those reported by Judzewitsch et al[389] and Jaspan et al,[398] based on the patients' age and duration of diabetes, the authors concluded that their patients may have had a smaller reversible component to their neuropathy than patients in the other two studies. The mean plasma sorbinil concentration, measured at the end of treatment in five of the 12 patients (10.6 ± 3.4 μg/mL, range, 6.3 to 14.5 μg/mL) was higher than that reported by Judzewitsch et al[389] (>4.0 μg/mL) after a daily dose of 250 mg, but similar to the mean peak drug concentration of 10.6 μg/mL found in healthy young subjects given 250 mg sorbinil daily for five consecutive days.[408]

Schouten et al[409-411] reported in three abstracts the results obtained in a three-month, double-blind, parallel treatment, placebo-controlled study in patients with diabetic neuropathy given 200 mg of sorbinil per day. Of 32 patients, 28, with mean age 50.8 years (range, 20 to 65) and with stable diabetes of 16.5 years' mean duration (range, 10 months to 41 years) have completed the study. When the results before and after sorbinil treatment were compared with the results before and after placebo, three of the ten measured nerve conduction variables improved significantly, specifically, the median MNCV, peroneal distal latency, and the Hoffman H-M interval. Sorbinil treatment had no effect on pain scores, vibratory perception threshold, or on the cardiovascular reflex test. Two patients receiving sorbinil have withdrawn because of drug-related fever and a generalized rash.[409,410]

Christensen et al[412] treated 37 patients with stable diabetes and abnormal vibratory perception threshold for four weeks with single daily doses of 50 mg or 200 mg of sorbinil in a double-blind, placebo-controlled study. No significant improvements in the right peroneal and median MNCV and vibratory perception threshold were noted when comparing the two treatment groups with each other or comparing each group for placebo periods with sorbinil periods. In addition, no significant improvement was observed in the function of the retina evaluated by nyctometry. An overall subjective improvement was recorded in the 200 mg group compared with the 50 mg group. The mean fasting plasma drug concentrations after three weeks of sorbinil administration (in μg/mL $\pm$ SD) were 2.95 $\pm$ 3.11 after 50 mg sorbinil and 7.98 $\pm$ 3.44 after 200 mg sorbinil.

A 24-week double-blind parallel group, placebo-controlled trial in male patients with symptomatic diabetic polyneuropathy of the distal, symmetrical sensorimotor type and with symptoms of sexual impotence was reported by Fagius et al.[413] Twenty-seven patients, aged 48.7 $\pm$ 10.4 years, with mean duration of diabetes of 20.7 $\pm$ 11.1 years and of polyneuropathy of 6.1 $\pm$ 4.6 years, receiving 250 mg sorbinil once daily, have completed the study. No major clinical benefit was seen in the sorbinil-treated patients, and no differences in sensory thresholds were observed. Only in MNCV of the posterior tibial nerve, F-wave latency, sensory distal latency of the ulnar nerve, and heart rate variation during deep breathing were significant differences between the patient groups seen to evolve in favor of sorbinil treatment. There was no evidence of continuing improvement throughout the treatment period, and beneficial effects observed were no greater than those seen in previous trials of considerably shorter treatment periods. The authors concluded that sorbinil treatment resulted in some improvement of peripheral nerve function in symptomatic diabetic polyneuropathy, but that the long-term effect may be of limited value.

In a 52-week double-blind study in IDDM patients with neuropathy, Christensen[414] treated 13 patients with 250 mg sorbinil per day and seven patients with placebo. Treatment produced no changes in MNCV of the peroneal and median nerve or in sensory conduction velocity of the sural and median nerve, in vibration and temperature perception on the upper and lower limb, and in beat-to-beat variation. No effect on retinal function was evident upon nyctometry, and no difference between the two treatments was shown by the patients' subjective assessment. The side effects were slight and transitory; in the sorbinil group they consisted of four cases of skin eruption, seven cases of skin itching, and seven patients complained of muscle pain.

Jaspan et al reported on the effects of sorbinil, given at a dose of 250 mg per day, on cardiac autonomic neuropathy[415] and on median nerve somatosensory evoked potentials[416] in 36 diabetic patients in a double-blind, parallel treatment, placebo-controlled study. The response was assessed by R-R interval ratios on electrocardiogram during expiration and inspiration at six breaths per minute. After six weeks of treatment, the subnormal R-R interval ratios and elevated heart rates were decreased, suggesting improvement in vagal function. At week 6 of treatment, serum sorbinil concentrations of 13.5 $\pm$ 1.3 μg/mL were found. Interestingly, linear regression analysis revealed no significant relationship between serum drug concentrations, decrease in erythrocyte sorbitol levels, and the degree of cardiac autonomic response.[417] Somatosensory-evoked potential data were regarded as being consistent with a drug-related improvement in peripheral nerve integrity, with no statistically significant changes in central conduction.[416]

Pfeifer et al[418] reported on the effect of sorbinil treatment on the cardiovascular performance in 14 diabetic patients in a double-blind placebo-controlled study. Before treatment, the resting and all stages of cardiac output, as well as the work-product (heart rate $\times$ systolic blood pressure), were lower in the diabetic patients ($p<0.03$) when compared with age-matched normal subjects. In contrast to the placebo-treated patients, treatment with sorbinil increased all stages of the work-product ($p<0.05$).

In an open-label pilot study in eight diabetic patients by Green et al,[419] treatment with sorbinil (250 mg/day) for six months resulted in improvements in bladder sensation and in decreased residual volume, while bladder motor function remained slightly subnormal. Preliminary results also suggest that AR inhibitors may improve somatic and autonomic neural dysfunction in the gastrointestinal tract of diabetic patients.[420]

Epalrestat (Sorbistat®)

Hotta et al[421] reported in abstract form the results obtained in 13 patients with diabetic peripheral neuropathy treated for 12 weeks with the AR inhibitor epalrestat at a daily dose of 300 mg. While a statistically significant increase in ulnar MNCV (+11.6%) was recorded, the effect on ulnar sensory conduction velocity was variable: compared with baseline, a 10.5% increase was obtained after four weeks of treatment, and a 5.3% decrease, after 12 weeks of treatment. Subjective assessment of pain and numbness was improved after two weeks of treatment.

In another study, reported by Okuno et al,[422] 13 diabetic patients with neuropathy accompanied by severe or moderate pain and/or paresthesia in distal upper and lower extremities were treated with epalrestat at a dose of 600 mg/day for eight weeks. While subjective improvement was reported in 87% of the treated patients, no correlation was obtained between subjective relief and motor, sensory, and mixed nerve conduction velocities in median and tibial nerves. The effects of epalrestat were compared with those obtained with 20 μg prostaglandin (PG) E_1 injected intravenously daily, for two weeks; it was concluded that epalrestat was more effective in objective measures.

In a ten-center open study, 152 diabetic patients (38 IDDM) with peripheral neuropathy manifested in sensory nerve disturbance and spontaneous pain were treated for four weeks with epalrestat given by mouth three times per day at daily doses of 300 mg (n=67) and 600 mg (n=85).[423] Subjective assessments were recorded for spontaneous pain, sensory nerve disturbance, and muscular and autonomic nerve disturbance. Objective assessments consisted of nervous function tests (patellar and Achilles' tendon reflex), vibration sensation, and motor and sensory nerve conduction velocity. Subjectively, moderate improvement was experienced by 38% and slight improvement by 71% of the patients receiving 600 mg/day, and by 22% and 69%, respectively, after 300 mg/day. The functional tests appeared to be less conclusive, since no effect on vibration sensation was detected and no clear dose-dependence was evident in the tendon reflexes or conduction velocity except in the sensory conduction velocity of the ulnar nerve. One case of urticaria was reported after 600 mg/day. The authors concluded that epalrestat was more effective when given at 600 mg/day for four weeks.

In another study by Okuno et al,[424] 17 patients with diabetic peripheral neuropathy were given epalrestat for eight weeks at a daily dose of 600 mg and the effects on the autonomic nervous system were evaluated by examining beat-to-beat variation during the test and by testing skin temperature and its recovery time after cold water exposure. Treatment increased beat-to-beat variation and relieved the symptoms (in 15 of 17 patients) but had no effect on MNCV. PGE_1, used as reference, was given to 16 patients by intravenous injection at a daily dose of 40 μg, for two weeks. PGE_1 relieved the symptoms in 12 of 16 patients, increased beat-to-beat variation, and shortened the recovery time of skin temperature.

Tolrestat (Alredase®)

An initial interim report on an ongoing long-term, open-label study in patients with painful or paresthetic diabetic distal, symmetrical peripheral neuropathy was presented by Koglin et al.[425] Nineteen patients are being treated with a daily dose of 200 mg tolrestat. Neurological evaluation, including subjective grading of the painful or paresthetic symptom, is being done at screening and at four- to eight-week intervals. After 24 weeks of treatment, no clinically significant abnormality in laboratory tests or adverse effects have been observed. As illustrated below, daily administration of 200 mg of tolrestat appears to reduce the symptoms of painful diabetic neuropathy; symptom improvement was noted after eight weeks of drug administration:

	Study week			
	4	8	16	24
Improved vs total*	3/13	7/13	7/9	7/8
Percentage improved	23	54	78	87.5

*Expressed in numbers of patients.

In a subsequent report[426] on patients that have completed 24 weeks of treatment, statistically significant increases in both ulnar and peroneal MNCV were attained at 24 weeks:

Nerve	MNCV (m/sec ± SE)		N	P
	Baseline	Week 24		
Ulnar	46.3 ± 5.0	48.0 ± 5.2	19	0.03
Peroneal	36.9 ± 4.6	40.1 ± 7.6	17	0.02

Pain scores, graded from 0 (absent) to 4 (incapacitating), improved after 24 weeks of treatment with tolrestat from a baseline score of 3.2 ± 0.9 to 2.0 ± 1.3 ($p<0.001$ for $n = 32$). No serious side effects were noted.

In a 19-center, one-year, double-blind study, reported by Boulton et al,[38] 550 patients with chronic painful/paresthetic neuropathy were randomly assigned to groups receiving tolrestat (50 mg, 100 mg, or 200 mg daily, or 100 mg twice daily) or placebo. MNCV was assessed in the peroneal, ulnar, tibial, and median nerves. Clinical responders were defined as patients showing improved MNCV and paresthetic symptoms. Compared with those taking placebo, patients taking 200 mg tolrestat once daily experienced statistically significant improvements in MNCV and paresthetic symptoms ($p<0.05$). Improvements in painful symptoms, however, were masked by a marked placebo response. Tolrestat, at a daily dose of 200 mg, was significantly better than placebo at 24 ($p = 0.02$), 42 ($p = 0.03$), and 52 weeks ($p = 0.04$) in producing concordant improvements in both MNCV and paresthetic symptom severity. A long-term clinical response was present at 24 weeks and maintained at 42 and 52 weeks in 28% of patients treated with tolrestat as compared with 5% receiving placebo ($p<0.002$).

In another 15-center, 8-week, double-blind study, reported by Ryder et al,[39] 260 patients with chronic painful diabetic neuropathy were randomized to one of three treatment groups receiving placebo, 400 mg tolrestat once daily, or 200 mg tolrestat twice daily. The 400 mg dose significantly increased the median MNCV ($p = 0.047$) as compared with placebo; peroneal MNCV was also increased, though the difference from placebo was not statistically significant. After four weeks, patients receiving 400 mg tolrestat daily experienced significantly greater improvement in the primary painful system compared to placebo ($p = 0.045$). By defining a clinical responder as a patient with concordant objective (mean MNCV) and subjective (painful symptom severity) improvement, compared with placebo, there were more clinical responders and fewer failures following administration of 400 mg tolrestat ($p = 0.023$).

These investigators have concluded that tolrestat administration can improve both MNCV and diabetic neuropathic painful/paresthetic symptoms at a dosage of 200 to 400 mg once daily.

The use of concordance analysis in the interpretation or results obtained with tolrestat in the two multi-center studies represents a major contribution to the method of evaluating the efficacy of treatment in studies seeking to show differences in response between populations in which many of the patients may be unresponsive, particularly when, as in diabetic neuropathy, relatively unsophisticated methods of assessment are used. The investigators consider concordance analysis as the most powerful and appropriate statistical approach because it takes into account the individual patient outcome, identifying patients with equivocal responses who tend to dilute overall group changes. Thus, in the tolrestat clinical trials, the results of the concordance analysis showed greater statistical significance at more time-points than when objective and subjective data were considered separately.

Diabetic keratopathy

The involvement of diabetes in the cornea was not considered seriously until the advent of vitreous surgery, when corneal complications became apparent.[427-429] During intraocular surgery in subjects with diabetes, the corneal epithelium often becomes edematous, thus obscuring intraoperative visualization of the posterior segment of the eye and necessitating removal of the corneal epithelium. While in non-diabetic patients re-epithelialization of the cornea occurs rapidly, in diabetic patients the epithelial defects heal slowly and incompletely,[427] and frequently require post-operative medical treatment.[429] It appears that when the diabetic cornea is stressed, as in vitrectomy, the mechanism maintaining fluid balance in the corneal epithelium is impaired, making the tissue incapable of maintaining normal hydration.[430,431] Other minor stress, such as contact lenses[432] and ocular manipulation during retinal photocoagulation,[433,434] is also less well tolerated by the diabetic cornea.[435]

The presence in the corneal epithelium of both aldose reductase and of an active pentose phosphate shunt (source of the necessary cofactor) raised the possibility that the epithelial abnormalities of the diabetic cornea could arise from the activity of aldose reductase. If so, then the complication could be controlled by inhibiting aldose reductase. This possibility was substantiated at the National Eye Institute by the use of AR inhibitors,[436] both in vitro[430] and in vivo.[430,431,437]

In preclinical studies, in vitro, the formation of xylitol by bovine corneal epithelium incubated in a xylose-containing medium was inhibited in the presence of the AR inhibitor alrestatin.[430,431] In vivo, the delay in the re-epithelialization of denuded corneas, shown to occur in both STZ-induced diabetic rats and in rats fed on a 50% galactose diet, was prevented by the topical application to the eye of seven structurally distinct AR inhibitors.[430] Regeneration of corneal epithelium was also accelerated in diabetic rats administered alrestatin (about 440 mg/kg) by intraperitoneal injection[431] and in galactosemic rats given sorbinil (about 60 mg/kg) with the diet.[433]

In vitro studies with rabbit cornea have shown that the pathogenesis of the diabetic corneal epithelium stems from the increased flux of glucose through the polyol pathway and the resultant decrease in NADPH availability. Sorbitol accumulation per se is therefore not a prerequisite for the diabetic complication of the cornea.[438]

The involvement of aldose reductase in human diabetic keratopathy is supported by the clinical report of improved corneal wound healing in a diabetic patient treated with the AR inhibitor sorbinil.[435] The report represents an extreme case of diabetic keratopathy in a 24-year-old woman with poorly controlled IDDM. After bilateral argon laser photocoagulation for extensive proliferative retinopathy and exudative maculopathy, the patient developed spontaneous bilateral central corneal erosions unresponsive to conventional treatment. In single-masked fashion, the patient's right eye was treated topically with sorbinil, five times daily. Over two months, the right eye responded slowly to treatment: the ocular inflammatory signs abated, and the epithelial defects lessened in size. In contrast, the placebo-treated left eye remained inflamed, ultimatly worsened and perforated, requiring keratoplasty. Five days after the operation, the characteristic diabetic epithelial defect occurred, and treatment with sorbinil was extended to the left eye. After one year of treatment with topical sorbinil five times per day, both eyes appear stable.[434]

According to Cobo,[435] the observed clinical effectiveness of an AR inhibitor in diabetic keratopathy may be produced by a two-pronged action: first, by decreasing or eliminating the accumulation of metabolites (formed by the polyol pathway) not commonly present in the non-diabetic corneal epithelium[439]; second, by a currently less easily documented effect of reversal or alleviation of the neuropathic complications of diabetes mellitus.

The demonstrations that aldose reductase is present in the corneal and conjunctive epithelium[440] and that AR inhibitors can influence the process of corneal re-epithelialization in both diabetic and galactosemic rats[431,437] and, apparently, in human diabetics,[435] indicate that aldose reductase is probably involved in the diabetes-induced abnormalities of corneal re-epithelialization and ulceration that may occur in diabetic patients when the cornea is stressed by operations such as vitrectomy and by techniques such as extended wear of contact lenses.[434,440]

Of importance are also observations that diabetic patients have greater incidence of corneal epithelial defects, particularly those with NIDDM; decreased tear production, and reduced corneal sensation.[441] Diabetic patients have also greater mean corneal thickness, particularly those with proliferative retinopathy[442] and persistent stromal edema,[429] suggesting some abnormality of the endothelial monolayer. Computer-assisted morphometric analysis of individual endothelial cells, as described by Matsuda et al,[443] showed that the corneal endothelium of diabetic patients,[444] alloxan-induced diabetic dogs,[445] and STZ-induced diabetic rats[446] had a marked variation in cell size (polymegathism) and cell shape (pleomorphism). The loss of a regular hexagonal cell pattern suggests that the diabetic endothelium is stressed, hence more vulnerable to surgical trauma. The degree of these endothelial changes appears to correspond directly to the level of glycemic control.[445] In view of the demonstration of aldose reductase in the corneal endothelium of animals[119,120] and humans,[124] it is possible that aldose reductase plays a role in the initiation of the endothelial cell changes in the diabetic cornea.[444] Evidence supporting the concept was obtained by decreasing such endothelial changes in 10-month STZ-induced diabetic rats by topical instillation of a 0.5% solution of an AR inhibitor, CT-112.[447] Pertinently, regeneration of the corneal endothelium was found to be delayed in galactosemic rats and was corrected by administration of another AR inhibitor, M-79,175.[448]

Retinopathy

Cunha-Vaz et al[449] have investigated the effect of sorbinil, given once daily at a dose of 250 mg, on the alteration of the blood-brain barrier in 32 NIDDM patients with no or minimal retinopathy, i.e., less than five microaneurysms in the posterior pole. In a double-blind, placebo-controlled study, the permeability of the blood-retinal barrier was measured by the penetration of intravenously-injected fluorescein into the posterior vitreous humor. After six months of treatment, based on results from 25 patients, the alteration of the blood-retinal barrier (expressed as the mean penetration ratio $\times 10^{-6}$/min, $\pm$ SD) increased significantly less in the sorbinil-treated group (-0.07 ± 1.18) compared with the placebo group (1.09 ± 1.35, $p<0.05$). A similar conclusion was reached by Cunha-Vaz et al[450] in a trial with sulindac.

Hotta et al[451] reported that in 45 diabetic patients with background or pre-proliferative retinopathy, treatment with epalrestat at a dose of 300 mg per day for three months resulted in improved electroretinograms and decreases in microaneurysms, exudates, and soft exudates. Further improvement was observed after 12 months of treatment, e.g., in fluorescein angiography.

Limited joint mobility

Stiffness of hands, associated with increased skin thickness in adult diabetics, was first reported by Lundbaek.[452] More recently, several reports have appeared on contractures of the finger joints in young patients with IDDM.[453-459] Finger joint contractures were also found to occur in older IDDM[460-462] and NIDDM patients.[460,462] A variety of terms have been used to describe the phenomenon, including "joint stiffness,"[453] "diabetic hand syndrome,"[463] and "juvenile diabetic cheiroarthropathy."[456] Since larger joints can also be involved, "limited joint mobility" has been suggested as a more appropriate term.[462] The use of this term has been questioned, however.[464] The subject is discussed in more detail in Chapter 1.

A role for aldose reductase in the pathogenesis of limited joint mobility in diabetes mellitus[457] was suggested by Eaton et al,[46] who achieved improvement in range of motion and in strength of digital flexion and extension in three diabetic subjects with adult limited joint mobility syndrome by treating them with the AR inhibitor sorbinil. Prompted by their finding, the authors have postulated that the syndrome was caused by osmotic swelling due to collagen hydration produced by sorbitol accumulation. The collagen constituents of periarticular tissues of the hands have thus been added to the list of tissues known or suspected to be vulnerable to polyol accumulation, hence controllable by treatment with AR inhibitors. The conclusion was questioned by Frank,[465] who argued that excessive hydration of collagen is extracellular, while aldose reductase, as a cytosolic enzyme, causes intracellular accumulation of polyols because of their limited capacity to traverse the cell's plasma membrane. Eaton[466] subsequently expanded his findings into the "collagen hydration hypothesis, a more general concept, in which increased hydration of collagen, independent of organ or tissue identity and in an extracellular as well as intracellular location, may represent a common pathophysiologic pathway contributing to secondary complications of diabetic hyperglycemia. Since collagen is ubiquitous in mammalian tissues, such a glycemia-intiated collagen hydration could lead to diabetic complications in virtually all tissues of the body."

Complete resolution of both skin and joint changes upon improved diabetic control in two patients with diabetic cheiroarthropathy was reported by Lister et al.[467] The finding does not support the view that these joint contractures are due to abnormal non-enzymatic glycation of collagen[468,469] since reversibility of such changes was not shown to occur (in tail collagen of diabetic rats) upon intensive insulin treatment by continuous subcutaneous infusion.[470]

Red blood cell sorbitol

The function of the mature red blood cell (RBC) depends entirely on the utilization of glucose. The mammalian erythrocyte is unique in that about 90% of its total energy requirement is provided by glycolysis. In humans, this limited metabolic capacity permits RBC survival for approximately 120 days, after which it is sequestered and phagocytozed in the reticuloendothelial system.[471] The hexokinase reaction is also rate-limiting in RBC glycolysis.[472] Among all the enzymes of the glycolytic pathway that show an age-dependent decrease in activity, hexokinase seems to be critical, with a half-life of 33 days. The decay of hexokinase activity as a function of cell age may be related to the decline in the RBC glycolytic rate.[471]

Under physiological conditions, the RBC metabolizes about 3% of the absorbed glucose via the polyol pathway.[171] Because of the very low affinity of the L-hexonate dehydrogenase for glucose (see Table 3), the conversion of glucose to sorbitol is attributed to aldose reductase.[171,174,179] Sorbitol penetrates cell membranes poorly,[172] resulting in higher RBC sorbitol levels than in the plasma.[171] Interestingly, in 34 IDDM patients the erythrocyte sorbitol dehydrogenase activity was significantly lower [0.219 $\pm$ 0.085 U/min per g Hb($\pm$SD)] than in normal blood donors [0.340 $\pm$ 0.094 U/min per g Hb].[473] In spite of the rapid uptake and conversion of glucose to sorbitol,[182,474,475] there is correlation between plasma glucose and RBC sorbitol concentrations, first reported by Morrison et al[171] and confirmed in several studies (Table 48), provided plasma glucose and RBC sorbitol levels are measured simultaneously,[479] or, at least within one hour.[477] Lapolla et al[478] reported that in a group of 62 insulin-treated diabetic patients, only 28% had RBC sorbitol levels above the normal range. The RBC sorbitol test is not suitable as an index of long-term glucose control.[182,477,478,480]

The observation that the RBC sorbitol levels in diabetic subjects are about twice as high as those in non-diabetic subjects[179] has been confirmed in a number of studies (Table 49). The dissimilarity in the absolute values reported from different laboratories is most likely attributable to methodological differences.[184] Usually, RBC sorbitol is determined enzymatically (Table 49) by measuring the appearance of NADH in the presence of sorbitol dehydrogenase by a procedure originally described by Clements et al[487] and modified by Malone et al.[179] If the enzymatic method is used, it is prudent to validate it by gas liquid chromatography.[179]

Table 48. Correlation between plasma glucose and red blood cell sorbitol concentration in human subjects.

No. of Subjects	Correlation		Ref. No.
	r	p	
10 ND, 19 D	0.90	—	171
30 ND, 155 D	0.59	<0.001	179
24 ND, 45 D	—	<0.001	181
30 ND 52 D	0.62	<0.001	182
114 ND, 114 D	0.33	<0.02	186
23 D[a]	0.55	<0.0001	476
90 D	0.48	<0.0001	477
62 D	0.73[b]	<0.001	478

ND = Non-diabetic, D = Diabetic
[a]Based on 159 observations
[b]Fasting plasma glucose

According to Rogers et al,[488] male subjects after puberty have two times higher RBC sorbitol levels than before puberty; in male subjects with diabetes, the RBC sorbitol levels after puberty are six times higher than before puberty. However, in postpubertal females with diabetes, the increase was only 50% vs controls.

The finding that the formation and accumulation of sorbitol in human RBC exposed to high ambient glucose concentrations was blocked by adding to the medium the AR inhibitor TMG[180] was confirmed in vivo by demonstrating that the elevated RBC sorbitol levels in diabetic rats and diabetic patients can be decreased by treatment with the AR inhibitor sorbinil.[183] The finding in diabetic patients was subsequently corroborated by several investigators using sorbinil, epalrestat (Table 50), tolrestat (Tables 51 and 52), or statil.[490,491]

There are two facets to the potential usefulness of the RBC sorbitol test: first, as suggested by Malone et al,[179,180] to serve as indicator of aldose reductase activity and its inhibition in other tissues containing aldose reductase, hence prone to diabetic complications[179] because of the increased flux of glucose through the polyol pathway, and second, to serve as indicator of systemic availability of an AR inhibitor. Both facets reflect the pharmacokinetics of an AR inhibitor, namely, its rates of absorption, presystemic elimination, uptake by the RBC, and elimination from the blood and RBC. In the proposal of Malone et al, the RBC-sorbitol test would reflect AR inhibitor uptake and elimination from a given tissue as compared with the RBC where the effect of the inhibitor is measured. The predictive value of the RBC-sorbitol test may depend, however, not only on differences in the rates of

Table 49. Sorbitol concentrations in red blood cells of non-diabetic and diabetic subjects.

Red blood cell sorbitol concentrations (nmol/g Hb ± SE, except where noted)	
Non-diabetic subjects	**Diabetic subjects**
5.2 ± 0.3 nmol/mL (GLC)[481]	13.1 ± 0.9 nmol/mL(GLC)[481]
5.8 ± 1.6 nmol/mL (±SD) (GLC)[482]	13.6 ± 5.1 nmol/mL (±SD) (GLC)[482]
5.9 ± 1.6 nmol/mL (±SD) (GLC)[184]	17.8 ± 8.2 nmol/mL (±SD) (GLC)[184]
10.1 ± 1.3 (Enz.)[179]	19.8 ± 2.3[405]
10.3 ± 0.8 (Enz.)[187,483]	21.7 ± 2.0[405]
16.9 ± 5.4 (±SD) (Enz.)[185]	22.7 ± 9.0 (±SD) (Enz.)[484,485]
17.0 ± 3.5 (Enz.)[182]	25.1 ± 4.0 (GLC)[476]
40.6 ± 8.8 (±SD) (Enz.)[186]	26.7 ± 3.7(GLC)[476]
41.8 ± 2.0 (Enz.)[478]	28.0 ± 18.9 (±SD) (Enz.)[179]
44.9 ± 3.2 (Enz.)[181]	28.8 ± 2.7 (Enz.)[183]
	31.8 ± 2.1 nmol/mL (Enz.)[182]
	36.6 ± 1.7 (Enz.)[187,483]
	37.4 ± 14.5 (±SD) (Enz.)[185]
	37.6 ± 18.6 (±SD) (Enz.)[486]
	66.1 ± 2.0 (Enz.)[478]
	90.8 ± 9.8 (Enz.) (NIDDM)[181]
	91.0 ± 6.4 (Enz.) (IDDM)[181]
	139.4 ± 90.0 (±SD) (Enz.)[186]

Enz. = Enzymatic method; GLC = Gas liquid chromatographic method. NB that 1 nmol sorbitol/ml red blood cell corresponds to approximately 3 nmol sorbitol/g Hb.[184]

AR inhibitor uptake and elimination from a given tissue as compared with the RBCs, but also on the differences in the tissue-specific role of aldose reductase in the development of localized biochemical, functional, and morphological changes. The postulate that the RBC-sorbitol test may be useful in monitoring the success of therapy with AR inhibitors,[183] e.g., in the nerve, was supported by results obtained in STZ-induced diabetic rats with sorbinil,[183,492] but not with epalrestat.[217] The results obtained with sorbinil[221] and statil[146] in galactosemic rats suggest that the potency of an AR inhibitor may vary between different tissues. Results obtained so far in diabetic patients do not support the postulate of Malone et al,[179,180,183,492,493] since no significant correlation was found between RBC sorbitol levels and the tactile and thermal perception thresholds for finger and toe.[494] Berger et al,[495] however, found an association between the severity of neuropathy and sorbitol accumulation in washed erythrocytes [incubated with 110 mM (1982 mg/dL) glucose] obtained from IDDM patients.

It is pertinent that, in contrast to the peripheral nerve, where an increased flux of glucose through the polyol pathway is associated with myoinositol depletion (see Chapter 2 for more detailed discussion), no association was found between myoinositol and sorbitol levels in erythrocytes of normal or diabetic subjects.[481,496-500] It is of interest that, in RBC of poorly controlled diabetic patients, Gronda et al[501] have found unchanged activity of Na/K-dependent ATPase but

Table 50. Effect of AR inhibitors on red blood cell sorbitol concentration in subjects with diabetes mellitus.

Subject population (n)	AR inhibitor (mg/day)	Duration of treatment (weeks)	RBC sorbitol (nmol/g Hb ± SE)		Ref. No.
			Nontreated	Treated	
Patients with IDDM (15)	Sorbinil (250)	2	28.8 ± 2.7	13.8 ± 2.4[a]	183
Diabetic patients with neuropathy (32)	Sorbinil (100)	4	22.7 ± 9.0[b]	12.4 ± 9.6[b]	484, 485
Patients with NIDDM or IDDM (7)	Sorbinil (250)	4	37.6 ± 18.6[b]	12.1 ± 1.7[b,a]	486
Diabetic patients with polyneuropathy (31)	Sorbinil (100)	4	21.7 ± 2.0 19.8 ± 2.3	12.6 ± 1.9 9.9 ± 2.3	405
Patients with NIDDM or IDDM (28)	Sorbinil (200)	4	13.1 ± 0.9[c]	3.5[c]	481
Patients with IDDM (15)	Sorbinil (200)	4	13.6 ± 5.1[b,c]	3.3 ± 1.2[b,c]	482
Diabetic patients with neuropathy (26)	Sorbinil (250)	6	49.4 ± 12.7	17.9 ± 3.2	417
Patients with diabetic peripheral neuropathy (13)	Epalrestat (300)	12	40.0 ± 6.3	23.1 ± 3.4	421
Patients with IDDM (30)	Statil (600)	2	8.6 ± 1.0[c,d]	4.5 ± 1.2[c,e]	488

AR = Aldose reductase; RBC = Red blood cell
[a]Effect observed after one week of treatment.
[b] ± SD.
[c]Expressed in nmol/mL RBC.
[d]Treated, pre-dose.
[e]3 hr after dosing.

Table 51. Effect of tolrestat on red blood cell sorbitol concentrations in subjects with diabetes mellitus.[489]

Period	RBC sorbitol (nmol/g Hb ± SE)			Plasma tolrestat (μg/mL ± SE)	
	Placebo (n = 12)	25 mg b.i.d. (n = 12)	100 mg b.i.d. (n = 11)	25 mg b.i.d.	100 mg b.i.d.
Pretreatment	22.4 ± 4.0	24.6 ± 3.3	25.8 ± 3.0	—	—
Treatment with tolrestat					
3 days	21.8 ± 2.9[a]	14.1 ± 3.3[b]	9.7 ± 1.3[c],***	0.51 ± 0.07	3.22 ± 0.68
7 days	21.9 ± 3.4	17.8 ± 3.0	8.9 ± 1.5***	0.47 ± 0.08	2.48 ± 0.33
13 days	26.2 ± 5.4	19.0 ± 5.6	10.3 ± 1.7[d]**	0.62 ± 0.21	2.63 ± 0.45
Mean ± SE	23.0 ± 3.5	18.6 ± 3.9*	10.0 ± 1.3***	0.51 ± 0.10	2.78 ± 0.37
Mean change, % ± SE	8.7 ± 10.3	−26.8 ± 7.8*	−61.1 ± 2.7***	—	—

No. of samples received: a = 11; b = 8; c = 10; d = 9.
*$p < 0.005$, **$p < 0.001$, ***$p < 0.0001$, as compared with pretreatment values.

Table 52. Effect of tolrestat on red blood cell sorbitol/plasma glucose ratios in subjects with diabetes mellitus.[489]

Period	RBC sorbitol (nmol/g Hb)/Plasma glucose (Mean ± SE)		
	Placebo (n = 12)	25 mg b.i.d. (n = 12)	100 mg b.i.d. (n = 11)
Pretreatment	1.96 ± 0.25	2.28 ± 0.30	2.78 ± 0.28[a]
Treatment with tolrestat	1.85 ± 0.24	1.63 ± 0.21**	1.35 ± 0.19***
Mean change, % ± SE	−4.1 ± 5.5	−26.5 ± 5.2 *	−50.3 ± 5.5 ***

*$p < 0.02$, **$p < 0.002$, ***$p < 0.0001$, as compared with pretreatment values.

significantly lower activity of the Ca-dependent ATPase. However, significantly lower activities of Na/K-, Ca-, and Mg-dependent ATPases in RBC of NIDDM patients were reported by Adamson et al.[502]

The usefulness of the RBC-sorbitol test as indicator of the systemic availability of an orally administered AR inhibitor is supported by the results obtained with several AR inhibitors in laboratory animals[152,183,212,233] and human subjects with diabetes.[183,405,421,475,476,481,482,484,486,489,490,500] A decrease in RBC sorbitol levels reflects the blood-level of the AR inhibitor and its uptake by the erythrocytes. This is illustrated by the results obtained in human diabetic patients treated with either 25 mg or 100 mg tolrestat, given twice daily.[489] As shown in Table 51, at the higher dose, tolrestat normalized RBC sorbitol levels after three days of treatment, when steady-state plasma tolrestat concentrations were attained, as expected from its plasma half-life of 10 to 12 hours.[503]

Because the RBC sorbitol levels will vary as a direct function of the plasma glucose concentrations (Table 48) and because the currently investigated AR inhibitors do not affect plasma glucose,[146,183,476,489] the RBC sorbitol levels can also be expressed as function of the coincident plasma glucose concentration, i.e., as the ratio of RBC sorbitol (in nmol/mg Hb) to plasma glucose (in nmol/L).[187] The ratio helps to correct the RBC sorbitol concentration for the influence of variable plasma glucose levels common to IDDM subjects.[187] The use of the RBC sorbitol/plasma glucose ratio in the evaluation of the effectiveness of tolrestat is illustrated in Table 52.

According to Srivastava et al,[98,191] upon incubation for 96 hours with high ambient glucose concentrations, the conformation of aldose reductase is altered, resulting in an activated form, with about ten times lower Km for glucose and increased maximal velocity. Interestingly, incubation with 30 mM concentration of other substrates, such as galactose, xylose, and glyceraldehyde, had no effect on AR activity. Activated aldose reductase was also found in the erythrocytes from diabetic patients with plasma glucose concentrations higher than 250 mg/dL (approximately 15 mM). Since in its activated form, aldose reductase was reported to be less sensitive to inhibition by alrestatin and sorbinil,[98,191] the authors speculated that diabetic patients may require higher systemic concentrations than expected from inhibitory values obtained with non-activated aldose reductase. In fact, as illustrated by results in Table 51, a 61% decrease in RBC sorbitol content in diabetic patients treated with tolrestat was associated with an average plasma total drug concentration of 2.8 ± 0.4 μg/mL,[489] corresponding to 19.5 ± 2.6 ng/mL of free drug, available for uptake by the RBC. This corresponds to an IC_{60} of 5.5×10^{-8}M, which is the same order of magnitude as the IC_{50} of 3×10^{-8} M obtained with human RBC in vitro.[152]

References

1. Marble A: Insulin—Clinical aspects: The first fifty years. *Diabetes* 1972;21(suppl 2): 632–636.
2. Marble A: Late complications of diabetes. A continuing challenge. *Diabetologia* 1976;12:193–199.
3. Ellenberg M: Chronic complications of diabetes mellitus. *NY State J Med* 1979: 2005–2014.
4. Cahill GF, Etzwiler DD, Freinkel N: "Control" and diabetes. *N Engl J Med* 1976;294: 1004–1005.
5. Cahill GF, Etzwiler DD, Freinkel N: Blood glucose control in diabetes. *Diabetes* 1976;25:237–239.
6. Holman RR, Mayor-White V, Orde-Peckar C, et al: Prevention of deterioration of renal and sensory-nerve function by more intensive management of insulin-dependent diabetic patients. A two-year randomized prospective study. *Lancet* 1983;1:204–208.
7. Lauritzen T, Frost-Larsen K, Larsen HW, Deckert T: Steno Study Group. Effect of 1 year of study of near-normal blood glucose levels on retinopathy in insulin-dependent diabetics. *Lancet* 1983;1:200–204.
8. KROC Collaborative Study Group: Blood glucose control and the evolution of diabetic retinopathy and albuminuria. A preliminary multicenter trial. *N Engl J Med* 1984; 311:365–372.
9. Lauritzen T, Frost-Larsen K, Larsen HW, Deckert T: Steno Study Group: Continuous subcutaneous insulin infusion. *Lancet* 1983;1:1445–1446.
10. Rosenstock J, Friberg T, Raskin P: Effect of glycemic control on microvascular complications in patients with Type I diabetes mellitus. *Am J Med* 1986;81: 1012–1018.
11. Pirart J: Diabète et complications dégénératives. Présentation d'une étude prospective portant sur 4400 cas observés entre 1947 et 1973. *Diab Metab* (Paris) 1977;3:97–107, 173–182. [For translation see *Diabetes Care* 1978;1:168–188.]
12. Gabbay KH: Hyperglycemia, polyol metabolism and complications of diabetes mellitus. *Ann Rev Med* 1975;26:521–535.
13. Weiner H, Wermuth B (eds): *Enzymology of carbonyl metabolism: Aldehyde dehydrogenase and aldo/keto reductase.* New York, AR Liss Inc, 1982, pp 398–400.
14. Wirth HP, Wermuth B: Immunohistochemical localization of aldehyde and aldose reductase in human tissues. Flynn TG, Weiner H (eds): *Enzymology of carbonyl metabolism 2: Aldehyde dehydrogenase, aldo-keto reductate, and alcohol dehydrogenase.* New York, AR Liss Inc, 1985, pp 231–239.
15. Cromlish JA, Flynn TG: Identification of pig brain aldehyde reductases with the High-Km aldehyde reductase, the Low-Km aldehyde reductase and aldose reductase, carbonyl reductase, and succinic semialdehyde reductase. *J Neurochem* 1985;44: 1485–1493.
16. Akagi Y, Kador PF, Kinoshita JH: Immunohistochemical localization for aldose reductase in diabetic lenses. *Invest Ophthalmol Vis Sci* 1987;28:163–167.
17. Gonzalez RG, Barnett P, Aguayo J, Cheng HM, Chylack LT Jr: Direct measurement of polyol pathway activity in the ocular lens. *Diabetes* 1984;33:196–199.
18. Kinoshita JH, Merola LO, Hayman S: Osmotic effects on the amino acid-concentrating mechanism in the rabbit lens. *J Biol Chem* 1965;240:310–315.
19. Van Heyningen R: Formation of polyols by the rat with "sugar" cataract. *Nature* 1959;184:194–195.

20. Sener A, Hutton JC, Schoonheydt J, et al: Relationship of endogenous to dietary sorbitol. A study in normal and diabetic rats. *Diab Metab* 1979;5:217–222.
21. Malaisse-Lagae F, Coutourier E, Dufrane SP, et al: Effect of a sorbitol-rich diet on plasma and erythrocyte sorbitol concentrations in normal and diabetic subjects. *Diabetes Res* 1984;1:209–211.
22. Kinoshita JH, Merola LO, Satoh K, Dikmak E: Osmotic changes caused by the accumulation of dulcitol in the lenses of rats fed with galactose. *Nature* 1962;194: 1085–1087.
23. Kinoshita JH, Merola LO, Dikmak E: Osmotic changes in experimental galactose cataracts. *Exp Eye Res* 1962;1:405–410.
24. Kinoshita JH: Cataracts in galactosemia. *Invest Ophthalmol* 1965;4:786–799.
25. Kinoshita JH: Mechanisms initiating cataract formation. *Invest Ophthalmol* 1974; 13:713–724.
26. Kinoshita JH, Dvornik D, Kraml M, Gabbay KH: The effect of an aldose reductase inhibitor on the galactose-exposed rabbit lens. *Biochim Biophys Acta* 1968;158: 472–475.
27. Dvornik D, Simard-Duquesne N, Kraml M, et al: Polyol accumulation in galactosemic and diabetic rats: Control by an aldose reductase inhibitor. *Science* 1973;182: 1146–1148.
28. Hutton JC, Schofield PJ, Williams JF, Hollows FC: The failure of aldose reductase inhibitor 3,3′-tetramethyleneglutaric acid to inhibit in vivo sorbitol accumulation in lens and retina in diabetes. *Biochem Pharmacol* 1974;23:2991–2998.
29. Beaumont P, Sosula L, Hollows FC: The effect of an inhibitor of the sorbitol pathway on (1) acute diabetic capillary ultrastructure and (2) on retinal glycogen accumulation in diabetic retinae. *IRCS Med Sci* 1975;3:120.
30. Beaumont P, Sosula L, Hollows FC: The effect of tetramethyleneglutarate (TMG) on diabetic rat retinal glycogen accumulation. *IRCS Med Sci* 1975;3:121.
31. Dvornik D: Chronic complications of diabetes. *Ann Rep Med Chem* 1978;13:159–166.
32. Kador PF, Robison WG, Kinoshita JH: The pharmacology of aldose reductase inhibitors. *Ann Rev Pharmacol Toxicol* 1985;25:691–714.
33. Williamson JR, Chang K, Rowold E, et al: Sorbinil prevents diabetes induced increases in vascular permeability but does not alter collagen cross-linking. *Diabetes* 1985;34:703–705.
34. Kador PF, Kinoshita JH: Diabetic galactosemic cataracts. *Human cataract formation. Ciba Foundation Symposium 106.* London, Pitman, 1984, pp 110–131.
35. Kinoshita JH, Kador P, Robison WG, et al: Aldose reductase and complications of diabetes. *Ann Int Med* 1984;101:82–91.
36. Tomlinson DR, Mayer HJ: Defects of axonal transport in diabetes mellitus—a possible contribution to the aetiology of diabetic neuropathy. *J Auton Pharmac* 1984;4:59–72.
37. Ward JD: Diabetic neuropathy, in Alberti KGMM, Krall LP (eds): *The Diabetes Annual 1.* Amsterdam, New York, Oxford, Elsevier Science Publishers, 1985, pp 288–308.
38. Boulton AJ for the Tolrestat in Neuropathy Study Group: Effects of tolrestat, a new aldose reductase inhibitor, on nerve conduction and paraesthetic symptoms in diabetic neuropathy. *Diabetologia* 1986;29:521A.
39. Ryder S for the Tolrestat in Painful Neuropathy Study Group: Objective (nerve conduction) and subjective (painful symptom) improvement in diabetic neuropathy following administration of tolrestat, a new aldose reductase inhibitor. *Diabetologia* 1986;29:588A.
40. Robison WG, Kador PF, Kinoshita JH: Retinal capillaries: Basement membrane thickening by galactosemia prevented with aldose reductase inhibitor. *Science* 1983;221:1177–1179.

41. Frank RN, Keirn RJ, Kennedy A, Frank KW: Galactose-induced retinal capillary basement membrane thickening: Prevention by sorbinil. *Invest Ophthalmol Vis Sci* 1983;24:1519–1529.
42. Shanks E, D'Amico DJ, Gragoudas ES: Experimental model of diabetic retinopathy in the rat: Effects of dietary galactose and sorbinil on retinal basement membranes. *Invest Ophthalmol Vis Sci* 1985;26(suppl):28.
43. Robison WG, Kador PF, Akagi Y, et al: Prevention of basement membrane thickening in retinal capillaries by a novel inhibitor of aldose reductase, tolrestat. *Diabetes* 1986;35:295–299.
44. Dvornik D, Millen J, Kemper C: Prevention by tolrestat of the biochemical and morphological changes in galactose-fed rats. *Diabetes* 1986;35(suppl 1):215A.
45. Kojima K, Matsubara H, Harada T, et al: Effects of aldose reductase inhibitor on retinal microangiopathy in streptozotocin-diabetic rats. *Jpn J Ophthalmol* 1985;29:99–109.
46. Eaton RP, Sibbitt WL, Harsh A: The effect of an aldose reductase inhibiting agent on limited joint mobility in diabetic patients. *JAMA* 1985;253:1437–1440.
47. Flynn TG: Aldehyde reductases: Monomeric NADPH-dependent oxidoreductases with multifunctional potential. *Biochem Pharmacol* 1982;31:2705–2712.
48. Flynn TG: Aldehyde reductases, in Weiner H, Wermuth B (eds): *Enzymology of carbonyl metabolism: Aldehyde dehydrogenase and aldo/keto reductase.* New York, AR Liss Inc, 1982, pp 169–182.
49. Flynn TG: Aldose and aldehyde reductase in animal tissues. *Metabolism* 1986;35(suppl 1):105–108.
50. Turner AJ: Aldehyde reductases: Enzymes in search of a function, in Weiner H, Wermuth B (eds): *Enzymology of carbonyl metabolism: Aldehyde dehydrogenase and aldo/keto reductase.* New York, AR Liss Inc, 1982, pp 183–195.
51. Srivastava SK, Ansari NH, Hair GA, Das B: Aldose and aldehyde reductases in human tissues. *Biochim Biophys Acta* 1984;800:220–227.
52. Turner AJ, Flynn TG: The nomenclature of aldehyde reductases, in Weiner H, Wermuth B (eds): *Enzymology of carbonyl metabolism: Aldehyde dehydrogenase and aldo/keto reductase.* New York, AR Liss Inc, 1982, pp 401–402.
53. Mano Y, Suzuki K, Yamada K, Shimazono N: Enzymic studies on TPN L-hexonate dehydrogenase from rat liver. *J Biochem* 1961;49:618–634.
54. Moonsammy GI, Stewart MA: Purification and properties of brain aldose reductase and L-hexonate dehydrogenase. *J Neurochem* 1967;14:1187–1193.
55. Turner AJ, Tipton KF: The characterization of two reduced nicotinamide-adenine dinucleotide phosphate-linked aldehyde reductases from pig brain. *Biochem J* 1972; 130:765–772.
56. Von Wartburg JP, Wermuth B: Aldehyde reductase from human tissues, in Wood WA (ed): *Methods of enzymology Vol 89: Carbohydrate metabolism, Part D* New York, Academic Press, 1982, pp 506–513.
57. Wermuth B: Aldo-keto reductases, in Flynn TG, Weiner H (eds): *Enzymology of carbonyl metabolism 2. Aldehyde dehydrogenase, aldo-keto reductase and alcohol dehydrogenase.* New York, AR Liss Inc, 1985, pp 209–230.
58. Branlant G, Biellman JF: Purification and properties of aldehyde reductases from pig liver. *Eur J Biochem* 1980;105:611–621.
59. Dons RF, Doughty CC: Isolation and characterization of aldose reductase from calf brain. *Biochim Biophys Acta* 1976;452:1–12.
60. Hoffmann PL, Wermuth B, Von Wartburg JP: Human brain aldehyde reductases: Relationship to succinic semialdehyde reductase and aldose reductase. *J Neurochem* 1980;35:354–366.

61. Flynn TG, Shires J, Walton DJ: Properties of the nicotinamide adenine dinucleotide phosphate dependent aldehyde reductase from pig kidney. *J Biol Chem* 1975; 250:2933–2940.
62. Wermuth B, Münch JDB, Von Wartburg JP: Purification and properties of NADPH-dependent aldehyde reductase from human liver. *J Biol Chem* 1977;252:3821–3828.
63. Ris MM, Von Wartburg JP: Heterogeneity of NADPH-dependent aldehyde reductase from human and rat brain. *Eur J Biochem* 1973;37:69–77.
64. O'Brien MM, Schofield PJ: Polyol pathway enzymes of human brain: Partial purification and properties of aldose reductase and hexonate dehydrogenase. *Biochem J* 1980;187:21–30.
65. Hers HG: Le méchanisme de la transformation de glucose en fructose par les vésicules séminates. *Biochim Biophys Acta* 1958;22:202–203.
66. Wermuth B, Von Wartburg JP: Aldose reductase from human tissues, in Wood WA (ed): *Methods in enzymology Vol 89: Carbohydrate metabolism, Part D* New York, Academic Press, 1982, pp 181–186.
67. Flynn TG, Cromlish JA: Pig muscle aldehyde reductase, in Weiner H, Wermuth B (eds): *Enzymology of carbonyl metabolism: Aldehyde dehydrogenase and aldo/keto reductase.* New York, AR Liss Inc, 1982, pp 209–222.
68. Boghosian RA, McGuinness ET: Affinity purification and properties of porcine brain aldose reductase. *Biochim Biophys Acta* 1979;567:278–286.
69. Levine L, Wu KY, Herrmann H: Decreased levels of an inhibitor of prostaglandin E 9-ketoreductase activity in chick dystrophic breast muscle. *Nature* 1976;260: 791–793.
70. Bernardo A, Burgos J, Martin R: Purification and properties of L-glycol dehydrogenase from hen's muscle. *Biochim Biophys Acta* 1981;659:189–198.
71. Crabbe MJC, Wolff S, Basak Halder A, Ting HH: Diabetic cataracts—is aldose reductase important? *Metab Pediatr Ophthalmol* 1981;5:33–38.
72. Wermuth B: Purification and properties of an NADPH-dependent carbonyl reductase from human brain. *J Biol Chem* 1981;256:1206–1213.
73. Hers HG: L'Aldose-réductase. *Biochim Biophys Acta* 1960;37:120–126.
74. Hayman S, Kinoshita JH: Isolation and properties of lens aldose reductase. *J Biol Chem* 1965;240:877–882.
75. Sheaff CM, Doughty CC: Physical and kinetic properties of homogeneous bovine lens aldose reductase. *J Biol Chem* 1976;251:2696–2702.
76. Crabbe MJC, Basak Halder A: Affinity chromatography of bovine lens aldose reductase and a comparison of some kinetic properties of the enzyme from lens and human erythrocyte. *Biochem Soc Trans* 1980;8:194–195.
77. Kador PF, Sharpless NE: Structure-activity studies of aldose reductase inhibitors containing the 4-oxo-4H-chromen ring system. *Biophys Chem* 1978;8:81–85.
78. Conrad SM, Doughty CC: Comparative studies on aldose reductase from bovine, rat and human lens. *Biochim Biophys Acta* 1982;708:348–357.
79. Herrmann RK, Kador PF, Kinoshita JH: Rat lens aldose reductase: Rapid purification and comparison with human placental aldose reductase. *Exp Eye Res* 1983; 37:467–474.
80. Tanimoto T, Fukuda H, Kawamura J: Purification and some properties of aldose reductase from rabbit lens. *Chem Pharm Bull* 1983;31:2395–2403.
81. Tanimoto T, Fukuda H, Kawamura J: Characterization of aldose reductase Ia and Ib from rabbit lens. *Chem Pharm Bull* 1984;32:1025–1031.
82. Gabbay KH, Cathcart ES: Purification and immunologic identification of aldose reductases. *Diabetes* 1974;23:460–468.

83. Chakrabarti S, Sima AAF, Yakigasha S: Aldose reductase in the BB rat; purification, immunological identification and localization in the retina and peripheral nerve. *Diabetes* 1986;35(suppl 1):101A.
84. Ryle CM, Dowling TG, Tipton KF: Purification and properties of low-Km aldehyde reductase from ox brain. *Biochim Biophys Acta* 1984;791:155–163.
85. Tipton KF, Ryle CM: Some properties of the "Low-K_m" aldehyde reductase from ox brain, in Flynn TG, Weiner H (eds): *Enzymology of carbonyl metabolism 2: Aldehyde dehydrogenase, aldo-keto reductase and alcohol dehydrogenase.* New York, AR Liss Inc, 1985, pp 241–250.
86. Wermuth B, Burgisser H, Bohren K, Von Wartburg JP: Purification and characterization of human-brain aldose reductase. *Eur J Biochem* 1982;127:279–284.
87. Attwood MA, Doughty CC: Purification and properties of calf liver aldose reductase. *Biochim Biophys Acta* 1974;370:358–368.
88. Petrash JM, Srivastava SK: Purification and properties of human liver aldehyde reductases. *Biochim Biophys Acta* 1982;707:105–114.
89. Gabbay KH, Kinoshita JH: Aldose reductase from mammalian tissues, in Wood WA (ed): *Methods in enzymology Vol 41: Carbohydrate metabolism, Part B.* New York, Academic Press, 1975, pp 159–165.
90. McKercher SR, Mathur SR, Grimshaw CE: Bovine kidney aldose reductase. *Fed Proc* 1985;44:472.
91. Dufrane SP, Malaisse WJ, Sener A: Aldose reductase activity in pancreatic islets. *Diabetologia* 1983;25:152.
92. Flynn TG, Finlayson SA, Morjana NA: Aldose reductase from human muscle. *Diabetes* 1985;34(suppl 1):184A.
93. Davidson WS, Murphy DG: Aldehyde reductases and their involvement in muscular dystrophy, in Flynn TG, Weiner H (eds): *Enzymology of carbonyl metabolism 2: Aldehyde dehydrogenase, aldo-keto reductase, and alcohol dehydrogenase.* New York, AR Liss Inc, 1985, pp 251–263.
94. Murphy DG, Davidson WS: Chicken muscle aldose reductase: Purification, properties and relationship to other chicken aldo/keto reductases. *Int J Biochem* 1986; 18:215–221.
95. Velle W: Aldose reductase from seminal vesicle and placenta of ruminants, in Wood WA (ed): *Methods in enzymology, Vol 41: Carbohydrate metabolism, Part B.* New York, Academic Press, 1975, pp 165–170.
96. Hastein T, Velle W: Purification and properties of aldose reductase from the placenta and the seminal vesicle of the sheep. *Biochim Biophys Acta* 1969;178:1–10.
97. Das B, Srivastava SK: Purification and properties of aldose reductase and aldehyde reductase II from human erythrocyte. *Arch Biochem Biophys* 1985;238:670–679.
98. Srivastava SK, Ansari NH, Hair GA, et al: Hyperglycemia-induced activation of human erythrocyte aldose reductase and alterations in kinetic properties. *Biochim Biophys Acta* 1986;870:302–311.
99. Hastein T, Velle W: Placental aldose reductase activity and foetal blood fructose during bovine pregnancy. *J Reprod Fert* 1968;15:47–52.
100. Kador PF, Carper D, Kinoshita JH: Rapid purification of human placental aldose reductase. *Anal Biochem* 1981;114:53–58.
101. Clements RS Jr, Winegrad AI: Purification of alditol: NADP oxidoreductase from human placenta. *Biochim Biophys Res Comm* 1972;47:1473–1479.
102. Kador PF, Merola LO, Kinoshita JH: Differences in the susceptibility of various aldose reductases to inhibition. *Docum Ophthalmol Proc Series* 1979;18:117–124.

103. Das B, Srivastava SK: Purification and properties of aldehyde reductases from human placenta. *Biochim Biophys Acta* 1985;840:324–333.
104. Brolin SE, Naeser P, Bodin B, Wentzel P, Eriksson UJ: Sorbitol may accumulate in early embryos, but does not seem to cause malformations. *Diabetologia* 1986; 29:522A.
105. Hod M, Star S, Passoneau JV, Unterman TG, Freinkel N: Effect of hyperglycemia on sorbitol and myo-inositol content of cultured rat conceptus: failure of aldose reductase inhibitors to modify myo-inositol depletion and dysmorphogenesis. *Biochem Biophys Res Comm* 1986;140:974–980.
106. Koh MS, Misch KJ, Yuen CT, Rhodes EL: Accumulation of sorbitol in endothelial cells—a possible cause of diabetic microangiopathy. *Diabetes Res* 1986;3:217–219.
107. Sheys GH, Arnold WJ, Watson JA, Hayashi JA, Doughty CC: Aldose reductase from Rhodotorula. *J Biol Chem* 1971;246:3824–3827.
108. Wirth HP, Wermuth B: Immunochemical characterization of aldo-keto reductases from human tissues. *FEBS Lett* 1985;187:280–282.
109. Cantor SM, Peniston AP: The reduction of aldoses at the dropping mercury cathode: Estimation of the aldehydo structure in aqueous solutions. *J Am Chem Soc* 1940; 62:2113–2121.
110. Inagaki K, Miwa I, Okuda J: Affinity purification and glucose specificity of aldose reductase from bovine lens. *Arch Biochem Biophys* 1982;216:337–344.
111. Grimshaw CE: Direct measurement of the rate of ring opening of D-glucose by enzyme-catalyzed reduction. *Carbohydr Res* 1986;148:345–348.
112. Dufrane SP, Malaisse WJ, Sener A: A micromethod for the assay of aldose reductase, its application to pancreatic islets. *Biochem Med* 1984;32:99–105.
113. Mallaisse-Lagae F, Malaisse WJ: Failure of aldose reductase inhibitors to affect insulin release. *IRCS Med Sci* 1986;14:242–243.
114. Clements RS, Weaver JP, Winegrad AI: The distribution of polyol NADP-oxidoreductase in mammalian tissues. *Biochim Biophys Res Comm* 1969;37: 347–353.
115. Das B, Srivastava SK: Activation of aldose reductase from human tissues. *Diabetes* 1985;34:1145–1151.
116. Gabbay KH: Purification and immunological identification of bovine retinal aldose reductase. *Isr J Med Sci* 1972;8:1626–1629.
117. Buzney SM, Frank RN, Varma SD, Tanishima T, Gabbay KH: Aldose reductase in retinal mural cells. *Invest Ophthalmol Vis Sci* 1977;16:392–396.
118. Ludvigson MA, Sorenson RL: Immunohistochemical localization of aldose reductase. I. Enzyme purification and antibody preparation. Localization in peripheral nerve, artery and testis. *Diabetes* 1980;29:438–449.
119. Ludvigson MA, Sorenson RL: Immunohistochemical localization of aldose reductase. II. Rat eye and kidney. *Diabetes* 1980;29:450–459.
120. Kern TS, Engerman RL: Distribution of aldose reductase in ocular tissues. *Exp Eye Res* 1981;33:175–182.
121. Kern T, Engerman RL: Immunohistochemical distribution of aldose reductase. *Histochem* 1982;14:507–515.
122. Akagi Y, Terubayashi H, Millen J, Kador PF, Kinoshita JH: Aldose reductase localization in dog retinal mural cells. *Curr Eye Res* 1986;5:883–886.
123. Akagi Y, Kador PF, Kuwabara T, Kinoshita JH: Aldose reductase localization in human retinal mural cells. *Invest Ophthalmol Vis Sci* 1983,24:1516–1519.
124. Akagi Y, Yajima Y, Kador PF, Kuwabara T, Kinoshita JH: Localization of aldose reductase in the human eye. *Diabetes* 1984;33:562–566.

125. Hoffmann PL, Wermuth B, Von Wartburg JP: Multiple aldehyde reductases of human brain. *Adv Exp Med Biol* 1980;132:749–759.
126. Wermuth B: Human carbonyl reductases, in Weiner H, Wermuth B (eds): *Enzymology of carbonyl metabolism: Aldehyde dehydrogenase and aldo/keto reductase.* New York, AR Liss Inc, 1982, pp 261–274.
127. Turner AJ, Illingworth JA, Tipton KF: Simulation of biogenic amine metabolism in the brain. *Biochem J* 1974;144:353–360.
128. Whittle SR, Turner AJ: Biogenic aldehyde metabolism in rat brain. Differential sensitivity of aldehyde reductase isoenzymes to sodium valproate. *Biochim Biophys Acta* 1981;657:94–105.
129. Monder C, Bradlow HL: Cortoic acids: Explorations at the frontier of corticosteroid metabolism. *Rec Progr Horm Res* 1980;36:345–400.
130. Lippman V, Monder C: Purification and properties of an NADPH-dependent 21-oxo-20-hydroxysteroid reductase (17 β-aldol reductase) from sheep liver. *J Biol Chem* 1978;253:2126–2131.
131. Wermuth B, Monder C: Aldose and aldehyde reductase exhibit isocorticosteroid reductase activity. *Eur J Biochim* 1983;131:423–426.
132. Kador PF, Millen J, Akagi Y, Kinoshita JH: Dog lens aldose reductase: Purification and comparison with rat lens enzyme. *Invest Ophthalmol Vis Sci* 1984;25(suppl):47.
133. Kador PF, Shiono T, Kinoshita JH: Studies with purified aldose reductase. *Invest Ophthalmol Vis Sci* 1983;24(suppl):267.
134. Walker Griffin B, McNatt LG: Characterization of the reduction of 3-acetylpyridine adenine dinucleotide phosphate by benzyl alcohol catalyzed by aldose reductase. *Arch Biochem Biophys* 1986;246:75–81.
135. Cheng HM, Gonzalez RB, Barnett PA, et al: Sorbitol/ fructose metabolism in the lens. *Exp Eye Res* 1985;40:223–229.
136. Jacobson M, Sharma YR, Cotlier E, Hollander JD: Diabetic complications in lens and nerve and their prevention by sulindac or sorbinil: Two novel aldose reductase inhibitors. *Invest Ophthalmol Vis Sci* 1983;24:1426–1429.
137. Williams WF, Odom JD: Study of aldose reductase inhibition in intact lenses by ^{13}C nuclear magnetic resonance spectroscopy. *Science* 1986;233:223–225.
138. Nakada T, Knee I: In vivo metabolism of 2-fluoro-2-deoxy-D-glucose in the aldose reductase sorbitol pathway in rat brain demonstrated by ^{19}F NMR spectroscopy. *Biochem Arch* 1986;2:53–61.
139. Terashima H, Hama K, Yamamoto R, et al: Effects of a new aldose reductase inhibitor on various tissues in vitro. *J Pharmacol Exp Ther* 1984;229:226–229.
140. Chaudhry PS, Cabrera J, Juliani HR, Varma SD: Inhibition of human lens aldose reductase by flavonoids, sulindac and indomethacin. *Biochem Pharmacol* 1983;32: 1995–1998.
141. Srivastava SK, Petrash JM, Sadana IJ, Ansari NH, Partridge CA: Susceptibility of aldehyde and aldose reductases of human tissues to aldose reductase inhibitors. *Curr Eye Res* 1983;2:407–410.
142. Maragoudakis ME, Wasvary J, Hankin H, Gargiulo P: Human placenta aldose reductase. Forms sensitive and insensitive to inhibition by alrestatin. *Mol Pharmacol* 1984;25:425–430.
143. Kinoshita JH, Fukushi S, Kador P, Merola LO: Aldose reductase in diabetic complications of the eye. *Metabolism* 1979;28(suppl 1):462–469.
144. Unpublished results from the National Eye Institute.
145. Terashima H, Hama K, Yamamoto R, et al: Effects of a new aldose reductase inhibitor on various tissues in vitro. *J Pharmacol Exp Ther* 1984;229:226–230.

146. Stribling D, Mirrlees DJ, Harrison HE, Earl DCN: Properties of ICI 128,436, a novel aldose reductase inhibitor, and its effects on diabetic complications in the rat. *Metabolism* 1985;34:336–344.
147. Kador PF, Kinoshita JH, Tung WH, Chylack LT Jr: Differences in the susceptibility of various aldose reductases to inhibition II. *Invest Ophthalmol Vis Sci* 1980;19:980–982.
148. Dvornik D, et al: Unpublished results from the Ayerst Laboratories Research; presented in part at the Cooperative Cataract Research Group meeting in Orlando, FL, May 4, 1980.
149. Müller P, Hockwin O, Ohrloff C: Comparison of aldose reductase inhibitors by determination of IC with bovine and rat lens extracts. *Ophthalmic Res* 1985; 17:115–119.
150. Tanimoto T, Fukuda H, Yamaha T, Tanaka C: Reaction and inhibition mechanisms for aldose reductase from rabbit lens. *Chem Pharm Bull* 1986;34:4183–4189.
151. Varma SD, Kinoshita JH: Inhibition of lens aldose reductase by flavonoids. Their possible role in the prevention of diabetic cataracts. *Biochem Pharmacol* 1976;25: 2505–2513.
152. Simard-Duquesne N, Greselin E, Dubuc J, Dvornik D: The effect of a new aldose reductase inhibitor (tolrestat) in galactosemic and diabetic rats. *Metabolism* 1985; 34:885–892.
153. Peterson MJ, Sarges R, Aldinger CE, MacDonald DP: CP-45,634: A novel aldose reductase inhibitor that inhibits polyol pathway activity in diabetic and galactosemic rats. *Metabolism* 1979;28(suppl 1):456–461.
154. Griffin BW, Chandler ML, Desantis L: Prevention of diabetic cataract and neuropathy in rats by two new aldose reductase inhibitors. *Invest Ophthalmol Vis Sci* 1984; 25(suppl):136.
155. Millen J, et al: Unpublished results from the Ayerst Research Laboratories.
156. Sredy J, Millen J, McCaleb ML, Tutwiler GF: Inhibition of polyol accumulation in lens, sciatic nerve and RBC by the aldose reductase inhibitor, tolrestat. *Fed Proc* 1986; 45:902.
157. Dvornik D, Millen J, Hicks D, Cayen M, Sredy J: The pharmacokinetics of aldose reductase inhibitors. Presented at the Internat Symposium on polyol pathway and its role in diabetic complications. Kashikojima, Japan Oct 28–30, 1986.
158. Poulson R: Inhibition of hexonate dehydrogenase and aldose reductase from bovine retina by sorbinil, statil, M79,175 and valproate. *Biochem Pharmacol* 1986;35:2955–2959.
159. Sato S, Kador PF, Kinoshita JH: Comparison of purified lens aldose reductase and kidney aldehyde reductase. Presented at the ARVO meeting, April 28–May 2, 1986, Sarasota, FL.
160. Skau K, Coats E, Tigar J, Schmidt J, Iyer L: Comparative inhibition of aldose and aldehyde reductase. Presented at the ASPET meeting, August 17–21, 1986, Baltimore, MD.
161. Kinsey VE, Wachtl C, Kuck JFR Jr, Reddy DVN: Current research on the culture of lenses. *Acta Conc Ophthalmol* 1958;18:865–872.
162. Levari R, Kornblueth W, Wertheimer E: The effect of insulin on the uptake of monosaccharides by the rat lens. *J Endocrin* 1961;22:361–369.
163. Kinoshita JH, Merola LO, Dikmak E: The accumulation of dulcitol and water in rabbit lens incubated with galactose. *Biochim Biophys Acta* 1962;62:176–178.
164. Kinoshita JH, Merola LO, Hayman S: Osmotic effects on the amino-acid concentrating mechanism in the rabbit lens. *J Biol Chem* 1965;240:310–315.
165. Hayman S, Lou MF, Merola LO, Kinoshita JH: Aldose reductase activity in the lens and other tissues. *Biochim Biophys Acta* 1966;128:474–482.

166. Kinoshita JH, Merola LO, Tung B: Changes in cation permeability in the galactose-exposed lens. *Exp Eye Res* 1968;7:80–90.
167. Kinoshita JH, Barber GW, Merola LO, Tung B: Changes in the levels of free amino acids and myoinositol in the galactose-exposed lens. *Invest Ophthalmol* 1969;8:625–632.
168. Chylack LT Jr, Kinoshita JH: A biochemical evaluation of a cataract induced in high-glucose medium. *Invest Ophthalmol* 1969;8:401–412.
169. Gabbay KH: Factors affecting the sorbitol pathway in diabetic nerve. *Diabetes* 1969;18(suppl 1):336–337.
170. Gabbay KH: The sorbitol pathway and the complications of diabetes. *N Engl J Med* 1973;288:832–836.
171. Morrison AD, Clements RS Jr, Travis SB, Oski F, Winegrad AI: Glucose utilization by the polyol pathway in human erythrocytes. *Biochem Biophys Res Comm* 1970; 40:199–205.
172. Lefevre PG, Davies RI: Active transport into the human erythrocyte: Evidence from comparative kinetics and competition among monosaccharides. *J Gen Physiol* 1951; 34:515–524.
173. Wick AN, Drury DR: Action of insulin on the permeability of cells to sorbitol. *Am J Physiol* 1951;166:421–423.
174. Travis SF, Morrison AD, Clements RS Jr, Winegrad AI, Oski FA: Metabolic alterations in human erythrocyte produced by increases in glucose concentration. The role of the polyol pathway. *J Clin Invest* 1971;50:2104–2112.
175. Garby L, Deverdier CH: Glucose metabolism in normal erythrocytes. I. Kinetics of the hexokinase reaction in intact cells. *Scand J Haematol* 1964;1:150–167.
176. Beutler E, Guinto E: The reduction of glyceraldehyde by human erythrocytes. L-hexonate dehydrogenase activity. *J Clin Invest* 1974;53:1258–1264.
177. Basak Halder A, Wolff S, Ting HH, Crabbe MJC: An aldose reductase from the human erythrocyte. *Biochem Soc Trans* 1980;8:644–645.
178. Crabbe MJC, Peckar CO, Basak Halder A, Cheng H: Erythrocyte glyceraldehyde-reductase levels in diabetics with retinopathy and cataract. *Lancet* 1980;2:1268–1270.
179. Malone JI, Knox G, Benford S, Tedesco TA: Red cell sorbitol. An indicator of diabetic control. *Diabetes* 1980;29:861–864.
180. Malone JI, Knox G, Benford S: Red cell sorbitol. An indicator of diabetic control. *Diabetes* 1979;28:386.
181. DeLeeuw I, Vertommen J, DeWinter P, Vanroelen W, Van Gaal L: Red blood cell sorbitol levels in normals and diabetics. *Diabetologia* 1981;21:263.
182. Sommers G, DePoorter I, Sener A, Malaisse WJ: Sorbitol concentration in the plasma and erythrocyte of diabetic subjects. *Diabetes Care* 1982;5:319–321.
183. Malone JI, Leavengood H, Peterson MJ, et al: Red blood sorbitol as an indicator of polyol pathway activity. Inhibition by sorbinil in insulin-dependent diabetic subjects. *Diabetes* 1984;33:45–49.
184. Popp-Snijders C, Lomecky M, DeJong AP: Determination of sorbitol in erythrocytes of diabetic and healthy subjects by capillary gas chromatography. *Clin Chim Acta* 1983;132:83–89.
185. Guillemin G, Boutroux V, Paolaggi F, et al: Determination du sorbitol erythrocytaire. *Ann Biol Clin* 1983;41:325–330.
186. Vertommen J, DeLeeuw I, Rillaerts M, Gijsels, Bekaert J: Discrepancy between insulin-dependent and non-insulin-dependent diabetes in the interrelationship between red-blood-cell sorbitol and glycaemia. *Diabetologia* 1984;27:343A.
187. Malone JI, Knox G, Harvey C: Sorbitol accumulation is altered in Type I (insulin-dependent) diabetes mellitus. *Diabetologia* 1984;27:509–513.

188. Barretto OC De-O, Ursich M, Nonoyama K: Reduced levels of erythrocyte sorbitol dehydrogenase activity in human diabetics. *Brazilian J Med Biol Res* 1985;18: 477–479.
189. Hotta N, Kakuta H, Fukasawa H, et al: Polyol pathway in retinae and erythrocytes: Regulation by hormones and aldose reductase inhibitor. *Diabetologia* 1986;29:550A.
190. Norris SC, Perkins CM, Bastain W, Mirrlees D, Yates RA: Studies on the pharmacokinetics and pharmacodynamics of "statil" (ICI-128,436), an aldose reductase inhibitor. *Clin Sci* 1985;69(suppl 12):22P.
191. Srivastava SK, Hair GA, Das B: Activated and unactivated forms of human erythrocyte aldose reductase. *Proc Natl Acad Sci* 1985;82:7222–7226.
192. Srivastava SK, Ansar NH, Hair GA, Aswasthi S, Das B: Activation of human erythrocyte, brain, aorta, muscle and ocular tissue aldose reductase. *Metabolism* 1986;35(suppl 1):114–119.
193. Bidot-Lopez P, Robertson S, O'Malley BC: Sorbitol accumulation in human diabetic and in normal platelets incubated in glucose. *Clin Res* 1979;27:363A.
194. O'Malley BC, Bidot-Lopez P, Lee EL, Robertson S: Sorbitol accumulation in human normal and diabetic platelets. *J Florida MA* 1982;69:460–462.
195. Hutton JC, Williams JF, Schofield PJ, Hollows FC: Polyol metabolism in monkey-kidney epithelial-cell cultures. Sorbitol synthesis. *Eur J Biochem* 1974;49:347–353.
196. Boot-Handford R, Heath H: The effects of aldose reductase inhibitors on the metabolism of cultured monkey kidney epithelial cells. *Biochem Pharmacol* 1981;30: 3065–3069.
197. Russel P, Merola LO, Yajima Y, Kinoshita JH: Aldose reductase in a cultured human retinal cell line. *Exp Eye Res* 1982;35:331–336.
198. Li W, Khatami M, Rockey J: The effects of glucose and an aldose reductase inhibitor on the sorbitol content and collagen synthesis of bovine retinal capillary pericytes in culture. *Exp Eye Res* 1985;40:439–444.
199. Li W, Shen S, Khatami M, Rockey JH: Stimulation of retinal capillary pericyte protein and collagen synthesis in culture by high-glucose concentration. *Diabetes* 1984;33: 785–789.
200. Li W, Chan LS, Khatami M, Rockey JH: Characterization of glucose transport by bovine retinal capillary pericytes in culture. *Exp Eye Res* 1985;41:191–199.
201. Hohman TC, Nishimura C, Robison WG Jr, Kinoshita JH: Aldose reductase in cultured human and canine retinal capillary pericytes. *Invest Ophthalmol Vis Sci* 1986; 27(suppl):328.
202. Kern TS, Engerman RL: Hexitol production by canine retinal microvessels. *Invest Ophthalmol Vis Sci* 1985;26:382–384.
203. Poulsom R, Heath H: Inhibition of aldose reductase in five tissues of the streptozotocin-diabetic rat. *Biochem Pharmacol* 1983;32:1495–1499.
204. Gabbay KH, Merola LO, Field RA: Sorbitol pathway: Presence in nerve and cord with substrate accumulation in diabetes. *Science* 1966;151:209–210.
205. Ward JD, Baker RWR, Davis BH: Effect of blood sugar control on the accumulation of sorbitol and fructose in nervous tissues. *Diabetes* 1972;21:1173–1178.
206. Quan-Ma R, Wells WW: The distribution of galactitol in tissues of rats fed galactose. *Biochim Biophys Res Comm* 1965;20:486–490.
207. Stewart MA, Kurien MM, Sherman WR, Cotlier EV: Inositol changes in nerve and lens of galactose fed rats. *J Neurochem* 1968;15:941–946.
208. Quan-Ma R, Wells HJ, Wells WW, Sherman FE, Egan TJ: Galactitol in the tissues of a galactosemic child. *Am J Dis Child* 1966;112:477–478.

209. Eklund H, Horjales E, Jörnvall H, Bränden CI, Jeffrey J: Molecular aspects of functional differences between alcohol and sorbitol dehydrogenases. *Biochemistry* 1985;24:8005–8012.
210. Simard-Duquesne N, et al: Unpublished results from the Ayerst Research Laboratories.
211. Giroix MH, Malaisse-Lagae F, Sener A, Malaisse WJ: Hexose metabolism in pancreatic islets. Galactose transport, phosphorylation and oxidation. *Mol Cell Biochem* 1985;66:61–64.
212. Hotta N, Kakuta H, Fukasawa H, et al: Effects of a fructose-rich diet and the aldose reductase inhibitor, ONO-2235, on the development of diabetic neuropathy in streptozotocin-treated rats. *Diabetologia* 1985;28:176–180.
213. Gonzalez AM, Sochor M, McLean P: The effect of an aldose reductase inhibitor (sorbinil) on the level of metabolites in lenses of diabetic rats. *Diabetes* 1983;32:482–485.
214. Beyer-Mears A, Cruz E: Reversal of diabetic cataract by sorbinil, an aldose reductase inhibitor. *Diabetes* 1985;34:15–52.
215. Tomlinson DR, Moriarty RJ, Mayer JH: Prevention and reversal of defective axonal transport and motor nerve conduction velocity in rats with experimental diabetes by treatment with the aldose reductase inhibitor sorbinil. *Diabetes* 1984;33:470–476.
216. Gillon KRW, Hawthorne JN, Tomlinson DR: Myo-inositol and sorbitol metabolism in relation to peripheral nerve function in experimental diabetes in the rat: The effect of aldose reductase inhibition. *Diabetologia* 1983;25:365–371.
217. Hu T, Merola LO Kuwabara T, Kinoshita JH: Prevention and reversal of galactose cataract in rats with topical sorbinil. *Invest Ophthalmol Vis Sci* 1984;25:603–605.
218. Sochor M, Kunjara S, McLean P: Sorbinil reduces kidney sorbitol and fructose concentrations in experimental diabetes. *Diabetologia* 1984;27:333A.
219. Beyer-Mears A, Ku L, Cohen MP: Glomerular polyol accumulation in diabetes and its prevention by oral sorbinil. *Diabetes* 1984;33:604–607.
220. Beyer-Mears A, Nicholas-Alexandre J, Cruz E: Sorbinil inhibition of renal aldose reductase. *Fed Proc* 1982; 41:858.
221. Yue DK, Hanwell MA, Satchell PM, Handelsman DJ, Turtle JR: The effects of aldose reductase inhibition on nerve sorbitol and myoinositol concentrations in diabetic and galactosemic rats. *Metabolism* 1984;33:1119–1122.
222. Akanuma H, Yamanouchi T, Ono H, Nomura K, Akanuma Y: Sorbitol determination by liquid chromatography: Application to red blood cells of diabetic rats. *J Biochem* 1985;97:579–588.
223. Ono H, Nozawa Y, Hayano S: Effects of M-79,175, an aldose reductase inhibitor, on experimental sugar cataracts. *Ganka Gakkai Zasshi* 1982;86:1343–1350.
224. Robey C, Dasmahapatra A, Cohen MP, Suarez S: Sorbinil prevents decreased erythrocyte (RBC) deformability in diabetes mellitus. *Diabetes* 1985;34(suppl 1):41A.
225. Robey C, Dasmahapatra A, Cohen MP: In vitro effects of hyperglycemia and sorbinil on erythrocyte (RBC) deformability. *Diabetes* 1986;35(suppl 1):108A.
226. Bareford D, Jennings PE, Stone PCW, et al: Effects of hyperglycaemia and sorbitol accumulation on erythrocyte deformability in diabetes mellitus. *J Clin Pathol* 1986;39:722–727.
227. Kern TS, Romang TC, Engerman RL: Erythrocyte filterability in alloxan-diabetes and in experimental galactosemia. *Clin Hemorheol* 1986;6:395–404.
228. Kemper C, Dvornik D: Prevention of neural myoinositol depletion in diabetic rats by aldose reductase inhibition with tolrestat. *Proc Soc Exp Biol Med* 1986;182:505–510.

229. Mayer HJ, Tomlinson DR, McLean GW: Slow orthograde axonal transport of radiolabelled protein in sciatic motoneurons of rats with short-term experimental diabetes: Effects of treatment with an aldose reductase inhibitor or myo-inositol. *J Neurochem* 1984;43:1265–1270.
230. Dvornik D, Sredy J, Hicks D, Sawicki D, Ackerman D: Polyol pathway and myoinositol (MI) content in peripheral nerve of long-term streptozocin (STZ) diabetic rats. *Diabetes* 1987;36(suppl 1):185A.
231. Okuda J, Yashima K, Inagaki K, Miwa I: Effects of an aldose reductase inhibitor, 1-[(p-bromophenyl)-sulfonyl] hydantoin, on cataract formation and tissue polyol levels in galactosemic rats. *Chem Pharm Bull* 1985; 33:2990–2995.
232. Millen J, Banknieder AR, Kemper C, Dvornik D: Effect of tolrestat in galactosemic dogs. *Diabetes* 1987;36(suppl 1):197A.
233. Kikkawa R, Hatanaka I, Yasuda H, et al: Effect of a new aldose reductase inhibitor, (E)-3-carboxymethyl-5-[(2E)-methyl-3-phenyl-propenylidene]rhodanine (ONO-2235) on peripheral nerve disorders in streptozotocin-diabetic rats. *Diabetologia* 1983;24: 290–292.
234. Asano T, Mochio S, Kuwata T, et al: Effect of aldose reductase inhibitor (ONO-2235) on somatic and autonomic nervous dysfunction in streptozotocin-induced diabetic rats. *J Japan Diab Soc* 1983;26:1105–1111.
235. Kikkawa R, Hatanaka I, Yasuda H, Kobayashi N, Shigeta Y: Prevention of peripheral nerve dysfunction by an aldose reductase inhibitor in streptozotocin-diabetic rats. *Metabolism* 1984;33:212–214.
236. Hotta N, Kakuta H: Pathogenesis of diabetic retinopathy from aspects of retinal metabolism. *J Japan Diab Soc* 1981;24:1100–1103.
237. Yoshida T, Nishioka H, Yoshioka K, et al: Effect of aldose reductase inhibitor ONO-2235 on reduced sympathetic nervous system activity and peripheral nerve disorders in STZ-induced diabetic rats. *Diabetes* 1987;36:6–13.
238. Yoshida T, Nishioka H, Kondo M, Terashima H: Restoration of decreased sympathetic (SNS) activity and of increased sorbitol (Sor) accumulation in streptozotocin (STZ) diabetic rats by treatment with aldose reductase inhibitor (ARI), ONO-2235. *Diabetes* 1985;34(suppl 1): 104A.
239. Poulsom R, Mirrlees DJ, Earl DCN, Heath H: The effects of an aldose reductase inhibitor upon the sorbitol pathway, fructose-1-phosphate and lactate in the retina and nerve of streptozotocin-diabetic rats. *Exp Eye Res* 1983;36:751–760.
240. Poulsom R, Boot-Handford RP, Heath H: The effects of long-term treatment of streptozotocin-diabetic rats with an aldose reductase inhibitor. *Exp Eye Res* 1983; 37:507–515.
241. Rillaerts EGL, Vertommen JJF, DeLeeuw IH: Effect of efficient aldose reductase inhibition on erythrocyte viscosity in vitro. *Diabetologia* 1986;29:586A.
242. Ericksson UJ, Naeser P, Brolin SE: Increased levels of sorbitol in offspring of manifest diabetic rats. *Acta Endocrinol* 1985;110(suppl 273):27.
243. Ericksson UJ, Naeser P, Brolin SE: Increased accumulation of sorbitol in offspring of manifest diabetic rats. *Diabetes* 1986;35:1356–1363.
244. Greene DA, DeJesus PV Jr, Winegrad AI: Effects of insulin and dietary myoinositol on impaired motor nerve conduction velocity in acute streptozotocin diabetes. *J Clin Invest* 1975;55:1326–1336.
245. Simmons DA, Winegrad AI, Martin DB: Significance of tissue myo-inositol concentrations in metabolic regulation in nerve. *Science* 1982;217:848–851.
246. Simmons DA, Winegrad AI, Martin DB: Significance of myo-inositol concentrations in metabolic regulation. *Trans Assoc Am Phys* 1982;95:292–298.

247. Cameron NE, Leonard MB, Ross IS, Whiting PH: The effects of sorbinil on peripheral nerve conduction velocity, polyol concentrations and morphology in the streptozocin-diabetic rat. *Diabetologia* 1986;29:168–174.
248. Meyer JH, Tomlinson DR: Prevention of defects of axonal transport and nerve conduction velocity by oral administration of myo-inositol or an aldose reductase inhibitor in streptozotocin-diabetic rats. *Diabetologia* 1983;25:433–438.
249. Gillon KRW, Hawthorne JN: Sorbitol, inositol and nerve conduction in diabetes. *Life Sci* 1983;32:1943–1947.
250. Finegold D, Lattimer SA, Nolle S, Bernstein M, Greene DA: Polyol pathway activity and myo-inositol metabolism. A suggested relationship in the pathogenesis of diabetic neuropathy. *Diabetes* 1983;32:988–992.
251. Hatanaka I: Studies on the pathogenesis of diabetic neuropathy using aldose reductase inhibitor, ONO-2235. *J Japan Diab Soc* 1985;28:901–908.
252. Kikkawa R, Hatanaka I, Shigeta Y: Preventive effect of aldose reductase inhibitor, ONO-2235, on peripheral nerve disorders in streptozotocin-diabetic rats, in Sakamoto N, Min HK, Baba S (eds): *Current topics in clinical and experimental aspects of diabetes mellitus.* New York, Elsevier Science Publishers, 1985, pp 365–369.
253. Mayer JH, Tomlinson DR: The influence of aldose reductase inhibition and nerve myo-inositol on axonal transport and nerve conduction velocity in rats with experimental diabetes. *J Physiol* 1983;340:25P–26P.
254. Fretten P, Tomlinson DR, Townsend J: Prevention of axonal transport defects, in vagus and sciatic nerves of diabetic rats, by aldose reductase inhibition. *Br J Pharmacol* 1984;82:265P.
255. Stewart MA, Sherman WR, Kurien MM, Moonsammy GI, Wisgerhof M: Polyol accumulation in nervous tissue of rats with experimental diabetes and galactosemia. *J Neurochem* 1967;14:1057–1066.
256. Dyck J: Current concepts in neurology. *N Engl J Med* 1982;307:283–286.
257. Gregersen G: Variations in motor conduction velocity produced by acute changes of the metabolic state in diabetic patients. *Diabetologia* 1968;4:273–277.
258. Eliasson SG: Nerve conduction changes in experimental diabetes. *J Clin Invest* 1964;43:2353–2358.
259. Preston GM: Peripheral neuropathy in the alloxan-diabetic rat. *J Physiol* 1967; 189:49P–50P.
260. Gabbay KH: Role of sorbitol pathway in neuropathy, in Camerini-Davalos RA, Cole HS (eds): *Vascular and neurological changes in early diabetes.* New York, Academic Press, 1973, pp 417–424.
261. Stewart MA, Passonneau JV: Identification of fructose in mammalian nerve. *Biochem Biophys Res Comm* 1964;17:536–541.
262. Stewart MA, Sherman WR, Anthony S: Free sugars in alloxan diabetic rat nerve. *Biochem Biophys Res Comm* 1966;22:488–491.
263. Gabbay KH, O'Sullivan JB: The sorbitol pathway: Enzyme localization and content in normal and diabetic nerve and cord. *Diabetes* 1968;17:239–243.
264. Gabbay KH, Snider JJ: Nerve conduction defect in galactose-fed rats. *Diabetes* 1972;21:295–300.
265. Sharma AK, Thomas PK, Baker RWR: Peripheral nerve abnormalities related to galactose administration in rats. *J Neurol Neurosurg Psychiatry* 1976;39:794–802.
266. Yue DK, Hanwell MA, Satchell PM, Turtle JR: The effect of aldose reductase inhibition on nerve conduction velocity in diabetic rats. *Diabetes* 1982;31:789–794.
267. Kikkawa R, Hatanaka I, Miyamoto Y, Kobayashi N, Shigeta Y: The effect of aldose reductase inhibitors on peripheral nerve disorders in chronic diabetic rats. *Diabetes Res Clin Pract* 1985;(suppl 1):S300.

268. Sima AAF: The development and structural characterization of the neuropathies in the spontaneously diabetic BB Wistar rat. *Metabolism* 1983;32(suppl 1):106–111.
269. Sima AAF, McEwen TAJ, Chakrabarti S: The effect of statil on early nerve dysfunction. *Diabetes* 1986; 35(suppl 1):206A.
270. Inserra JJ, Fossile A, Notvest RO, Keim K: Auditory-evoked brainstem response (ABR) as a measure of nerve transmission time in rats. *Fed Proc* 1986;45:463.
271. Notvest RO, Inserra JJ: Tolrestat, an aldose reductase inhibitor, prevents nerve dysfunction in conscious diabetic rats. *Diabetes* 1987;36:500–504.
273. Zahnd GR, Wuarin-Bierman L, Kaufmann F, Adler J: Hyperalgesia in spontaneous and experimental animal models of diabetic neuropathy. *Diabetologia* 1986;29:609A.
274. Fagius J: Autonomic neurophysiology in long-term diabetes. *Clin Physiol* 1985;5(suppl 5):74–78.
275. Droz B, Koenig HL: The turnover of proteins in axons and nerve endings. *Symp Int Soc Cell Biol* 1969;8:35–50.
276. Lasek RJ: Protein transport in neurons. *Int Rev Neurobiol* 1970;13:289–324.
277. Weiss PA, Hiscoe HB: Experiments on the mechanism of nerve growth. *J Exp Zool* 1948;107:315–395.
278. Grafstein B, Forman DS: Intracellular transport in neurons. *Physiol Rev* 1980;60:1167–1283.
279. Tomlinson DR, Willars GB, Robinson JR: Prevention of defects of axonal transport in experimental diabetes by aldose reductase inhibitors. *Drugs* 1986;32(suppl 2): 15–18.
280. Schmidt RE, Matschinsky FM, Godfrey DA, Williams AD, McDougal DB: Fast and slow axoplasmic flow in sciatic nerve of diabetic rats. *Diabetes* 1975;24:1081–1085.
281. Tomlinson DR, Holmes PR, Mayer JH: Reversal, by treatment with an aldose reductase inhibitor, of impaired axonal transport and motor nerve conduction velocity in experimental diabetes mellitus. *Neurosci Lett* 1982;31:189–193.
282. Mayer JH, Tomlinson DR: Axonal transport of cholinergic transmitter enzymes in vagus and sciatic nerves of rats with acute experimental diabetes mellitus; correlation with motor nerve conduction velocity and effects of insulin. *Neurosci* 1983;9:951–957.
283. Robinson JR, Tomlinson DR: Impaired axonal transport of choline-containing lipids in rats with experimental diabetes mellitus and its prevention by sorbinil, an aldose reductase inhibitor. *J Physiol* 1985;369:158P.
284. Mayer JH, Tomlinson DR: Slow orthograde axonal transport in experimental diabetes in the rat: Effects of an aldose reductase inhibitor. *J Physiol* 1984;351:16P.
285. Tomlinson DR, Sidenius P, Larsen JR: Slow component-a of axonal transport, nerve myoinositol, and aldose reductase inhibition in streptozocin-diabetic rats. *Diabetes* 1986;35:398–402.
286. Robinson JR, Whiteley SJ, Tomlinson DR: Influence of aldose reductase on slow axonal transport in diabetes and galactosemia. *J Neurochem* 1985;44(suppl):S–121.
287. Tomlinson DR, Townsend J: Protection by the aldose reductase inhibitor "statil" (ICI 128,436) against loss of an axonally transported enzyme in nerve terminals of diabetic rats. *Diabetes* 1985;34(suppl 1):202A.
288. Tomlinson DR, Townsend J, Fretten P: Prevention of defective axonal transport in streptozocin-diabetic rats by treatment with "statil" (ICI 128,436), an aldose reductase inhibitor. *Diabetes* 1985;34:970–972.
289. Mayer JH, Herberg L, Tomlinson DR: Axonal transport and nerve conduction and their relation to nerve polyol and myoinositol levels in spontaneously diabetic BB/D rats. *Neurochem Pathol* 1984;2:285–293.
290. Greene DA: Metabolic abnormalities in diabetic peripheral nerve: Relation to impaired function. *Metabolism* 1983;32(suppl 1):112–123.

291. Ritchie JM: The oxygen consumption of mammalian nonmyelinated nerve fibers at rest and during activity. *J Physiol* 1967;188:309–329.
292. Das PK, Bray GM, Aguayo AJ, Rasminsky M: Diminished quabain-sensitive, sodium-potassium ATPase activity in sciatic nerves of rats with streptozotocin-induced diabetes. *Exp Neurol* 1976;53:285–299.
293. Clements RS Jr: Diabetic neuropathy—New concepts of its etiology. *Diabetes* 1979; 28:604–611.
294. Greene DA, Lattimer SA: Impaired rat sciatic nerve sodium-potassium adenosine triphosphatase in acute streptozocin diabetes and its correction by dietary myo-inositol supplementation. *J Clin Invest* 1983;72:1058–1063.
295. Greene DA, Lattimer SA: Impaired energy utilization and Na,K-ATPase in diabetic peripheral nerve. *Am J Physiol* 1984;246:E311–E318.
296. Greene DA, Lattimer S, Ulbrecht J, Carroll P: Glucose-induced alterations in nerve metabolism: Current perspective on the pathogenesis of diabetic neuropathy and future directions for research and therapy. *Diabetes Care* 1985;8:290–299.
297. Greene DA, Yagihashi S, Lattimer SA, Sima AAF: Nerve Na ,K -ATPase, conduction, and myo-inositol in the insulin-deficient BB rat. *Am J Physiol* 1984;247:E534–539.
298. Mizisin AP, Myers RR, Powell HC: Endoneurial sodium accumulation in galactosemic rat nerves. *Muscle Nerve* 1986;9:440–444.
299. Powell HC, Costello ML, Myers RR: Galactose neuropathy: permeability studies, mechanism of edema, and mast cell abnormalities. *Acta Neuropathol* 1981;55:89–95.
300. Myers RR, Costello ML, Powell HC: Increased endoneurial fluid pressure in galactose neuropathy. *Muscle Nerve* 1979;2:299–303.
301. Mizisin AP, Powell HC, Myers RR: Edema and increased endoneurial sodium in galactose neuropathy. Reversal with an aldose reductase inhibitor. *J Neurol Sci* 1986; 74:35–43.
302. Simpson CMF, Hawthorne JN: Myo-inositol metabolism and (Na +K)-ATPase activity in relation to peripheral nerve function in rats with streptozotocin-induced diabetes. *Biochem Soc Trans* 1986;14:364–365.
303. Greene DA, Lattimer SA: Relationship of polyol (sorbitol) pathway inhibition to a myo-inositol-mediated defect in sodium-potassium ATPase activity. *Diabetes* 1984;33:712–716.
304. Greene DA, Lattimer SA, Finegold DN, Tamres LK: Impaired Na-dependent amino acid uptake in diabetic peripheral nerve. Correction by aldose reductase inhibition or myoinositol supplementation. *Clin Res* 1985;33:431A.
305. Wells AM, Greene DA: A sorbinil responsive myoinositol-related Na/K-ATPase defect in diabetic rat superior cervical ganglion. *Diabetes* 1985;34:102A.
306. Greene DA, Mackway AM: Decreased myo-inositol content and Na/K-ATPase activity in superior cervical ganglion of STZ-diabetic rat and prevention by aldose reductase inhibition. *Diabetes* 1986;35:1106–1108.
307. Cohen MP, Dashmahapatra A, Shapiro E: Reduced glomerular sodium/potassium adenosine triphosphatase activity in acute streptozocin diabetes and its prevention by oral sorbinil. *Diabetes* 1985;34:1071–1074.
308. Cohen MP, Klepser H: Binding of an aldose reductase inhibitor to renal glomeruli. *Biochem Biophys Res Comm* 1985;129:530–535.
309. Willow M, Kuenzel EA, Catterall WA: Inhibition of voltage-sensitive sodium channels in neuroblastoma cells and synaptosomes by the anticonvulsant drugs diphenyl-hydantoin and carbamazepine. *Mol Pharmacol* 1984;25:228–234.
310. Cohen MP, Klepser H, Cua E: Effect of diabetes and sorbinil treatment on phospholipid metabolism in rat glomeruli. *Biochim Biophys Act* 1986;876:226–232.

311. Garner MH, Spector A: Glucose-6-phosphate modification of bovine renal Na,K-ATPase: A model for changes occurring in the human renal medulla. *Biochem Biophys Res Comm* 1985;131:1206–1211.
312. Garner MH, Spector A: Native and glucosylated Na,K-ATPase: The effects of an aldose reductase inhibitor. *Invest Ophthalmol Vis Sci* 1986;27(suppl):136.
313. McCormack AJ, Gitelman HJ, Finn WF: Effects of aldose reductase inhibition on early changes in renal function in diabetic rats. *Clin Res* 1986;34:549A.
314. Goldfarb S, Simmons DA, Kern E: Amelioration of glomerular hyperfiltration in acute experimental diabetes by dietary myo-inositol and by an aldose reductase inhibitor. *Clin Res* 1986;34:725.
315. Varagiannis E, Beyer-Mears A, Cruz E: Diminished proteinuria by an aldose reductase inhibitor, sorbinil. *Diabetes* 1984;33(suppl 1):43A.
316. Beyer-Mears A, Cruz E, Edelist T, Varagiannis E: Diminished proteinuria in diabetes mellitus by sorbinil, an aldose reductase inhibitor. *Pharmacology* 1986;32:52–60.
317. Beyer-Mears A, Del Val M, Varagiannis E: Effect of sorbinil on proteinuria and hypertension in diabetic nephropathy. *Diabetes* 1986;35(suppl 1):203A.
318. Beyer-Mears A, Cruz E, Dillon P, Tanis D, Roche M: Diabetic renal hypertrophy diminished by aldose reductase inhibition. *Fed Proc* 1983;44:505.
319. Kilzer P, Chang K, Marvel J, et al: Albumin permeation of new vessels is increased in diabetic rats. *Diabetes* 1985;34:333–336.
320. Chang K, Tomlinson M, Jeffrey JR, et al: Galactose ingestion increases vascular permeability and collagen solubility in normal male rats. *J Clin Invest* 1987; 79:367–373.
321. Williamson JR, Chang K, Rowold E, Kilo C, Lacy PE: Islet transplants in diabetic Lewis rats prevent and reverse diabetes-induced increases in vascular permeability and prevent but do not reverse collagen solubility changes. *Diabetologia* 1986;29: 392–396.
322. Williamson JR, Rowold E, Chang K, et al: Sex steroid-dependency of diabetes-induced changes in polyol metabolism, vascular permeability and collagen crosslinking. *Diabetes* 1986;35:20–27.
323. Chang K, Veigel C, Jeffrey JR, Tilton RG, Kilo C: Diabetes-induced increased albumin permeation in the eye: Prevention by inhibitors of aldose reductase. *Diabetes* 1986;35(suppl 1):101A.
324. Lorenzi M, Toledo S, Lane M: Polyol and glucose accumulation by human endothelial cells cultured in high glucose are not prevented by sorbinil. *Clin Res* 1985;33:63A.
325. MacGregor LC, Rosecan LR, Laties AM, Matschinsky FM: Microanalysis of total lipid, glucose, sorbitol, and myo-inositol in individual retina layers of normal and alloxan rabbits. *Diabetes* 1984;33(suppl 1):89A.
326. MacGregor LC, Matschinsky FM: Correlation of biochemical and electrophysiological abnormalities in retinas of experimentally diabetic animals. *Diabetes* 1985;34(suppl 1):13A.
327. MacGregor LC, Matschinsky FM: Treatment with aldose reductase inhibitor or with myo-inositol arrests deterioration of the electroretinogram of diabetic rats. *J Clin Invest* 1985;76:887–889.
328. Campochiaro PA, May E, Blaydes S, Vinores SA: Aldose reductase induction and progressive ultrastructural degeneration in diabetic retinal pigment epithelium. *Soc Neurosci Abstr* 1986;12:638.
329. Kinoshita JH, Kador P, Datiles M: Aldose reductase in diabetic cataracts. *JAMA* 1981;246:257–261.

330. Simard-Duquesne N, Dvornik D: Galactitol accumulation and irreversible lens opacities in galactosemic rats. *Invest Ophthalmol* 1973;12:82–83.
331. Fukushi S, Merola LO, Kinoshita JH: Altering the course of cataracts in diabetic rats. *Invest Ophthalmol Vis Sci* 1980,19.313–315.
332. Chiou SH, Chylack LT Jr, Bunn HF, Kinoshita JH: Role of nonenzymatic glycosylation in experimental cataract formation. *Biochem Biophys Res Comm* 1980;95:894–901.
333. Datiles M, Fukui H, Kuwabara T, Kinoshita JH: Galactose cataract prevention with sorbinil, an aldose reductase inhibitor: A light microscopic study. *Invest Ophthalmol Vis Sci* 1982;22:174–179.
334. Poulsom R, Boot-Handford RP, Heath H: Some effects of aldose reductase inhibition upon the eyes of long-term streptozotocin-diabetic rats. *Curr Eye Res* 1983;2:351–355.
335. Cotlier E: Hypophysectomy effect on lens epithelium and galactose development in rats. *Arch Ophthalmol* 1962;67:476–482.
336. Sippel TO: Change in the water, protein, and glutathion contents in the lens in the course of galactose cataract development in rats. *Invest Ophthalmol* 1966;5:568–575.
337. Simard-Duquesne N, Greselin E, Gonzalez R, Dvornik D: Prevention of cataract development in severely galactosemic rats by the aldose reductase inhibitor, tolrestat. *Proc Soc Exp Biol Med* 1985;178:599–605.
338. Varma SD, Kinoshita JH: Topical treatment of galactose cataracts. *Docum Ophthalmol Proc Series* 1976;8:305–309.
339. Parmar NS, Ghosh MN: Effect of gossypin, a flavonoid, on the formation of galactose-induced cataracts in rats. Exp Eye Res 1979;29:229–232.
340. Beyer-Mears A, Farnsworth PN: Diminished sugar cataractogenesis by quercetin. *Exp Eye Res* 1979;28:709–716.
341. Waterbury LD, Mahoney JM, Pfister JR: Inhibition of lens aldose reductase (A.R.) by 7-dimethylsulfamoyl-xanthone-2-carboxylic acid (RS 7535). *Fed Proc* 1979: 38:254.
342. Unakar NJ, Tsui Y: Inhibition of galactose-induced alterations in ocular lens with sorbinil. *Exp Eye Res* 1983;36:685–694.
343. Hu TS, Datiles M, Kinoshita JH: Reversal of galactose cataract with sorbinil in rats. *Invest Ophthalmol Vis Sci* 1983;24:640–644.
344. Kelly K, Cruz E, Tanis D, Beyer-Mears A: Reversal of Stage II galactose cataract by combination of sorbinil and normal diet. *Invest Ophthalmol Vis Sci* 1984;25:269.
345. Beyer-Mears A, Kelly K, Cruz E: Synergism of sorbinil and normal diet on reversal of Stage-II cataract. *Pharmacology* 1985;31:170–179.
346. Varma SD, Mizuno A, Kinoshita JH: Diabetic cataracts and flavonoids. *Science* 1977;195:205–206.
347. Beyer-Mears A, Del Val M, Cruz E: Reversal of Stage II diabetic cataract by sorbinil. *Invest Ophthalmol Vis Sci* 1986;27(suppl):136.
348. Beyer-Mears A, Cruz E, Varagiannis E: Reversal of Stage-I sugar cataract by sorbinil, an aldose reductase inhibitor. *Pharmacology* 1985;31:88–96.
349. Keiding S, Mellemgaard L: Dose dependence of galactose cataract in the rat. *Acta Ophthalmol* 1972;50:174–182.
350. Rohrbach, DH, Martin GR: Structure of basement membrane in normal and diabetic tissue. *Ann NY Acad Sci* 1982;401:203–211.
351. Lubec G: Definition of the glomerular basement membrane. *Renal Physiol* 1984;7:1–2.
352. Williamson JR, Kilo C: Current status of capillary basement-membrane disease in diabetes mellitus. *Diabetes* 1977;26:65–75.
353. Siperstein MD, Unger RH, Madison LL: Studies of muscle capillary basement membranes in normal subjects, diabetic and prediabetic patients. *J Clin Invest* 1968; 47:1973–1999.

354. Osterby R: Morphometric studies of the peripheral glomerular basement membrane in early juvenile diabetes. I. Development of initial basement membrane thickening. *Diabetologia* 1972;8:84–92.
355. Kilo C, Vogler N, Williamson JR: Muscle capillary basement membrane changes related to aging and diabetes mellitus. *Diabetes* 1972;21:881–905.
356. Siperstein MD: Capillary basement membranes and diabetic microangiopathy. *Adv Intern Med* 1972;18:325–344.
357. Siess EA, Nathke HE, Dexel T, et al: Dependency of muscle capillary basement membrane thickness on the duration of diabetes. *Diabetes Care* 1979;2:472–478.
358. Williamson JR, Kilo C: Capillary basement membranes in diabetes. *Diabetes* 1983;32(suppl 2):96–100 and references cited.
359. Bloodworth JMB Jr, Engerman RL, Powers KL: Experimental diabetic microangiopathy. *Diabetes* 1969;18:455–458.
360. Bloodworth JMB Jr, Engerman RL, Camerini-Davalos RA, Powers KL: Variations in capillary basement membrane width produced by aging and diabetes mellitus. *Adv Metab Disord* 1970; (suppl I):279–287.
361. Engerman R, Bloodworth JMB Jr, Nelson S: Relationship of microvascular disease in diabetes to metabolic control. *Diabetes* 1977;26:760–769.
362. Engerman RL, Kern TS: Experimental galactosemia produces diabetic-like retinopathy. *Diabetes* 1984;33:97–100.
363. Efimov AS, Gordienko VM, Tkachuk YV, et al: Use of naphthylimidoacetic acid in rats with experimental diabetes. *Probl Endokrinol* 1980;26:69–72.
364. Kern TS, Engerman RL: Hexitol production by canine retinal microvessels. *Invest Ophthalmol Vis Sci* 1984;25(suppl):159.
365. Robison WG, Hohman T, Katz M, Drea C: Retinal capillaries: Characterization of the thickened basement membranes in diabetic, galactosemic, and senescent rats. *Invest Ophthalmol Vis Sci* 1985;26(suppl):327.
366. Robison WG, Kador PF, Akagi Y, Kinoshita JH: Basement membrane thickening in ocular vessels of galactosemic rats prevented with aldose reductase inhibitors. *Invest Ophthalmol Vis Sci* 1984;25(suppl):66.
367. Nagata M, Robison WG Jr, Kador PF, Kinoshita JH: Differential basement membrane thickening in ocular and nonocular tissues of animal models of diabetes. *Invest Ophthalmol Vis Sci* 1986;27(suppl):255.
368. Sarges R, Howard HR, Kelbaugh PR: Synthesis of optically active spirohydantoins by asymmetric induction. Hydantoin formation from amino nitriles and chlorosulfonyl isocyanate, *J Org Chem* 1982;47:4081–4085.
369. Sestanj K, Bellini F, Fung S, et al: N-[[5-(Trifluoromethyl)-6-methoxy-1-naphthalenyl]thioxo-methyl]-N-methylglycine (tolrestat), a potent, orally active aldose reductase inhibitor. *J Med Chem* 1984;27:255–256.
370. Robison WG Jr, Hohman TC, Kador PF, et al: Prevention of retinal microangiopathy in long-term diabetic models by aldose reductase inhibitors. *Invest Ophthalmol Vis Sci* 1986;27(suppl):255.
371. Griffin BW, Chandler ML, Desantis L: Prevention of diabetic cataract and neuropathy in rats by two new aldose reductase inhibitors. *Invest Ophthalmol Vis Sci* 1984;25(suppl):136.
372. Chandler ML, Shannon WA, Desantis L: Prevention of retinal capillary basement membrane thickening in diabetic rats by aldose reductase inhibitors. *Invest Ophthalmol Vis Sci* 1984;25(suppl):159.
373. Stribling DR, Harrison HE, Gaschen F, Rossi GL: Effect of aldose reductase inhibition with statil (ICI-128,436) on retinal capillary basement membrane thickening in streptozotocin diabetic rats. *Diabetologia* 1986;29:597A.

374. Cohen AM, Teitelbaum A, Saliternik R: Genetics and diet as factors in development of diabetes mellitus. *Metabolism* 1972;21:235–240.
375. Rosenmann E, Yanko L, Cohen AM: Comparative study of the pathology of sucrose-induced diabetes in the rat and adult-onset diabetes in man. *Isr J Med Sci* 1975;11:753–761.
376. Yanko L, Rosenmann E, Cohen AM: A correlative study on the occurrence of retinopathy and nephropathy in sucrose-fed diabetic rats. *Acta Diabet Lat* 1975;12:52–65.
377. Papachristodoulou D, Heath H, Kang SS: The development of retinopathy in sucrose-fed and streptozotocin-diabetic rats. *Diabetologia* 1976;12:367–374.
378. Boot-Handford R, Heath H: Identification of fructose as the retinopathic agent associated with the ingestion of sucrose-rich diets in the rat. *Metabolism* 1980;29: 1247–1252.
379. Heath H, Hamlett YC: The sorbitol pathway: Effect of streptozotocin induced diabetes and the feeding of a sucrose-rich diet on glucose, sorbitol and fructose in the retina, blood and liver of rats. *Diabetologia* 1976;12:43–46.
380. Hotta N, Kakuta H, Fukasawa H, et al: Prevention of diabetic retinopathy by aldose reductase inhibitor in fructose-fed streptozotocin-diabetic rats. *Diabetes Res Clin Pract* 1985;(suppl 1):S251.
381. Sato H, Oikawa S, Suzuki H, et al: Effect of aldose reductase inhibitor (M 79,175) on thickness of renal glomerular basement membrane in galactose-fed STZ (streptozotocin) induced diabetic rats. *Diabetes Res Clin Pract* 1985;(suppl 1):S494.
382. Boulton AJM, Ward JD: Diabetic neuropathies and pain. *Clin Endocrinol Metab* 1986;15:917–931.
383. Gillon KRW, King RHM, Thomas PK: The pathology of diabetic neuropathy and the effects of aldose reductase inhibitors. *Clin Endocrinol Metab* 1986;15:837–853.
384. Gabbay KH, Spack N, Loo S, Hirsch H, Ackil AA: Aldose reductase inhibition: Studies with alrestatin. *Metabolism* 1979;28(suppl 1):471–476.
385. Culebras A, Alio J, Herrera JL, Lopez-Fraile IP: Effect of an aldose reductase inhibitor on diabetic peripheral neuropathy. *Arch Neurol* 1981;38:133–134.
386. Handelsman DJ, Turtle JR: Clinical trial of an aldose reductase inhibitor in diabetic neuropathy. *Diabetes* 1981;30:459–464.
387. Fagius J, Jameson S: Effects of aldose reductase inhibitor treatment in diabetic polyneuropathy—a clinical and neurophysiological study. *J Neurol Neurosurg Psychiatry* 1981;44:991–1001.
388. Pitts NE, Gundersen K, Mehta DJ, et al: Aldose reductase inhibitors in clinical practice. Preliminary studies on diabetic neuropathy and retinopathy. *Drugs* 1986;32(suppl 1):30–35.
389. Judzewitsch R, Jaspan JB, Polonsky KS, Halter JB, et al: Aldose reductase inhibition improves nerve conduction velocity in diabetic patients. *N Engl J Med* 1983;308: 119–125.
390. Winegrad AI, Simmons DA, Martin DB: Has one diabetic complication been explained? *N Engl J Med* 1983;308:152–154.
391. Graf RJ, Halter JB, Halar E, Porte D Jr: Nerve conduction abnormalities in untreated maturity-onset diabetes. *Ann Intern Med* 1981;90:298–303.
392. Graf RJ, Halter JB, Pfeifer MA, et al: Glycemic control and nerve conduction abnormalities in non-insulin-dependent subjects. *Ann Intern Med* 1981;94:307–311.
393. Pfeifer MA: Effects of glycemic control and aldose reductase inhibition on nerve conduction velocity. *Am J Med* 1985;79(suppl 5A):19–23.
394. Young RR, Shahani BT: Nerve conduction velocity in diabetes (letter to editor). *N Engl J Med* 1983;309:190–191.

395. Brzezinski WA, Recker RR: Nerve conduction velocity in diabetes (letter to editor). *N Engl J Med* 1983;309:191.
396. O'Neill WC: Nerve conduction velocity in diabetes (letter to editor). *N Engl J Med* 1983;309:191.
397. Halter JB, Halar EM, Porte D, Weinberg CR, Jaspan JB: Nerve conduction velocity in diabetes (letter to editor). *N Engl J Med* 1983;309:191–192.
398. Jaspan J, Maseli R, Herold K, Bartkus C: Treatment of severely painful diabetic neuropathy with an aldose reductase inhibitor: Relief of pain and improved somatic and autonomic nerve function. *Lancet* 1983;2:758–762.
399. Young RJ, Matthews DM, Clarke BF, Martyne CN, Ewing DJ: Aldose reductase inhibition for diabetic neuropathy. *Lancet* 1983;2:969.
400. Abraham RR, Abraham RM, Wynn V: Aldose reductase inhibition for diabetic neuropathy. *Lancet* 1983;2:969.
401. Young RJ, Ewing DJ, Clarke BF: A controlled trial of sorbinil, an aldose reductase inhibitor, in chronic painful diabetic neuropathy. *Diabetes* 1983;32:938–942.
402. Rosenstock J, Challis P, Raskin P: The effect of sorbinil on severe painful diabetic neuropathy. *Diabetes* 1986;35(suppl 1):101A.
403. Lehtinen J, Partanen J, Hyvonen SK, Uusitupa M: The effect of aldose reductase inhibitor (sorbinil) on nerve conduction variables. *Acta Endocrinol* 1983; 103(suppl 257):Abstract 41.
404. Lehtinen J, Hyvonen K, Kilpelainen H, et al: The effect of small dose of aldose reductase inhibitor (sorbinil) on diabetic neuropathy. *Acta Neurol Scand* 1984;69(suppl 98):198–199.
405. Lehtinen JM, Hyvonen SK, Uusitupa M, Puhakainen E: The effect of an aldose reductase inhibitor (sorbinil) on diabetic neuropathy. *Diabetologia* 1984;27:303A.
406. Lehtinen JM, Hyvonen SK, Uusitupa M, et al: The effect of sorbinil treatment on red cell sorbitol levels and clinical and electrophysiological parameters of diabetic neuropathy. *J Neurol* 1986;233:174–177.
407. Lewin IG, O'Brien IAD, Morgan MH, Corrall RJM: Clinical and neurophysiological studies with the aldose reductase inhibitor, sorbinil, in symptomatic diabetic neuropathy. *Diabetologia* 1984;26:445–448.
408. Foulds G, O'Brien MM, Bianchine JR, Gabbay KH: Kinetics of an orally absorbed aldose reductase inhibitor, sorbinil. *Clin Pharmacol Ther* 1981;30:693–700.
409. Heimans JJ, Schouten JA, Van Der Veen EA, Visser SL: Treatment of diabetic neuropathy with an aldose reductase inhibitor. *Clin Neurol Neurosurg* 1984;86:317.
410. Schouten JA, Heimans JJ, Popp-Snijders C, et al: A three-month placebo-controlled efficacy study of sorbinil for diabetic neuropathy. *Neth J Med* 1985;28:216.
411. Schouten JA, Heimans JJ, Popp-Snijders C, et al: A 3-month, placebo-controlled, efficacy study of sorbinil for diabetic neuropathy. *Diabetologia* 1984;27:329A.
412. Christensen JEJ, Varnek L, Gregersen G: The effect of an aldose reductase inhibitor (Sorbinil) on diabetic neuropathy and neural function of the retina: A double-blind study. *Acta Neurol Scand* 1985;71:164–167.
413. Fagius J, Brattberg A, Jameson S, Berne C: Limited benefit of treatment of diabetic polyneuropathy with an aldose reductase inhibitor: A 24-week controlled trial. *Diabetologia* 1985;28:323–329.
414. Christensen JEJ: Missing effect of sorbinil at long-term treatment of diabetic neuropathy. *Diabetes Res Clin Pract* 1985;(suppl 1):S100–S101.
415. Jaspan J, Herold K, Bartkus C: Improvement in cardiac autonomic nerve dysfunction in diabetic patients with aldose reductase inhibitor therapy. *Clin Res* 1985;33:433A.

416. Jaspan JB, Towle VL, Maselli R, Herold K: Clinical studies with an aldose reductase inhibitor in the autonomic and somatic neuropathies of diabetes. *Metabolism* 1986;35(suppl 1):83–92.
417. Jaspan JB, Herold K, Bartkus C: Effect of sorbinil therapy in diabetic patients with painful peripheral neuropathy and autonomic neuropathy. *Am J Med* 1985;79(suppl 5A):24–37.
418. Pfeifer M, Snider H, Peterson H, et al: Improvement in cardiovascular performance by sorbinil in diabetics. *Diabetes* 1986;35(suppl 1):102A.
419. Green A, Jaspan J, Kavin H, et al: Influence of aldose reductase inhibitor (ARI) on neurogenic vesical dysfunction in diabetes. *Diabetes* 1986;35(suppl 1):102A.
420. Kavin H, Jaspan J, Green A: Diabetic gastrointestinal (GI) neuropathy: Effect of aldose reductase inhibitor (ARI). *Gastroenterology* 1986;90:1486.
421. Hotta N, Kakuta H, Kimura M, et al: Experimental and clinical trial of aldose reductase inhibitor in diabetic neuropathy. *Diabetes* 1983;32:98A.
422. Okuno G, Oki A, Tako H, Kawakami F, Yamazaki T: Recent progress in the treatment of diabetic neuropathy: A comparative study between prostaglandin E and a new aldose reductase inhibitor ONO-2235, in Baba S, Gould MK, Zimmet P (eds): *Diabetes mellitus.* Australia, Academic Press, 1984, pp 191–199.
423. Goto Y, Oikawa N, Akanuma Y, et al: Clinical study of a new aldose reductase inhibitor (ONO-2235) in diabetic neuropathy. A multicenter study. *J Japan Diab Soc* 1985;28:89–99.
424. Okuno G, Oki A, Yamazaki T, et al: The effects of aldose reductase inhibitor, ONO-2235 and prostaglandin E1 on diabetic neuropathy. *Diabetes Res Clin Pract* 1985;(suppl 1):S240.
425. Koglin L, Clark C, Ryder S, Mullane JF: The results of the long-term open-label administration of Alredase in the treatment of diabetic neuropathy. *Diabetes* 1985; 34(suppl 1):202A.
426. Koglin L, Kincaid J, Fineberg N, et al: The aldose reductase inhibitor tolrestat increases peripheral nerve conduction velocities and decreases neuropathic pain in patients with symptomatic, peripheral diabetic neuropathy. *Diabetes* 1986;35 (suppl 2):118A (1986).
427. Perry HD, Foulks GN, Thoft RA, Tolentino FI: Corneal complications after closed vitrectomy through the pars plana. *Arch Ophthalmol* 1978;96:1401–1403.
428. Brightbill FS, Myers FL, Bresnick GN: Postvitrectomy keratopathy. *Am J Ophthalmol* 1978;85:651–655.
429. Foulks GN, Thoft RA, Perry HD, Tolentino FI: Factors related to corneal epithelial complications after closed vitrectomy in diabetics. *Arch Ophthalmol* 1979; 97:1076–1078.
430. Kinoshita JH, Fukushi S, Kador P, Merola LO: Aldose reductase in diabetic complications of the eye. *Metabolism* 1979;28(suppl 1):462–469.
431. Fukushi S, Merola LO, Tanaka M, Datiles M, Kinoshita JH: Re-epithelization of denuded corneas in diabetic rats. *Exp Eye Res* 1980;31:611–621.
432. Eichenbaum JW, Feldstein M, Podos SM: Extended-wear aphakic soft contact lenses and corneal ulcers. *Br J Ophthalmol* 1982;66:663–666.
433. Pfister RR, Schepens CL, Lemp MA, Webster RG: Photocoagulation keratopathy: Report of a case. *Arch Ophthalmol* 1971;86:94–96.
434. Kanski JJ: Anterior segment complications of retinal photocoagulation. *Am J Ophthalmol* 1975;79:424–427.

435. Cobo M: Aldose reductase and diabetic keratopathy, pp 87–89, in Cogan DG (moderator): Aldose reductase and complications of diabetes. *Ann Intern Med* 1984;101:82–91.
436. Kador PF, Robison GF, Kinoshita JH: The pharmacology of aldose reductase inhibitors. *Ann Rev Pharmacol Toxicol* 1985;25:691–714.
437. Datiles MB, Kador PF, Fukui HN, Hu TS, Kinoshita JH: Corneal re-epithelialization in galactosemic rats. *Invest Ophthalmol Vis Sci* 1983;24:563–569.
438. Hay A, Cheng HM, Gonzalez RG, Kenyon KR: Activation of the sorbitol pathway in the cornea. *Invest Ophthalmol Vis Sci* 1986;27(suppl):31.
439. Faulborn J, Conway BP, Machemer R: Surgical complications of pars plana vitreous surgery. *Ophthalmology* 1978;85:116–125.
440. Kupfer C: Conclusions, pp 59–91. Cogan DG (moderator). Aldose reductase and complications. *Ann Intern Med* 1984;101:82–91.
441. Schultz RO, Van Horn DL, Peters MA, Klewin KM, Schutten WH: Diabetic keratopathy. *Trans Am Ophthalmol Soc* 1981;79:180–199.
442. Busted N, Olsen T, Schmitz O: Clinical observations on the corneal thickness and the corneal endothelium in diabetes mellitus. *Br J Ophthalmol* 1981;65:687–690.
443. Matsuda M, Suda T, Matanabe R: Quantitative analysis of corneal endothelial changes in anterior keratoconus. *Am J Ophthalmol* 1984;98:43.
444. Schultz RO, Matsuda M, Yee RW, Edelhauser HF, Schultz, KJ: Corneal endothelial changes in Type I and Type II diabetes mellitus. *Am J Ophthalmol* 1984;98:401–410.
445. Yee RW, Matsuda M, Kern TS, Engerman RL, Edelhauser HF: Corneal endothelial changes in diabetic dogs. *Curr Eye Res* 1985;4:759–766.
446. Meyer LA, Foley KM, Ubels JL, Edelhauser HF: Diabetes-induced corneal endothelial changes in rats. *Invest Ophthalmol Vis Sci* 1986;27(suppl):175.
447. Matsuda M, Awata T, Ohashi Y, et al: The effects of aldose reductase inhibitor on the diabetic corneal endothelium. Presented at the Internat Symp on polyol pathway and its role in diabetic complications. Kashikojima, Japan Oct 28–30, 1986.
448. Akagi Y, Majima K, Takahashi Y, et al: Repair of corneal endothelium in galactosemic rat. Presented at the Internat Symp of polyol pathway and its role in diabetic complications. Kashikojima, Japan Oct 28–30, 1986.
449. Cunha-Vaz JC, Mota C, Leite EC, Abreu JRF, Ruas MA: Effect of sorbinil on blood-retinal barrier in early diabetic retinopathy. *Diabetes* 1986;35:574–578.
450. Cunha-Vaz JC, Mota C, Leite EC, Abreu JR, Ruas MA: Effect of sulindac on the permeability of the blood-retinal barrier in early diabetic retinopathy. *Arch Ophthalmol* 1985;103:1307–1311.
451. Hotta N, Kakuta H, Fukasawa H, et al: The clinical trial of aldose reductase inhibitor on diabetic retinopathy. *Diabetes* 1986;35(suppl 1):213A.
452. Lundbaek K: Stiff hands in long-term diabetes. *Acta Med Scand* 1957;158:447–451.
453. Rosenbloom AL, Frias JL: Diabetes mellitus, short stature and joint stiffness. *Clin Res* 1974;22:92A.
454. Grgic A, Rosenbloom AL, Weber FT, et al: Joint contracture—common manifestation of childhood diabetes mellitus. *J Pediatr* 1976;88:584–588.
455. Trasiman HS, Traisman ES, Marr TJ, Wise J: Joint contractures in patients with juvenile diabetes and their siblings. *Diabetes Care* 1979;1:360–361.
456. Benedetti A, Noacco C, Macor S, Pittaro I: Joint lesions in diabetes. *N Engl J Med* 1975;292:1033–1034.
457. Rosenbloom AL, Silverstein JH, Lezotte DC, Richardson K, McCallum M: Limited joint mobility in childhood diabetes mellitus indicates risk for microvascular disease. *N Engl J Med* 1981;305:191–194.

458. Brice JEH, Johnston DI, Noronha JL: Limited finger joint mobility in diabetes. *Arch Dis Child* 1981;57:879–881.
459. Edidin DV: Cutaneous manifestations of diabetes mellitus in children. *Pediatr Dermatol* 1985;2:161–179.
460. Lawson PM, Maneschi F, Kohner EM: The relationship of hand abnormalities to diabetes and diabetic retinopathy. *Diabetes Care* 1983;6:140–143.
461. Campbell RR, Hawkins SJ, Maddison PJ, Reckless JPD: Limited joint mobility in diabetes mellitus. *Ann Rheum Dis* 1985;44:93–97.
462. Slama G, Letanoux M, Thibult N, et al: Quantification of early subclinical limited joint mobility in early diabetes. *Diabetes Care* 1985;8:329–332.
463. Jung Y, Hohmann TC, Novak J, et al: Diabetic hand syndrome. *Metabolism* 1971;20: 1008–1015.
464. Rosenbloom AL: Sorbinil and limited joint mobility in diabetes. *JAMA* 1985;254:1452 (letter).
465. Frank RN: Sorbinil and limited joint mobility in diabetics. *JAMA* 1985;254:1452 (letter).
466. Eaton RP: The collagen hydration hypothesis: a new paradigm for the secondary complications of diabetes mellitus. *J Chron Dis* 1986;39:763–766.
467. Lister DM, Graham-Brown RAC, Borden A: Resolution of diabetic cheiroanthropathy. *Br Med J* 1986;293:1537.
468. Buckingham BA, Uitto J, Sanborg C, et al: Scleroderma-like syndrome and the non-enzymatic glucosylation of collagen in children with poorly controlled insulin dependent diabetes (IDDM). *Pediatr Res* 1981;15:626.
469. Buckingham BA, Vitto J, Sandborg C, et al: Scleroderma-like changes in insulin-dependent diabetes mellitus: Clinical and biochemical studies. *Diabetes Care* 1984;7:163–169.
470. McLennan S, Yue DK, Marsh M, et al: The prevention and reversibility of tissue non-enzymatic glycosylation in diabetes. *Diabetic Medicine* 1986;3:141–146.
471. Fornaini G, Magnani M, Fazi A, et al: Regulatory properties of human erythrocyte hexokinase during cell ageing. *Arch Biochem Biophys* 1985;239:352–358.
472. Jacobasch G, Minakami S, Rapoport SM: Glycolysis of erythrocyte, in Yoshikawa H, Rapoport M (eds): *Cellular and molecular biology of erythrocytes.* Baltimore, University Park Press, 1974, pp 55–92.
473. Barretto OC De-O, Ursich M, Nonoyama K: Reduced levels of erythrocyte sorbitol dehydrogenase activity in human diabetics. *Brazilian J Med Biol Res* 1985;18: 477–479.
474. Hubinont C, Sener A, Malaisse WJ: Sorbitol content of plasma and erythrocytes during induced short-term hyperglycemia. *Clin Biochem* 1981;14:19–20.
475. Kamon N, Mabuchi H, Takeda R: Effects of an aldose-reductase inhibitor on short-term changes of human red cell sorbitol in vivo. *Diabetes Res Clin Pract* 1985; (suppl 1): S281–S282.
476. Raskin P, Rosenstock J, Challis P, et al: Effect of tolrestat on RBC sorbitol levels subjects with diabetes. *Clin Pharmacol Ther* 1985;38:625–630.
477. Price DE, Grant PJ, Strickland M, et al: The relationship between red cell sorbitol and blood glucose concentration in diabetes during hyperglycemic clamp studies and in out-patients. *Clin Sci* 1986;70(suppl 13):18P–19P.
478. Lapolla A, Poli T, Valerio A, Fedele D: Is red cell sorbitol content a good marker of glycemic control in diabetic patients? *Diabetes Res* 1985;2:283–286.
479. Akgun S, Ertel NH, Kemp FW: Red cell sorbitol and diabetic control. *Horm Metab Res* 1985;17:355–357.

480. Verschoor L, Wolffenbuttel BHR, Weber RFA, Van Koetsveld PM: Sorbitol content in erythrocytes not useful as an indicator of metabolic control in IDDM? *Diabetes Res Clin Pract* 1985;(suppl 1):S582.
481. Popp-Snijders C, Lomecky-Janousek MZ, Schouten JA, Van Der Veen EA: Myo-inositol and sorbitol in erythrocytes from diabetic patients before and after sorbinil treatment. *Diabetologia* 1984;27:514–516.
482. Popp-Snijders C, Lomecky-Janousek MZ, Schouten JA, Van Der Veen EA: Red cell sorbitol determined by capillary gas chromatography in Type 1 (insulin-dependent) diabetic patients before and after sorbinil treatment. *Diabetologia* 1983;25:187.
483. Malone JI, Harvey RC, Putnam JC: Sorbitol, inositol and phosphatidylinositol (PI) elevated in diabetic red cells. The influence of sorbinil. *Diabetes* 1983;32:161A.
484. Kilpelainen H, Puhakainen E, Saamanen AM, Lehtinen J, Riekkinen PJ: The effect of aldose reductase inhibitor (sorbinil) on erythrocyte sorbitol concentration in diabetic neuropathy. *J Neurochem* 1983;41(suppl)S27.
485. Puhakainen E, Saamanen AM, Lehtinen J, Kilpelainen H: The effect of aldose reductase inhibitor (sorbinil) on erythrocyte sorbitol concentration in diabetic neuropathy. *Acta Endocrinol* 1983;103(suppl 257):Abstract 56.
486. Wright J, Collier J, Stevenson D, English J, Passas R, et al: Sorbinil lowers erythrocyte sorbitol concentration in diabetes. *Clin Sci* 1984;66:44P.
487. Clements RS Jr, Morrison AD, Winegrad AI: Polyol pathway in aorta: Regulation by hormones. *Science* 1969;166:1007–1008.
488. Rogers DG, Deren S, Sherman WR, White NH, Santiago JV, et al: Sex and puberty related differences in red blood cell polyol levels (RBC-P) in Type I diabetics. *Diabetes* 1986;35(suppl 1):105A.
489. Dvornik D, Gonzalez R, Hicks D, Smith T, Ryder S, et al: Effect of tolrestat on RBC sorbitol levels in subjects with diabetes mellitus. *Diabetes Res Clin Pract* 1985; (suppl 1):S146.
490. Price D, Kemp J, Perkins M, Bastain W, Airey M, et al: The pharmacokinetics of ICI-128,436 and its effect on red cell sorbitol level in diabetic patients. *Diabetes* 1986;35(suppl 1):142A.
491. Price DE, Kemp J, Perkins CM, Bastain W, Airey CM, et al: The pharmacokinetics of ICI 128,436 and its effects on erythrocyte sorbitol level in diabetic patients. *Diabetologia* 1986;29:584A.
492. Peterson MJ, Page MG, Just LJ, Aldinger CE, Malone JI: Applicability of red blood cell sorbitol measurements to monitor the clinical activity of sorbinil. *Metabolism* 1986;35(suppl 1):93–95.
493. Malone JI: Sorbitol and plasma glucose. *Diabetes Care* 1982;5:648–649.
494. Broadstone VL, Pfeifer MA: Lack of correlations between RBC-sorbitol levels and diabetic neuropathy. *Clin Res* 1985;33:849A.
495. Berger W, Lehner D, Fluckiger R: Heterogeneity of sorbitol accumulation in glucose incubated erythrocytes: a possible explanation for the inherent susceptibility to neural complications in diabetic patients. *Diabetologia* 1986;29:517A.
496. Malone JI, Harvey RC, Putnam JC: Sorbitol, inositol and phosphatidylinositol (PI) elevated in diabetic red cells. The influence of sorbinil. *Diabetes* 1983; 32:161A.
497. Malone JI, Lowitt S, Harvey HC, Mandlow S: The effect of sorbinil (an aldose reductase inhibitor) upon red cell sorbitol and inositol. *Diabetes* 1984;33(suppl 1) :172A.
498. Wright J, Passas R, Stevenson D, Collier J: The effect of oral sorbinil at two doses on erythrocyte sorbitol and myoinositol concentration in diabetes. *Diabetes Res Clin Pract* 1985;(suppl 1):S–609.

499. Martyn CN, Matthews DM, Popp-Snijders C, Tucker J, Ewing DJ, et al: Effects of sorbinil treatment on erythrocytes and platelets of persons with diabetes. *Diabetes Care* 1986;9:36–39.
500. Popp-Snijders C, Lomecky-Janousek MZ, Schouten JA, Van Der Veen EA: Myo-inositol and sorbitol in erythrocytes from diabetic patients before and after sorbinil treatment. *Neth J Med* 1986;28:67–68.
501. Gronda C, Rossi JPFC, Cedola NV, Gagliardino JJ: Decreased Ca^{2+}-ATPase activity in erythrocyte membranes from diabetic patients. *IRCS Med Sci* 1986;14:476.
502. Adamson I, Okafor C, Abu-Bakare A: Erythrocyte membrane ATPases in diabetes: effect of dikanut (*Irvingia gabonensis*). *Enzyme* 1986;34(suppl 1):118A.
503. Hicks DR, Kraml M, Cayen MN, Dubuc J, Ryder S, et al: Tolrestat kinetics. *Clin Pharmacol Ther* 1984;36:493–499.

Chapter 5

The Medicinal Chemistry of Aldose Reductase Inhibitors

by Leslie Humber, Ph.D.

SYNOPSIS

This chapter is a survey of aldose reductase (AR) inhibitors that are in clinical development or that have been reported to be active in experimental animals upon oral administration. The scientific and patent literature has been reviewed from 1965 through 1986. Among compounds in clinical development, two main structural types of inhibitors are identified: the acetic acids such as tolrestat, epalrestat and statil, and the spirohydantoins and related compounds such as sorbinil, methosorbinil, alconil, CT-112 and ADN-138.

Contents

INTRODUCTION

Insulin therapy is effective for the primary control of glucose levels and has considerably reduced mortality from the acute effects of diabetes. However, the development of complications such as neuropathy, nephropathy, retinopathy and cataracts usually proceeds in spite of insulin administration, probably because of the difficulty in completely normalizing plasma glucose. Since the tissues involved (nerve, kidney, retina and lens) do not require insulin for glucose uptake, they are exposed to a high glucose concentration that enters the polyol pathway and is reduced by aldose reductase (AR) to sorbitol. As discussed in Chapter 4, increased flux of glucose through the polyol pathway has been linked to the development of some complications of chronic diabetes, and consequently, inhibition of the enzyme AR may provide a pharmacological approach to the control of these complications.

The enzyme AR was first characterized by Hayman and Kinoshita[1] in 1965; since then, hundreds of compounds have been synthesized and tested as AR inhibitors. This chapter will review the development of the AR inhibitors that are in clinical development as well as those that have demonstrated in vivo activity. Readers are referred to a recent article by Humber[2] for a comprehensive review of aldose reductase inhibitors.

THE DEVELOPMENT OF ALRESTATIN AND TOLRESTAT (ALREDASE®)

Alrestatin (AY-22,284), *1*, the first AR inhibitor to be clinically investigated, was developed at the Ayerst Research Laboratories. In 1966, work on AR inhibitors was

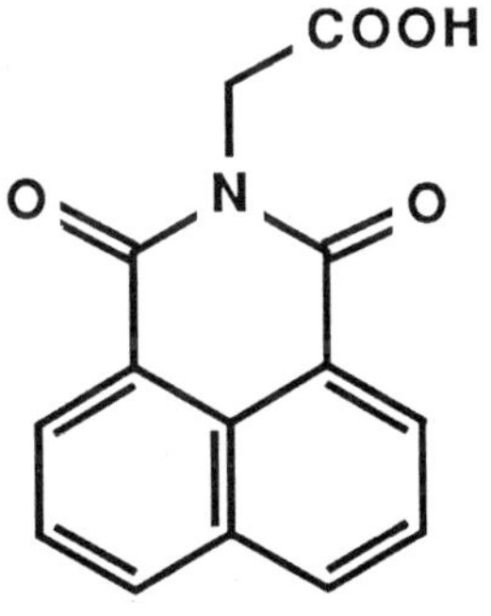

1

initiated at Ayerst, after Hayman and Kinoshita[1] observed that, in vitro, the enzyme was inhibited by a variety of aliphatic and keto acids, octanoic acid being one of the most potent, although cytotoxic, causing 59% inhibition at 1×10^{-4}M. The program at Ayerst, using a partially purified enzyme preparation isolated from calf lens, involved the systematic screening of various straight-chain carboxylic acids. For aliphatic carboxylic acids containing one to 23 carbon atoms there was a relationship between chain length and inhibitory activity; maximal activity was associated with a chain length of eight to 12 carbon atoms. Straight-chain α, ω-dicarboxylic acids showed a similar relationship, with inhibitory activity being maximal between the C_7 and C_{12} acids.

A series of dicarboxylic acids was synthesized in which the chain separating the carboxylic acid groups was substituted by a ring. The most active was found to be AY-20,037, tetramethyleneglutaric acid, *2* (TMG), which inhibited calf lens AR by 30% at 1×10^{-6}M. TMG was used to validate in vitro the hypothesis that AR was involved in the initiation and development of galactose cataracts,[3] although it was inactive when administered orally.[4,5]

A series of pyridylanilines was next investigated; N-(3-nitro-2-pyridyl)-3-trifluoromethylaniline, *3* (AY-20,263) was found to inhibit calf lens AR by 56% at 1×10^{-5}M, and was the first AR inhibitor to be demonstrated active upon injection into the vitreous cavity of the eye of rats fed a high galactose diet, by reducing galactitol levels in the lens by 53%, and delaying the onset of cataract.[6]

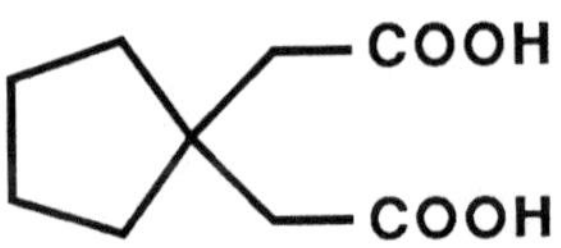

2

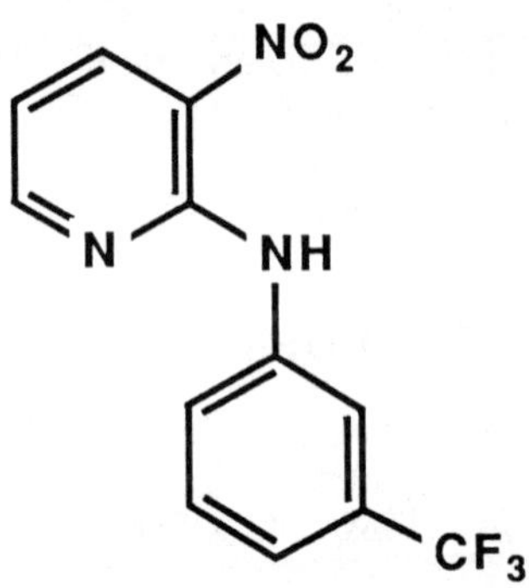

3

Hundreds of compounds were subsequently tested. Phthaloylglycine, *4*, was found to be potent in vitro ($IC_{50} = 2.5 \times 10^{-6}$M) but was inactive upon oral administration. This was attributed to a facile opening of the five-membered ring, giving the corresponding phthalamic acid, *5*, which had virtually no effect on AR in vitro. In order to retain structural features of phthaloylglycine, but in a molecular framework that would be resistant to hydrolysis, alrestatin (AY-22,284), *1*, a compound first described in 1931,[7] was synthesized,[8] tested, and found to be active in vitro ($IC_{50} = 3.5 \times 10^{-6}$M). It was also the first AR inhibitor to be effective upon oral administration, decreasing polyol accumulation in both streptozocin-induced diabetic rats and in rats fed galactose, and delaying cataract formation in the latter model.[4]

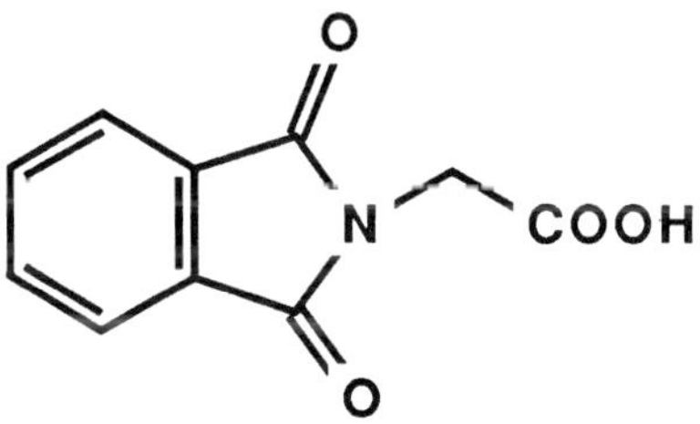

4

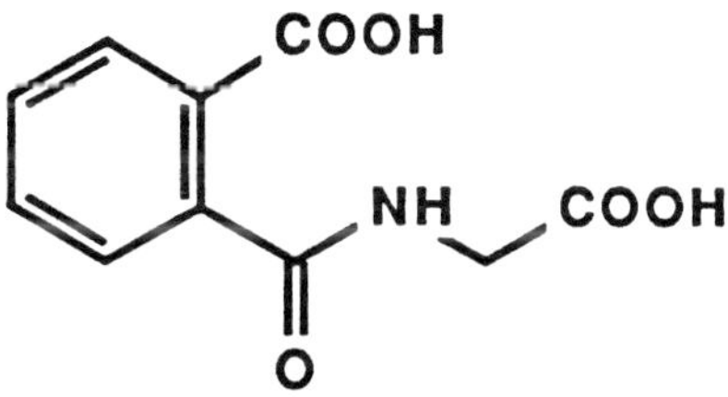

5

Alrestatin was remarkably stable in vivo, being excreted unchanged in several species, and after extensive pharmacological studies, alrestatin was tested in man at high dosage in diabetic patients with clinical signs of neuropathy[9] and impaired nerve conduction velocity.[10]

Since alrestatin, albeit at relatively high doses, showed clinical efficacy in the treatment of chronic complications of diabetes,[9,10] Ayerst Research Laboratories continued the search for another, more potent, orally-active AR inhibitor. Initial attempts were directed toward analogs of alrestatin, and a series were synthesized.[11] The thio analog *6*, upon oral administration, was about six times more potent than alrestatin in lowering galactitol levels in the lens and sciatic nerve of galactosemic rats.[11] Since the thio analog tends to undergo hydrolysis to alrestatin, it served only as a prototype for further molecular modifications. One type involved the deletion of the oxo function to generate thionaphthostyrilacetic acids.[12] Halogen derivatives of this system showed high activity both in vitro and in vivo, and were considerably more potent than the thio analog of alrestatin. Thus, the 6-bromothionaphthostyrilacetic acid derivative, *7*, inhibited AR by 79% at 1×10^{-7}M, and in vivo at an oral dose of 131 mg/kg, lowered nerve galactitol levels in the galactosemic rat by 80%.[12] However, compounds containing the naphthostyril nucleus were colored and produced staining of animal tissue.

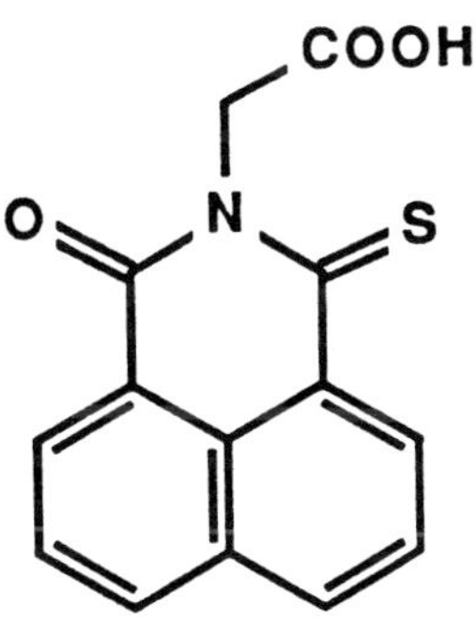

6

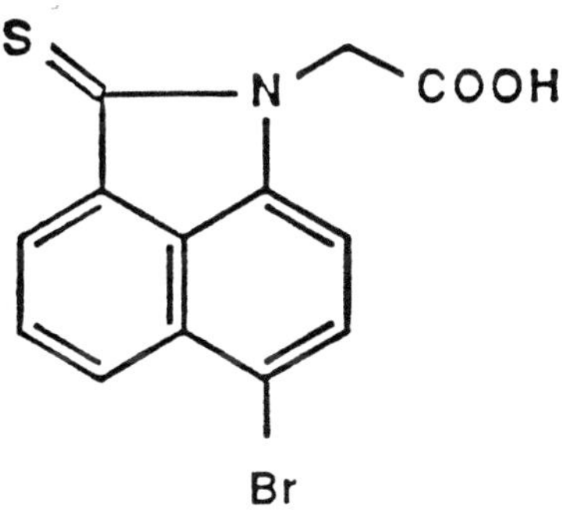

7

Further molecular modifications, were generated by cleaving the five-membered ring of the naphthostyril nucleus to afford a naphthoylglycine.[13–16] The unsubstituted naphthoylglycine had only moderate activity, however, after the investigation of numerous analogs, it was established that the N-methyl-5-trifluoromethyl-6-methoxy analog, *8*, tolrestat, was one of the most potent in this series. Tolrestat inhibited calf lens AR with an IC_{50} of 3.5×10^{-8}M, and on oral administration in the four-day galactosemic rat model[4] it decreased galactitol accumulation in the sciatic nerve with an ED_{50} of 7.3 mg/kg.[17] After extensive pharmacological and biochemical studies,[17–25] tolrestat was selected for clinical development.

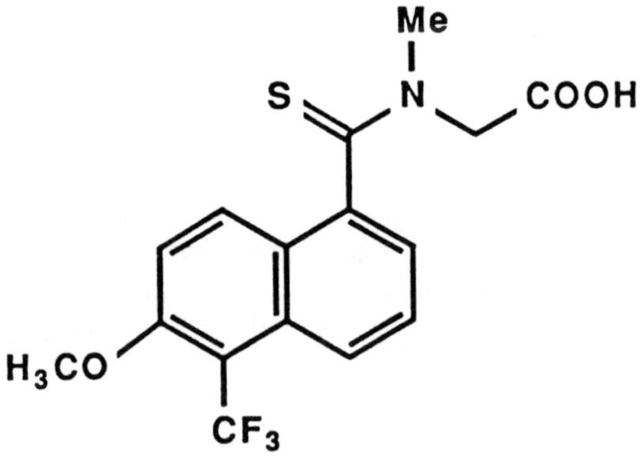

8

Although tolrestat is a highly crystalline compound, crystals suitable for crystallographic analysis could not be obtained. Suitable crystals, however, were obtained for the analog in which the trifluoromethyl group was replaced by a trifluoromethylthio group, giving a compound that was equipotent to tolrestat in vitro. Fig 1 shows a computer-generated projection of this compound derived from its crystallographic coordinates.[26] The energy-minimized conformation of tolrestat obtained by molecular mechanics calculations using the SIMPLEX algorithm is shown in Fig 2, while Fig 3 is a superpositioning of Figs 1 and 2. The conformations of the side chains on both molecules are virtually identical in the crystal and as obtained by minimization, and it is probable that the conformation seen in Fig 3, or a very similar low-energy conformation, may represent the conformations of these compounds at the receptor site.

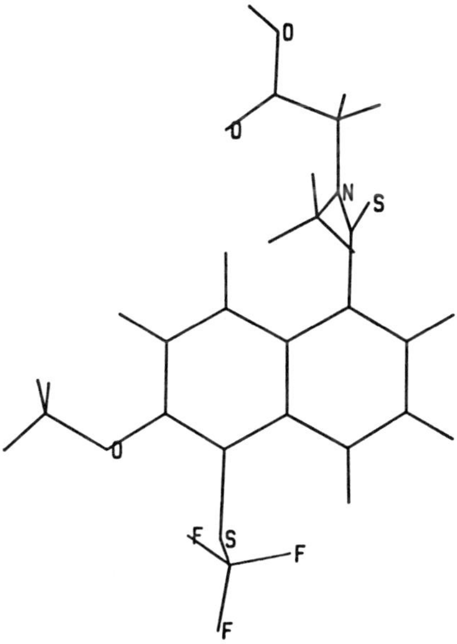

Figure 1. X-ray structure of trifluoromethylthio analog of tolrestat.

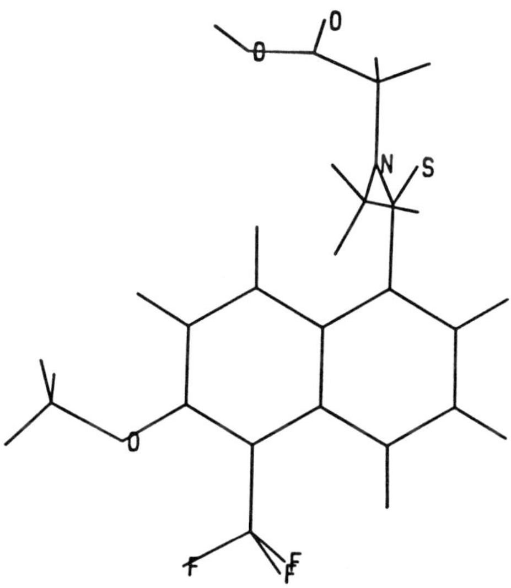

Figure 2. Energy-minimized computer generated conformation of tolrestat.

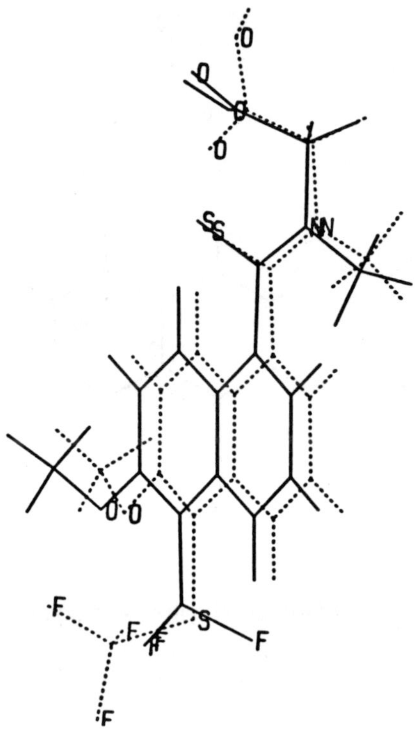

Figure 3. Superimposition of energy-minimized structure of tolrestat and X-ray structure of trifluoromethylthio analog of tolrestat.

SPIROHYDANTOINS AND RELATED STRUCTURES

AR inhibitors containing a spirohydantoin or related system have been studied by several groups. Sorbinil (CP-45,634; (S) (+)-6-fluoro-2,3-dihydrospiro [4H-1-benzopyran-4,4′-imidazolidine]-2′,5′-dione, *9*), was first disclosed in 1978[27] and is the best known member of this class and is being developed by Pfizer. Its absolute configuration was elucidated by x-ray crystallographic studies,[28,29] which show that in the crystal, the pyran ring of sorbinil adopts a pseudochair conformation (Fig 4) such that the N3′ nitrogen is attached pseudoequatorially. The alternative pseudochair, with the N3′ nitrogen pseudoaxially attached, was found, by molecular mechanics calculations, to be only 0.57 kcal/mol less stable than the solid-state conformation. Nuclear magnetic resonance (NMR) studies indicate the existence of both conformers in solution,[29] therefore these studies do not provide a basis for identifying the conformation that interacts with the enzyme.

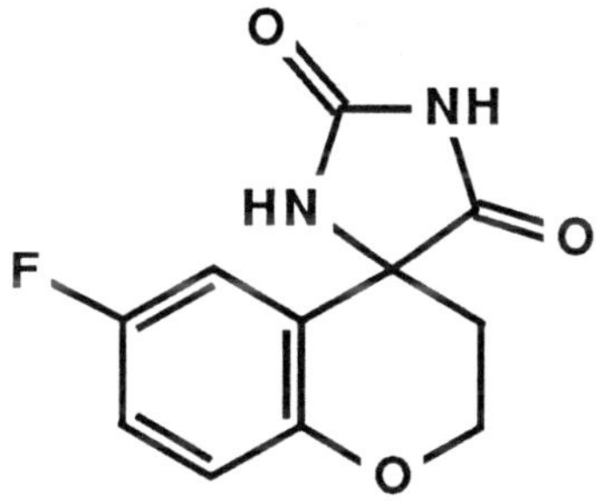

9

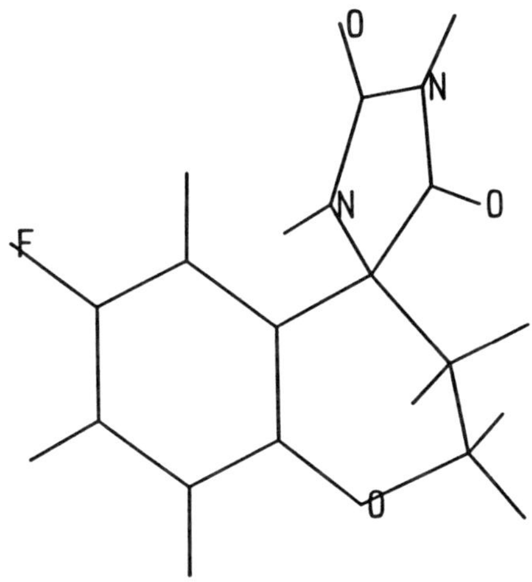

Figure 4. X-ray structure of sorbinil.

The effects of sorbinil, its enantiomer, and the racemic form on calf lens AR in vitro, and in vivo on sorbitol accumulation in the sciatic nerve of diabetic rats, are shown in Table 1. At 1×10^{-6}M, (−)-sorbinil was only marginally active (23%), while (+)-sorbinil caused 98% inhibition. A limited number of sorbinil analogs with different substitution patterns have been disclosed; they are shown in Table 1 together with their activities in vitro and in vivo.[30-33] The racemic 6,7-dichloro, 6,8-dichloro, and 6-chloro analogs (Nos. 5, 6 and 7) are more potent in vitro than racemic sorbinil (No. 1); this is also the case in vivo for the 6,8-dichloro and the 6-chloro analogs which inhibit sorbitol accumulation by 82 and 64%, compared with 45% for (±)-sorbinil, at an oral dose of 0.75 mg/kg in the streptozocin-induced diabetic rat. Bulky substituents at position-6 such as phenyl or phenoxy (Nos. 9 and 11) lead to compounds that are inactive in vivo while the 8-phenyl

Table 1. In vitro and in vivo AR inhibitory activities of 2,3-dihydro[4H]-1-benzopyran-4,4′-imidazolidine-2′,5′-diones.

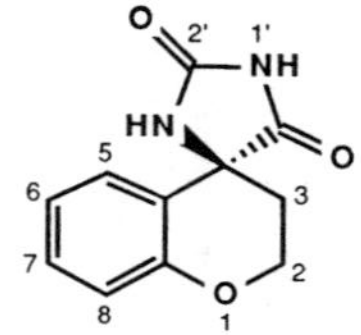

No.	Reference	Substitution	% Inhibition of AR (conc.)[a]			% Decrease of Sorbitol accumulation in vivo (dose. mg/kg[b])					
			10^{-5}M	10^{-6}M	10^{-7}M	0.25	0.75	1.5	2.5	5.0	10.0
1; (±)	27	6-F	58	52	3	19	45	72			
2; (+) (Sorbinil)	27	6-F	100	98	39	47	78				
3; (−)	27	6-F	63	23			19		6	22	
4	30	6–0Me	92	35	7				24		
5	30	6,7-Cl_2	96	91	84			64			
6	30	6,8-Cl_2	90	78	81		82				
7	30	6-Cl	81	77	64		64	84			
8	30	8-Cl	85	52	6			30			
9	31	6-C_6H_5	$IC_{50} < 1 \times 10^{-4}$M					0			
10	31	8-C_6H_5	$IC_{50}\,1 \times 10^{-6}$M								54
11	31	6-OC_5H_5	$IC_{50}\,1 \times 10^{-5}$M					0			
12	32	6-Cl, 8-NH_2		58[c]		17					
13	32	6-F, 8-NH_2		40[c]		40					
14 (Methosorbinil)	33	2-Me, 6-F	$IC_{50}\,6.5 \times 10^{-8}$M								

[a]A partially purified calf lens AR was used unless indicated otherwise.
[b]Rats were made diabetic with streptozocin and compounds were administered orally at 4, 8 and 24 hr following streptozocin administration. Sorbitol levels in the sciatic nerve were measured and compared to controls.
[c]Human placenta AR was used.

derivative (No. 10) retains moderate in vivo potency. An account of the development of sorbinil, and additional structure-activity relationships in that series, have recently appeared.[34] Methosorbinil (M-79,175), the 2-methyl analog of sorbinil (Table 1, No. 14), of unknown stereochemistry, was reported to have an IC_{50} of 6.5 $\times 10^{-8}$M using a rabbit lens AR.[33] Sorbinil, tested under the same conditions, had an IC_{50} of 1.1 $\times 10^{-7}$M.[33] Methosorbinil was also reported to markedly reduce sorbitol levels in the lens of streptozocin-induced diabetic rats upon oral administration of doses of 0.1 to 1.0 mg/kg.[35] Methosorbinil is reported to be in development by Eisai.

The 2,3-dihydro[4H]-1-benzopyran nucleus of sorbinil has been replaced by a wide variety of other rings; the most potent representatives are shown in Table 2 with reported AR inhibitory activities in vitro and in vivo. Of 15 systems reported, four representatives had IC_{50}'s of 1 $\times 10^{-7}$M or less: the thiochroman, No. 3; the spiroindolinone, No. 14; and the fluorenone derivatives, No. 15 (alconil, AL-1567) and No. 16 (AL-1576). AR inhibitory activities of 20 analogs of alconil were recently reported.[44] Alconil and AL-1576 have been extensively studied in vivo; on oral administration they reduced sciatic nerve sorbitol levels in the streptozocin-induced diabetic rat and prevented cataract formation.[45]

The spirohydantoin moiety, in turn, can be replaced by other systems containing an acidic hydrogen; representative examples with their AR inhibitory activities are collected in Table 3. The spiro-oxazolidinedione, No. 1,[46] had an IC_{50} of 1 $\times 10^{-7}$M (calf lens AR), while the spiro-thiazolidinedione, No. 2,[47] was more potent, with an IC_{50} of 8 $\times 10^{-9}$M. In vivo data have been reported for the spirosuccinimide No. 3.[48]

Five-membered heterocycles that contain an acidic hydrogen but which are not spiro-fused were also investigated. The phenylsulfonylhydantoin No. 4 was the best of 54 analogs tested.[49] It reduced galactitol accumulation in the galactosemic rat model at oral doses 50 mg/kg, and decreased cataract formation in rats at the same dose.[53] In a series of phenyl-substituted thiazolidinediones, No. 5 was the most effective, inhibiting sorbitol accumulation in sciatic nerve by 83% at a dose of 25 mg/kg.[50] The 3-ethoxy-4-pentyloxy-thiazolidinedione No. 6[51] (CT-112) was reported to be in development by the Takeda Company. In vitro, CT-112 inhibited human placental AR by 35% at 1 $\times 10^{-6}$M. The spiro-[pyrrolidine-3,1′[4H]-pyrrolo[3,2,1-ij]quinoline]2,2′,5(1′H)trione, No. 7, had an IC_{50} of 4 $\times 10^{-7}$M for inhibition of rat lens AR.[52] After oral administration to rats at 25 mg/kg, blood was taken and 0.5 mL of serum was added to the in vitro incubation mixture containing rat lens AR; after five hours, AR was inhibited by 68.5%.[52] No. 7, phenytoin and sorbinil were evaluated for inhibition of pentylenetetrazol-induced convulsions in mice; the results (see Fig 5) show that, in contrast to phenytoin and sorbinil, No. 7 is devoid of anticonvulsant activity.[52]

No. 8 (ADN-138), a 1,4-benzoxazine analog of No. 7, had an IC_{50} of 6 $\times 10^{-7}$M for inhibition of rat lens AR[52]; it was shown to reduce sorbitol levels in the nerve, and to increase impaired motor nerve conduction velocity in streptozocin-induced diabetic rats at oral doses of 5 mg/kg/day and 20 mg/kg/day for three weeks.[54] ADN-138 is reported to be in development by the Kyorin Pharmaceutical Co.

Table 2. In vitro and in vivo AR inhibitory activities of miscellaneous spiro-imidazolidine-2′, 5′-diones.

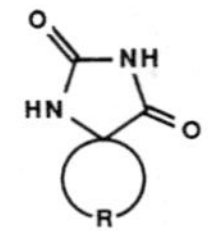

No.	Reference	R	% Inhibition of A.R. (Conc)[a]	% Inhibition of sorbitol accumulation in vivo (dose)[b]
1.	30	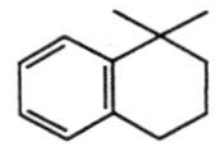	34% (1×10^{-5}M)	3% (5 mg/kg)
2.	30	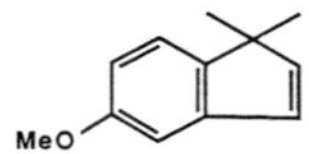	81% (1×10^{-5}M)	33% (5 mg/kg)
3.	27	(+) 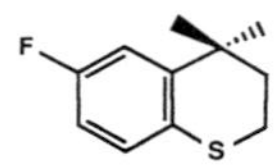	74% (1×10^{-7}M)	55% (0.75 mg/kg)
4.	36	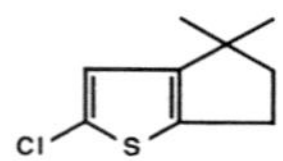	55% (1×10^{-5}M)	20% (2.5 mg/kg)
5.	36	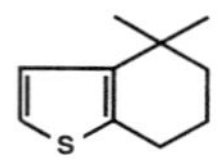	52% (1×10^{-4}M)	56% (25 mg/kg)

6.	37	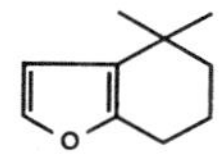	50% (1×10^{-4}M)	46% (25 mg/kg)
7.	38	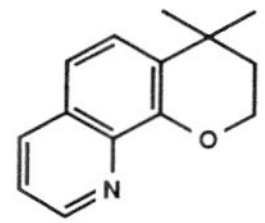	75% (1×10^{-4}M)	27% (1.5 mg/kg)
8.	38	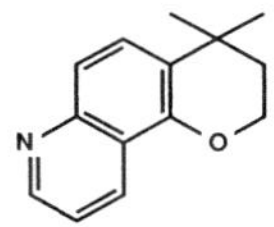	94% (1×10^{-4}M)	92% (10 mg/kg)
9.	39	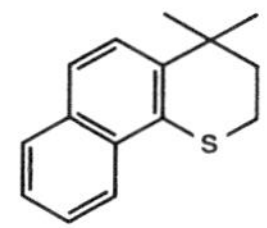	100% (1×10^{-4}M)	32% (1.5 mg/kg)
10	39	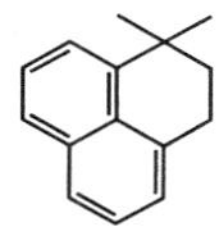	71% (1×10^{-4}M)	28% (5 mg/kg)
11.	39	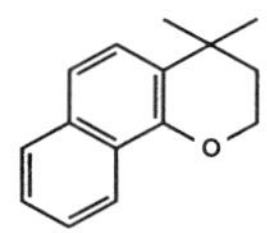	72% (1×10^{-4}M)	30% (1.5 mg/kg)

[a]A calf lens AR was used unless otherwise indicated.
[b]See footnote b, Table 1, for details.
[c]Rat lens AR.

Table 2. (continued)

No.	Reference	R	% Inhibition of A.R. (Conc)[a]	% Inhibition of sorbitol accumulation in vivo (dose)[b]
12.	40	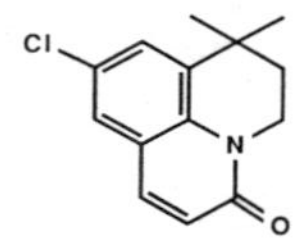	94% (1×10^{-6}M)	32% (1.5 mg/kg)
13.	41	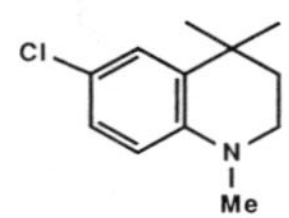	IC_{50}: 1×10^{-6}M	80% (10 mg/kg)
14.	42	(+) 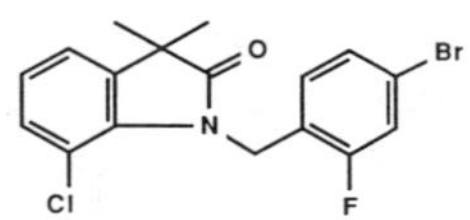	IC_{50}: 9.8×10^{-9}M	ED_{50}: 0.62 mg/kg
15. (Alconil)	43	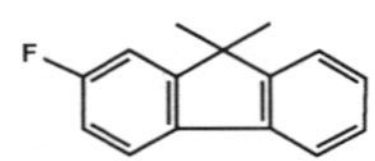 (AL-1567)	IC_{50}: 4.3×10^{-8}M[c]	—
16.	43	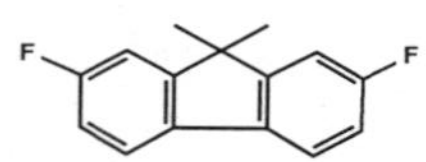 (AL-1576)	IC_{50}: 2.4×10^{-8}M[c]	—

[a]A calf lens AR was used unless otherwise indicated. [b]See footnote b, Table 1, for details. [c]Rat lens AR.

Table 3. AR inhibitors containing acidic heterocycle other than a spirohydantoin.

No.	Reference	Structure	% Inhib. of AR[a] (Conc.)	% Decrease of sorbitol accumulation in vivo[b] (dosage)
1.	46	(−) 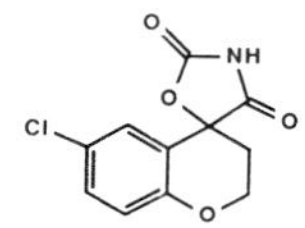	Ic_{50}: 1×10^{-7}M	ED_{50}: 1.5-2.5 mg/kg
2.	47	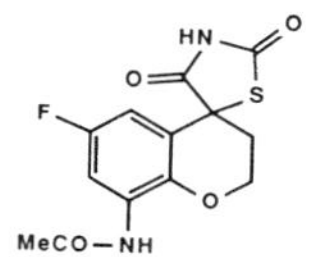	IC_{50}: 8×10^{-9}M	—
3.	48	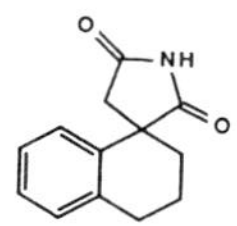	—	46% (5 mg/kg)
4.	49	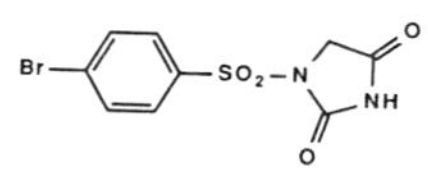	IC_{50}: 3.7×10^{-7}M	—

[a]Partially purified calf lens AR was used except where indicated.
[b]See footnote b, Table 1 for details.
[c]Human placenta AR.
[d]Rat lens AR.

Table 3. (continued)

No.	Reference	Structure	% Inhib. of AR[a] (Conc.)	% Decrease of sorbitol accumulation in vivo[b] (dosage)
5.	50	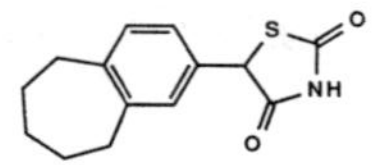	34% (1×10^{-6}M)[c]	83% (25 mg/kg)
6. (CT-112)	51	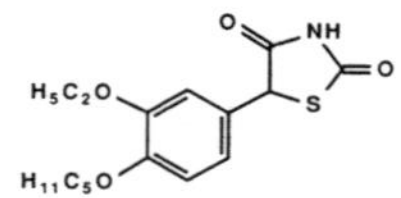	35% (1×10^{-6}M)[c]	—
7.	52	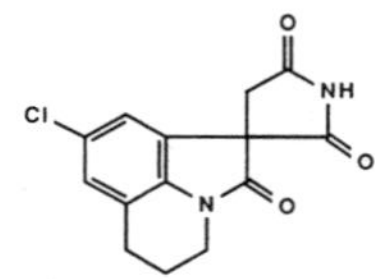	IC_{50}: 4×10^{-7}M[d]	—
8. (ADN-138)	52	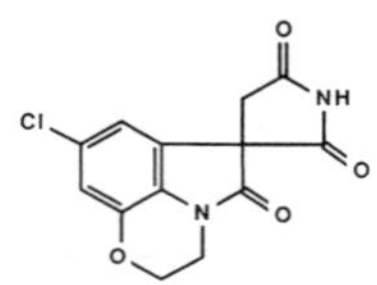	IC_{50}: 6×10^{-7}M[d]	

[a]Partially purified calf lens AR was used except where indicated.
[b]See footnote b, Table 1 for details.
[c]Human placenta AR.
[d]Rat lens AR.

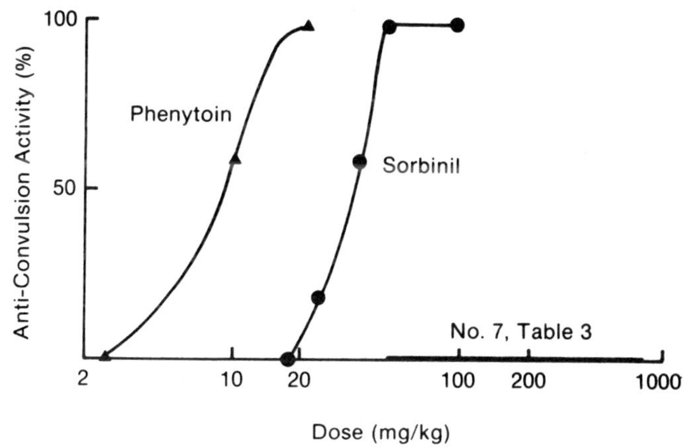

Figure 5. Anticonvulsant activities of phenytoin, sorbinil and No. 7, Table 3. (Reproduced from reference 52).

HETEROCYCLIC ALKANOIC ACIDS

Several potent AR inhibitors have been developed which, structurally, are heterocyclic alkanoic acids. Of a large series of rhodanine derivatives,[55,56] (E)-3-carboxymethyl-5-[(2E)-methyl-3-phenylpropenylidene]rhodanine (ONO-2235), *10*, epalrestat, has been selected for clinical development. Epalrestat has an IC_{50} of 1×10^{-8}M with AR from rat lens and an IC_{50} of 2.6×10^{-6}M with human placental AR.[57]

The quinolineacetic acid *11* (ICI-105,552)[58] and the phthalazinoneacetic acid *12* (statil; ICI-128,436)[59] have been studied in laboratory animals. In vitro, at 5×10^{-5}M, ICI-105,552 prevented sorbitol accumulation in monkey kidney epithelial

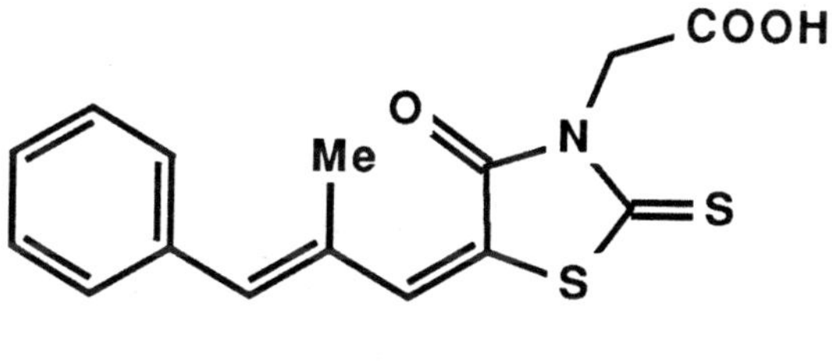

10

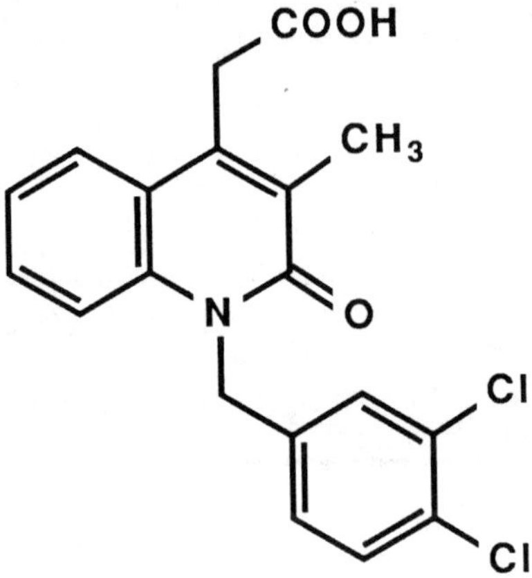

11

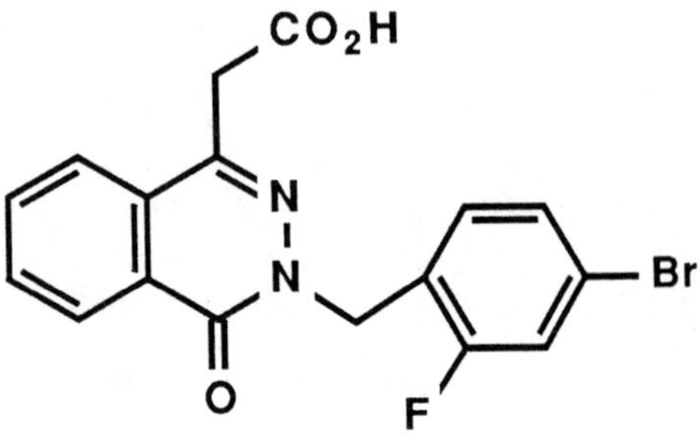

12

cells cultured in a glucose-containing medium[60]; in vivo, it caused an 86% reduction of sorbitol levels in the sciatic nerve of streptozocin-induced diabetic rats upon oral administration of 50 mg/kg/day.[58] Statil inhibited human lens AR with an IC_{50} of 2×10^{-8}M,[61] and on treatment of streptozocin-induced diabetic rats for three weeks at oral doses of 25 mg/kg/day, elevated sciatic nerve sorbitol levels were reduced to levels found in non-diabetic controls.[62] A review of structure-activity relationships in compounds related to *11* and *12* was recently presented.[63]

The furanone propionic acid, *13* (FR-51785), isolated from cultures of *Chaetomella raphigera*, inhibited rabbit lens AR with an IC_{50} of 1.6×10^{-7}M.[64] A number of synthetic analogs of FR-51785 were investigated, the most potent being the 3,4-dichlorophenyl analog with an IC_{50} of 3.1×10^{-7}M and which was active in vivo, inhibiting sorbitol accumulation in the streptozocin-induced diabetic rat by 41% at 10 mg/kg, orally.[65]

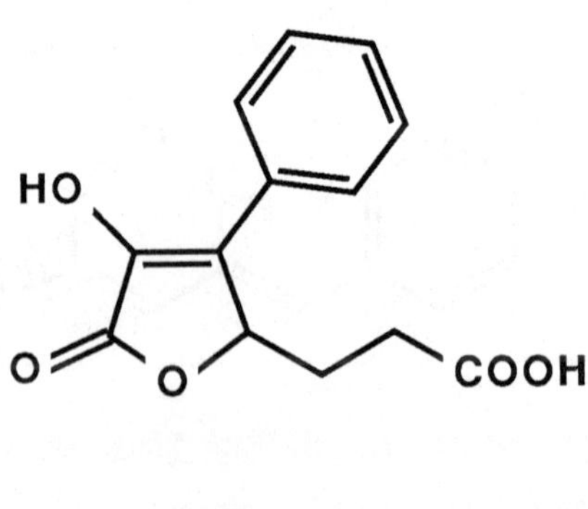

13

A group of seven coumarin-4-acetic acid derivatives were tested[66] at 1×10^{-4}M against calf lens AR and found to be active (65% to 100% inhibition). Compound *14* inhibited the enzyme by 81% at 1×10^{-4}M, and caused a 21% inhibition of sciatic nerve sorbitol accumulation in the streptozocin-induced diabetic rat upon oral administration of 25 mg/kg given three times daily. The same group studied a series of benzopyran- and benzothiopyran-carboxylic acids[67]; compound *15* was found to inhibit AR by 80% at 1×10^{-4}M and to block sorbitol accumulation by 28% using the same model and dosage schedule.

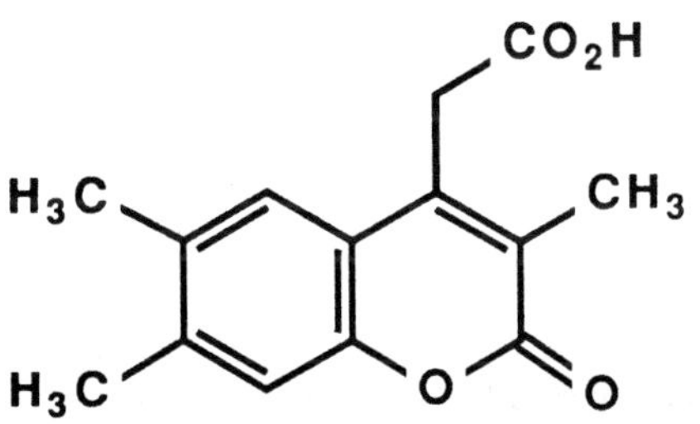

14

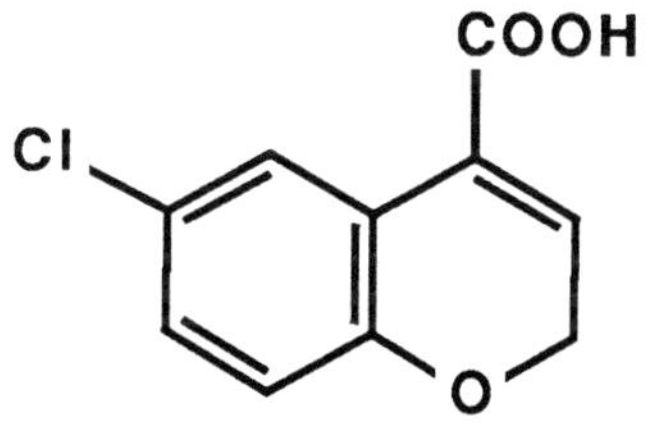

15

MISCELLANEOUS AR INHIBITORS

In vivo-active AR inhibitors have been uncovered in various other chemical classes. Several hundreds of naturally occurring flavonoids have been studied and many are active in vitro (see Reference 2 for a review), but only quercitrin, which inhibited rat lens AR by 55% at 1×10^{-7}M[68] was tested orally.

Administration of quercitrin, *16*, in the diet, to the streptozocin-induced diabetic degu (*Octodon degus*), decreased lens sorbitol accumulation by 50% and delayed the onset of cataracts.[69] The degu, a rodent native to the South American Andes, was selected for the study because its lens AR activity is three to four times higher than the rats, and as a consequence it develops lens opacities within ten to 12 days, rather than in the three to four months required for the rat after induction of diabetes. Based on an estimated food intake of 10 g/day, the total administered dose of quercitrin was between 3.2 and 3.5 g/kg/day. This high oral dose of quercitrin required to elicit an effect in vivo, compared with its high in vitro potency as an AR inhibitor, reflects the poor systemic availability of orally administered quercitrin.

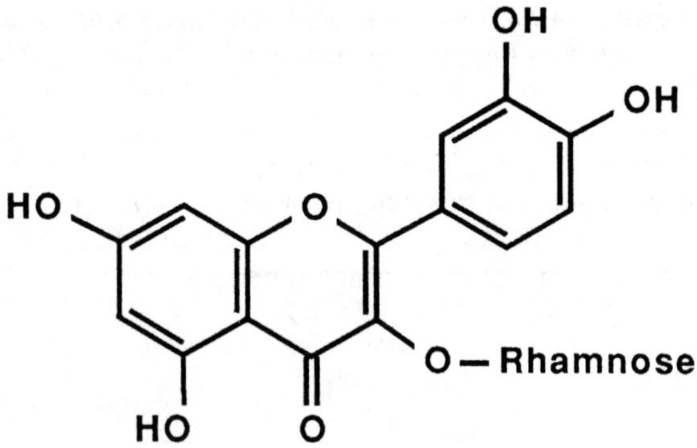

16

A series of synthetic flavones has been described[70] of which 7-methylsulfonamido-3-propylflavone-4-carboxylic acid, *17*, was the most potent, having an IC_{50} of 1.3×10^{-7}M with calf lens AR. At 100 mg/kg/day for two days in the streptozocin-induced diabetic rat, *17* lowered sorbitol levels in the sciatic nerve by 57%, and inositol levels by 28%. The route of administration was not specified. The same group have prepared the 3-methanesulfonyl derivative of quercetin, *18*, and found it to inhibit calf lens AR with an IC_{50} of 1.6×10^{-7}M, and in the same in vivo rat model used above,[70] to lower sorbitol levels in the sciatic nerve by 41% at a dose of 100 mg/kg, again by an unspecified route of administration.[71]

Compound *19* (70-A-196), 2,2′,4,4′-tetrahydroxybenzophenone, inhibited rat lens AR with an IC_{50} of 1×10^{-7}M; in streptozocin-induced diabetic rats given a 35% xylose diet, it also inhibited cataract formation upon oral administration.[72]

A series of 29 substituted xanthone-2-carboxylic acids, which had been prepared as anti-allergy agents, were studied as AR inhibitors by Pfister et al.[73] The dimethylaminosulfamoyl derivative *20*, a water insoluble compound, inhibited rabbit lens AR by 67% at 1×10^{-6}M and was reported to be active both topically and orally in delaying the appearance of cataracts in rats receiving a diet containing 35% galactose.

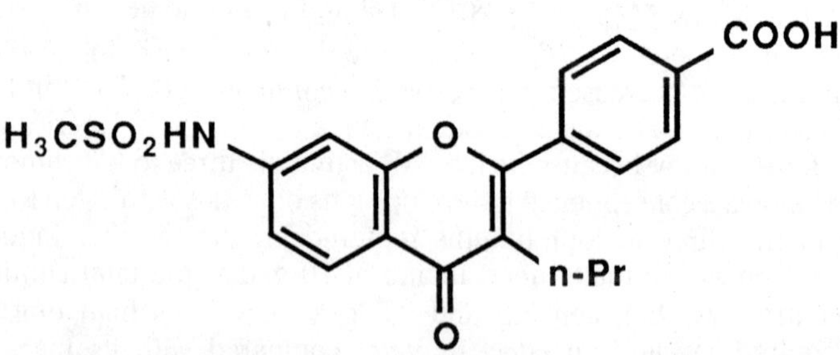

17

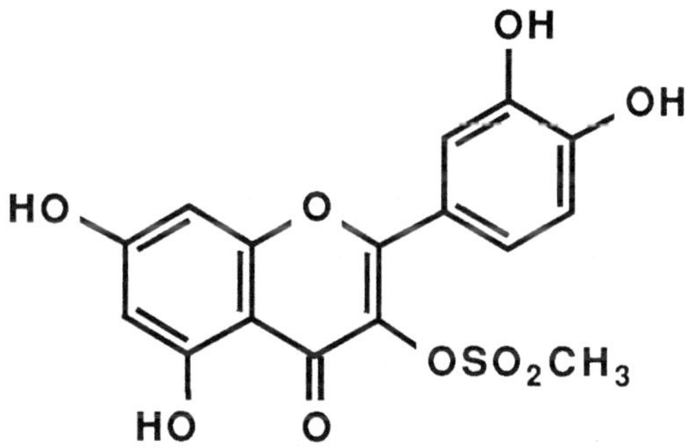

18

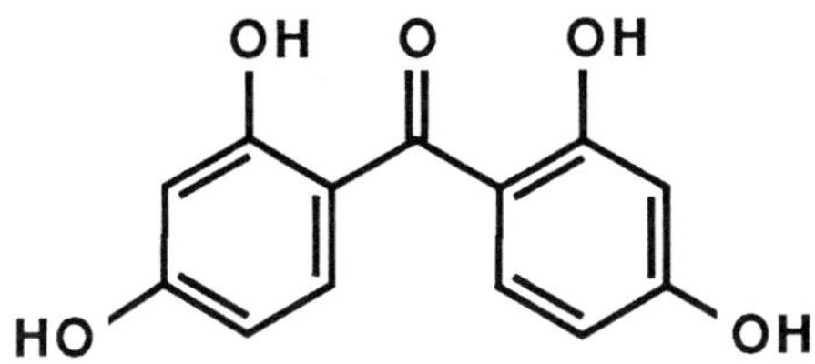

19

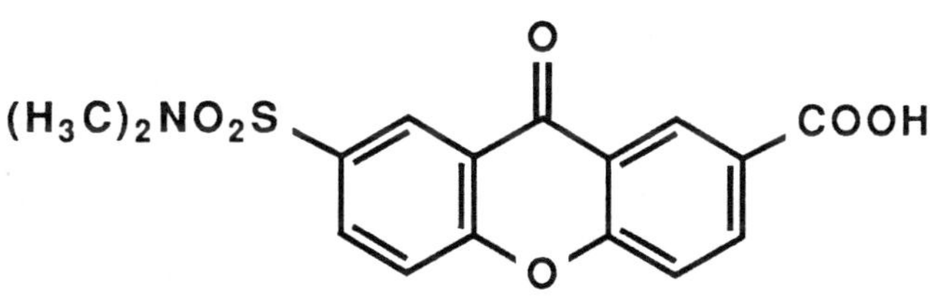

20

The pyrroloquinolinedione *21* (AHR-5191) had an IC_{50} of 8×10^{-5}M with calf lens AR and caused a 43% decrease in rat lens galactitol levels when orally administered at 100 mg/kg/day for three days.[74]

The nonsteroidal anti-inflammatory agent sulindac was found to inhibit calf lens AR with an IC_{50} of 1×10^{-7}M,[75] and human lens AR with an IC_{50} of 4×10^{-7}M.[76] In the four-day galactosemic rat model described by Simard-Duquesne et al,[18] sulindac was weakly active, preventing galactitol accumulation in the lens and the

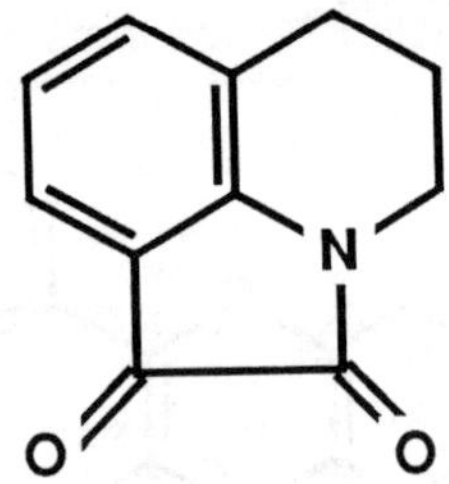

21

sciatic nerve at 62 mg/kg/day, the highest dose tested. Many other drugs of this class have been tested and found to be inactive or only marginally active as inhibitors of AR in vitro.[2]

A MODEL OF THE AR INHIBITOR SITE

Numerous studies on the kinetics of AR inhibition by several inhibitors show that they do not compete for the substrate binding site on the enzyme (see Reference 2 for a review); other studies show that they do not compete for the nucleotide cofactor binding site.[77,78]

Kador and Sharpless[78] have suggested that a wide range of AR inhibitors bind at a common inhibitor site on the enzyme. Based on this, plus observed correlation between their lowest empty molecular orbitals (LEMO) and inhibitory potencies, and the identification of a polarizable carbonyl group in each of the inhibitors, these investigators have proposed a model for the superpositioning of these inhibitors in which the polarizable carbonyl groups lie in a common region. This led further to a proposal of a model of the inhibitor binding site which comprises planar lipophilic regions, hydrogen bonding sites, and a sterically constrained charge-transfer pocket. They have also presented evidence supporting the presence of a tyrosine residue in close proximity to the inhibitor binding site, and the hydroxyl group of the tyrosine is presumed to be the nucleophile which reversibly participates in an interaction with a polarizable carbonyl group of the inhibitors. Kador and Sharpless[78] believe they have described the minimal structural features required for AR inhibition and have suggested that their proposal may permit the rational design of more potent and specific inhibitors of AR. But while such a model can be of value, it should be pointed out that of the AR inhibitors which are currently being studied clinically (see Table 4), only the spirohydantoin type has been considered in the development of the model.[78] If the compounds in Table 4 should indeed act at the same site on the enzyme, incorporation of features derived from an analysis of the structures of all of these compounds could generate a modified model of the AR inhibitory site which may be of even greater value. At this writing, one series of compounds, 2-(arylamino)-4(3H)-quinazolinones, have been designed as AR inhibitors based exclusively on requirements of the model, however, in vitro results were disappointing.[79]

Table 4. AR inhibitors undergoing clinical trials.

Structure	Name	Company
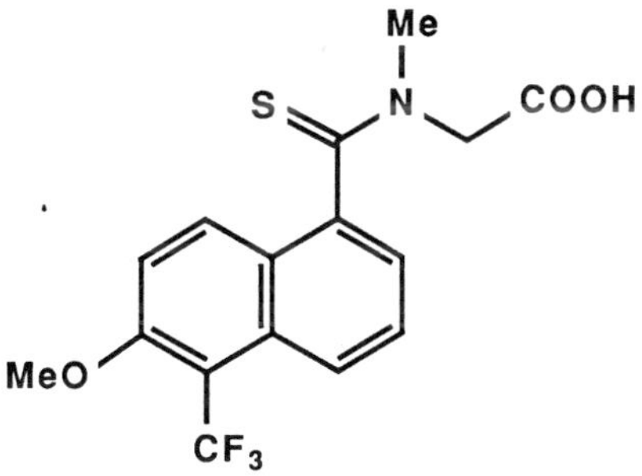	AY-27,773 Tolrestat Alredase	Ayerst
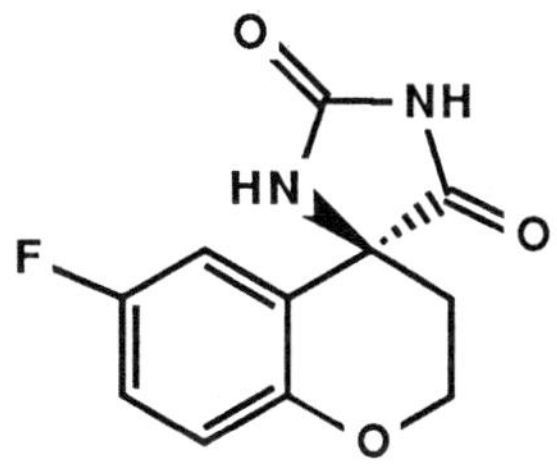	CP-45,634 Sorbinil	Pfizer
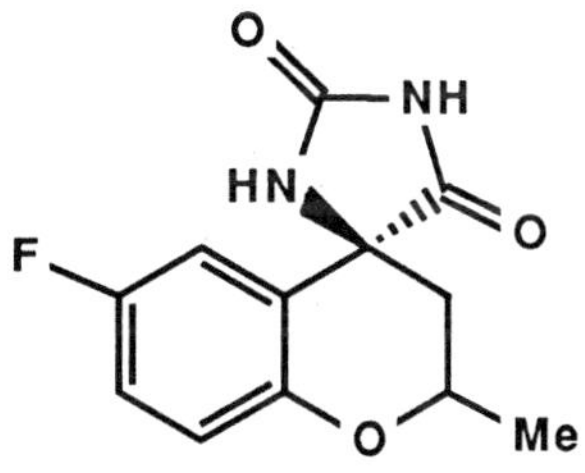	M-79,175 Methosorbinil	Eisai
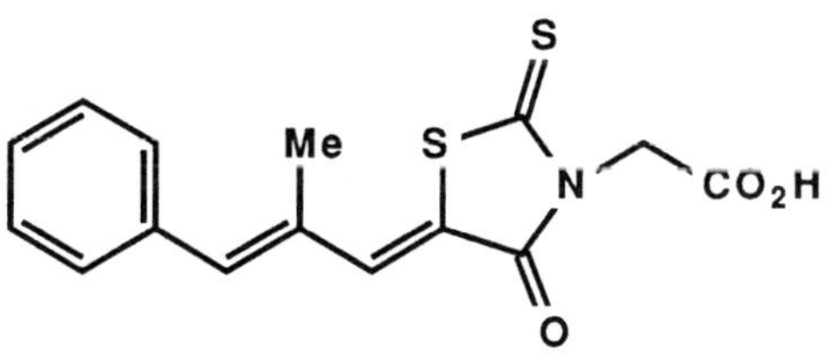	ONO-2235 Epalrestat	Ono

Table 4. AR inhibitors undergoing clinical trials.

Structure	Compound	Company
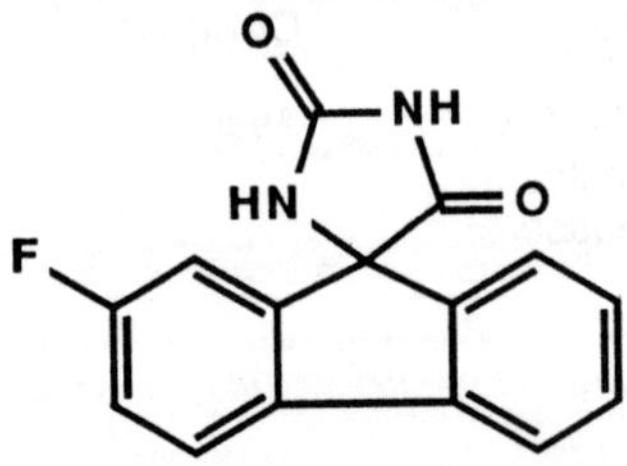	AL-1567 Alconil	Alcon
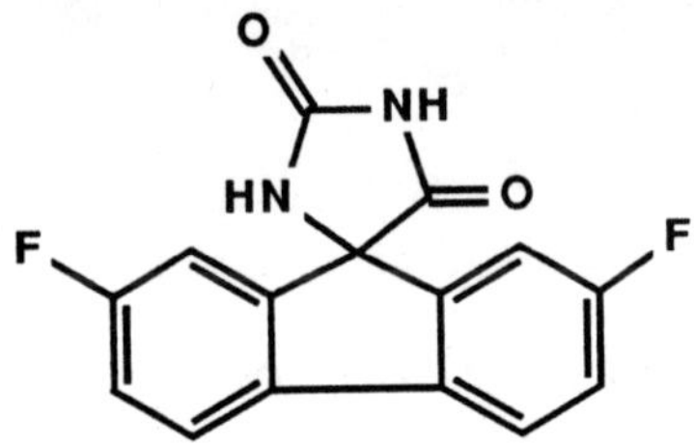	AL-1576	Alcon
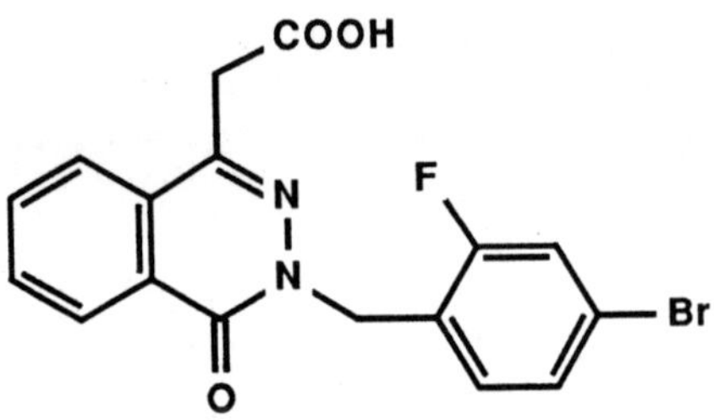	ICI-128,436	I.C.I.
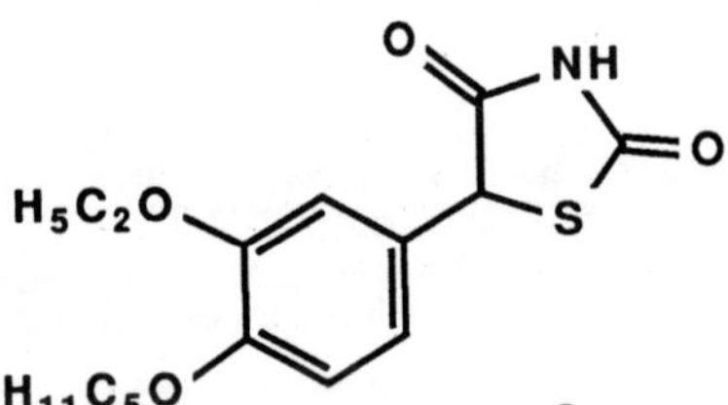	CT-112	Takeda
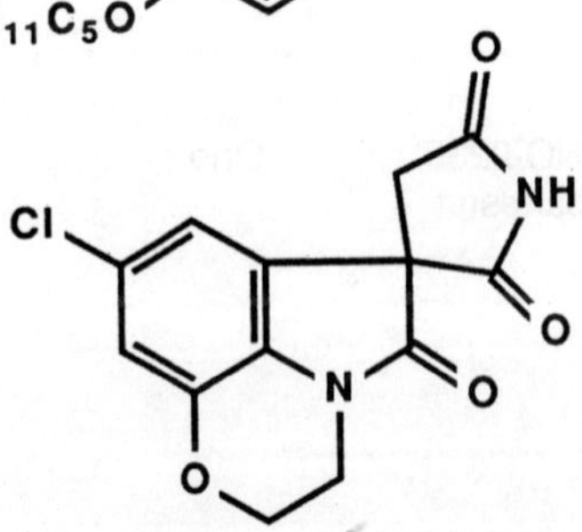	ADN-138	Kyorin

SUMMARY

Since the partial purification of AR in 1965[1] and the elaboration of a role for this enzyme in the pathogenesis of some of the complications of chronic diabetes, thousands of compounds, both natural products and synthetic molecules, have been tested as AR inhibitors in various laboratories. Many compounds have been found to be active in vitro, and it appears that in vitro AR inhibitory activity can be readily found.[2] High in vitro activity is, however, not the only prerequisite for oral activity in vivo. Not only must the drug be absorbed, but it must also reach sufficiently high levels in the target organ or tissue to effectively inhibit AR. Clearly, the structural and physicochemical requirements for effective in vivo inhibition of AR at the desired sites are unique and are met by relatively few compounds. The discovery of clinically useful AR inhibitors has depended less on the finding of high in vitro activity than on the identification of compounds with suitable pharmacokinetics and tissue distribution patterns.

References

1. Hayman S, Kinoshita JH: Isolation and properties of lens aldose reductase. *J Biol Chem* 1965;240:877–882.
2. Humber L: The medicinal chemistry of aldose reductase inhibitors. Ellis GP, West GB (eds): *Progress in Medicinal Chemistry*. Amsterdam, Elsevier, 1987;24:299–343.
3. Kinoshita JH, Dvornik D, Kraml M, Gabbay KH: The effect of an aldose reductase inhibitor on the galactose-exposed rabbit lens. *Biochim Biophys Acta* 1968; 158:472–475.
4. Dvornik D, Simard-Duquesne N, Kraml M, et al: Polyol accumulation in galactosemic and diabetic rats: Control by an aldose reductase inhibitor. *Science* 1973;182: 1146–1148.
5. Hutton JC, Schofield PJ, Williams JF, Hollows FC: The failure of aldose reductase inhibitor 3,3′-tetramethyleneglutaric acid to inhibit in vivo sorbitol accumulation in lens and retina in diabetes. *Biochem Pharmacol* 1974;23:2991–2998.
6. Kinoshita JH: Mechanisms initiating cataract formation. *Invest Ophthalmol* 1974;13:713–724.
7. Stephen H: A new synthesis of phthalimidoacetonitriles and a note on aminoacetonitrile sulphates. *J Chem Soc* 1931;871–875.
8. Sestanj K, Simard-Duquesne N, Dvornik D: Compositions for and a method of treating diabetic complications. United States Patent 3,821,383; published on June 28, 1974.
9. Fagius J, Jameson S: Effects of aldose reductase inhibitor treatment in diabetic polyneuropathy—a clinical and neurophysiological study. *J Neurol Neurosurg Psychiatry* 1981;44:991–1001.
10. Culebras A, Alio J, Herrera JL, Lopez-Fraile IP: Effect of an aldose reductase inhibitor on diabetic peripheral neuropathy. *Arch Neurol* 1981;38:133–134.
11. Sestanj K: Thioxo-1H-benz[de]isoquinoline-2(3H)-acetic acid derivatives and antidiabetic use thereof. United States Patent 4,254,108; published on March 3, 1981.
12. Sestanj K: 2-Thioxobenz[cd]indole-1(2H)-acetic acid derivatives. United States Patent 4,369,188; published on January 18, 1983.

13. Sestanj K, Abraham NA, Bellini F, Treasurywala A: N-Naphthalenylthioxomethyl-aminoacid derivatives. United States Patent 4,391,816; published on July 5, 1983.
14. Bellini F, Sestanj K, Humber LG: N-[[6-(Lower alkoxy)-5-(trifluoromethylthio)-1-naphthalenyl]thioxomethyl]-N-(lower alkyl)glycines. United States Patent 4,391,825; published on July 5, 1983.
15. Sestanj K, Abraham NA, Bellini F, Treasurywala A: N-Naphthoylglycine derivatives. United States Patent 4,439,617; published on March 27, 1984.
16. Sestanj K, Abraham NA, Bellini F, Treasurywala A: N-naphthoylglycine derivatives. United States Patent 4,568,693; published on February 4, 1986.
17. Sestanj K, Bellini F, Fung S, et al: N-[[5-(trifluoromethyl)-6-methoxy-1-naphthaleny]-thioxomethyl]-N-methylglycine (Tolrestat), a potent, orally active aldose reductase inhibitor. *J Med Chem* 1984;27:255–256.
18. Simard-Duquesne N, Greselin E, Gonzalez R, Dvornik D: Prevention of cataract development in severely galactosemic rats by the aldose reductase inhibitor, tolrestat. *Proc Soc Exp Biol Med,* 1985;178:599–605.
19. Dvornik D, Simard-Duquesne N, Greselin E, et al: AY-27,773: A novel orally active inhibitor of aldose reductase. *Diabetes* 1983;32(suppl 1):164A.
20. Robison WG Jr, Kador PF, Akagi Y, Kinoshita JH: Basement membrane thickening in ocular vessels of galactosemic rats prevented with aldose reductase inhibitors. *Invest Ophthalmol Vis Sci* 1984;25(suppl 2):66.
21. Hicks DR, Kraml M, Cayen MN, et al: Tolrestat kinetics. *Clin Pharmacol Ther* 1984; 36:493–499.
22. Cayen MN, Hicks DR, Ferdinandi ES, et al: Metabolic disposition and pharmacokinetics of the aldose reductase inhibitor tolrestat in rats, dogs, and monkeys. *Fed Proc* 1984;43:750.
23. Simard-Duquesne N, Greselin E, Dubuc J, Dvornik D: The effects of a new aldose reductase inhibitor (Tolrestat) in galactosemic and diabetic rats. *Metabolism* 1985;34: 885.
24. Kemper C, Huslin L, Dvornik D: The effect of the aldose reductase inhibitor tolrestat on the nerve polyol levels of streptozotocin diabetic rats. *Fed Proc* 1985;44:1392.
25. Robison WG, Kador PF, Akagi Y, et al: Prevention of basement membrane thickening in retinal capillaries by a novel inhibitor of aldose reductase, tolrestat. *Diabetes* 1986;35:295–299.
26. Varughese KI, Przybylska M, Sestanj K, Bellini F, Humber LG: The crystal structure of N-[[6-methoxy-5-(trifluoromethyl)thio-1-naphthalenyl]thioxomethyl]-N-methyglycine, $C_{16}\ H_{14}\ F_3\ NO_3\ S_2$. *Can J Chem* 1983;61:2137–2140.
27. Sarges R: Hydantoin therapeutic agents. United States Patent 4,130,714; published on December 19, 1978.
28. Kissinger CR, Adman ET, Clark JI, Stenkamp RE: Crystal structure of sorbinil, $C_{11}\ H_9\ FN_2\ O_3$, *Acta Cryst* 1985;41: 988–990.
29. Sarges R, Bordner J, Dominy BW, Peterson MJ, Whipple EB: Synthesis, absolute configuration, and conformation of the aldose reductase inhibitor sorbinil. *J Med Chem* 1985;28:1716–1720.
30. Sarges R: Hydantoin derivatives as therapeutic agents. United States Patent 4,117,230; published on September 26, 1978.
31. Sarges R: Phenyl or phenoxy substituted spiro-imidazolidinedione derivatives. United States Patent 4,181,729: published on January 1, 1980.
32. Sarges R, Schnur RC: Treating diabetes-associated complications with hydantoin amines. United States Patent, 4,248,882; published on February 3, 1981.

33. Nakai N, Fujii Y, Kobashi K, Nomura K: Aldose reductase inhibitors: flavonoids, alkaloids, acetophenones, benzophenones, and spirohydantoins of chroman. *Arch Biochem Biophys* 1985;239:491–496.
34. Sarges R, Peterson MJ: Sorbinil: A member of the novel class of spirohydantoin aldose reductase inhibitors. *Metabolism* 1986;35(suppl 1):101–104.
35. Ono H, Nozawa Y, Hayano S: Effects of M79175, an aldose reductase inhibitor, on experimental sugar cataracts. *Nippon Ganka Gakkai Zasshi (Acta Soc Ophthalmol Jpn)* 1982;86:1343–1350.
36. Sarges R, Schnur RC: Thienohydantoin derivatives. United States Patent 4,127,665; published on November 28, 1978.
37. Kelbaugh PR, Sarges R: Spiro-furanohydantoin derivatives. United States Patent 4,147,797; published on April 3, 1979.
38. Schnur RC: Spiro-quinolylhydantoins. United States Patent 4,176,185; published on November 27, 1979.
39. Sarges R, Belletire JL: Spiro-polycyclicimidazolidinedione derivatives. United States Patent 4,181,728; published on January 1, 1980.
40. Schnur RC: Spiro-quinolone hydantoins. United States Patent 4,193,996; published on March 18, 1980.
41. Sarges R: Hydantoin derivatives, anti-diabetic compositions thereof, and method of use thereof. United States Patent 4,273,775: published on June 16, 1981.
42. Brittain, DR, Wood R: Indoline derivatives. European Patent 125,090; published on November 14, 1984.
43. Griffin BW, Chandler ML, Desantis L: Prevention of diabetic cataract and neuropathy in rats by two new aldose reductase inhibitors. *Invest Ophthalmol Vis Sci* 1984;25(suppl 2):136.
44. York B: Treatment of diabetic complications with certain spiro-imidazolidine-diones. United States Patent 4,540,700; published on September 10, 1985.
45. Griffin BW, Chandler ML, Desantis L: Prevention of diabetic cataract and neuropathy in rats by two aldose reductase inhibitors. *Invest Ophthalmol Vis Sci* 1984;25(suppl 2):159.
46. Schnur RC, Sarges R, Peterson MJ: Spirooxazolidinedione aldose reductase inhibitors. *J Med Chem* 1982;25:1451–1454.
47. Hegler H, Schneider F, Lederer F: Thiazolidine derivatives, their preparation, intermediates and pharmaceutical compositions. European Patent 129,747; published on January 2, 1985.
48. Belletire JL, Sarges R: Method for lowering sorbitol levels using spiro-imides. United States Patent 4,307,108; published on December 22, 1981.
49. Inagaki K, Miwa I, Yashiro T, Okuda J: Inhibition of aldose reductase from rat and bovine lenses by hydantoin derivatives. *Chem Pharm Bull* 1982;30:3244–3254.
50. Kawamatsu Y, Fugita T, Yamamoto Y: Thiazolidine derivatives and production thereof. United States Patent 4,486,594; published on December 4, 1984.
51. Sohda T, Mizuno K, Imamiya E, et al: Studies on antidiabetic agents. III. 5-arylthiazolidine-2,4-diones as potent aldose reductase inhibitors. *Chem Pharm Bull* 1982;30:3601–3616.
52. Irikura T, Takagi K, Fujimori S, Hirata Y: Novel class of spiro-linked pyrrolidine-2,5-diones and preparation thereof. European Patent 147,805; published on July 10, 1985.
53. Okuda J, Yashima K, Inagaki K, Miwa I: Effects of an aldose reductase inhibitor, 1-[(p-bromophenyl)-sulfonyl]hydantoin, on cataract formation and tissue polyol levels in galactosemic rats. *Chem Pharm Bull* 1985;33:2990–2995.

54. Hirata Y, Fugimori S, Okamura K, Takagi K, Masuzawa K: Effect of ADN-138, a new aldose reductase inhibitor, on experimental diabetic neuropathy, abstract. Paper presented at the International Symposium on Polyol Pathway and Its Role in Diabetic Complications, Kashikojima, Japan, October 28 to 30, 1986, p 44.
55. Tadeo T, Satoghi S, Masanori K, et al: Rhodanine derivatives, a process for their preparation and aldose reductase inhibitors containing such derivatives. European Patent 045,165; published on February 3, 1982.
56. Tadeo T, Masanori K, Akio A, et al: Rhodanine derivatives, a process for their preparation, and aldose reductase inhibitor containing the rhodanine derivatives as active ingredient. European Patent 047,109; published on March 10, 1982.
57. Terashima H, Hama K, Yamamoto R, et al: Effects of a new aldose reductase inhibitor on various tissues in vitro. *J Pharmacol Exp Ther* 1984; 229:226–230.
58. Poulsom R, Heath H: Inhibition of aldose reductase in five tissues of the streptozotocin-diabetic rat. *Biochem Pharmacol* 1983;32:1495–1499.
59. Stribling D, Mirrlees DJ, Earl DCN: The effect of ICI-128,436, a novel aldose reductase inhibitor, on the development of diabetic complications in the rat. *Diabetologia* 1983;25:196.
60. Boot-Handford R, Heath H: The effects of aldose reductase inhibitors on the metabolism of cultured monkey kidney epithelial cells. *Biochem Pharmacol* 1981;30: 3065–3069.
61. Stribling D, Mirrlees DJ, Harrison HE, Earl CN: Properties of ICI-128,436, a novel aldose reductase inhibitor, and its effects on diabetic complications in the rat. *Metabolism* 1985;34:336–344.
62. Fretten P, Tomlinson DR, Townsend J: Prevention of axonal transport defects, in vagus and sciatic nerves of diabetic rats, by aldose reductase inhibition. *Br J Pharmacol* 1984;82:265P.
63. Brittain DR: Aldose reductase inhibitors: structure, activity, and their potential for therapy in diabetic complications, in Lambert RW (ed): *Proceedings of the Third SCI-RSC Medicinal Chemistry Symposium*. London, Royal Society of Chemistry, 1986, p 210.
64. Okamoto M, Uchida I, Umehara K, Kohsaka M, Imanaka H: New furanone derivatives, process for the preparation thereof and use thereof. European Patent 099,692; published on February 2, 1984.
65. Ito Y, Kitaura Y, Oku T, et al: New furanone derivatives and pharmaceutically acceptable salts useful for the treatment of diabetic complications. Japanese Patent 60-178,879; published on September 12, 1985.
66. Sarges R, Belletire JL, Schnur RC: Pharmaceutical preparations containing coumarin carboxylic acid derivatives. United States Patent 4,210,667; published on July 1, 1980.
67. Belletire JL: Halogen substituted benzopyran and benzothiopyran-4-carboxylic acids. United States Patent 4,210,663; published on July 1, 1980.
68. Varma SD, Mikuni I, Kinoshita JH: Flavonoids as inhibitors of lens aldose reductase. *Science* 1975;188:1215–1216.
69. Varma SD, Mizuno A, Kinoshita JH: Diabetic cataracts and flavonoids. *Science* 1977;195:205–206.
70. Creuset MH, Feniou C, Guichard F, et al: 7-Acylamino- or sulfamoyl-flavone-4'-carboxylic acid derivatives inhibit aldose reductase and are used for ocular and nervous complications in diabetes and as diuretics and antihypertensives. French Patent 2,543,140; published on September 28, 1984.
71. Creuset MH, Feniou C, Guichard F, et al: New derivatives of tetrahydroxy-3′,4′,5,7-flavone, their method of preparation and their therapeutic use. European Patent 121,489; published on October 10, 1984.

72. Ono H, Ohtsuka I, Kawase H, et al: 2,2′,4,4′-Tetrahydroxybenzophenone as a new aldose reductase inhibitor. *Jpn J Ophthalmol* 1982;26:114.
73. Pfister JR, Wymann WE, Mahoney JM, Waterbury LD: Synthesis and aldose reductase inhibitory activity of 7-sulfamoylxanthone-2-carboxylic acids. *J Med Chem* 1980; 23:1264–1267.
74. Munson HR Jr: Compounds and methods for treating diabetic complications. United States Patent 4,198,414; published on April 15, 1980.
75. Dvornik D, Simard-Duquesne N: Aldose reductase inhibition by (Z)-5-fluoro-2-methyl-1-[[4-(methylsulfinyl)phenyl]methylene]-1-H-indene-3-acetic acid. United States Patent 4,307,114; published on December 22, 1981.
76. Chaudhry, PS, Cabrera J, Juliani HR, Varma SD: Inhibition of human lens aldose reductase by flavonoids, sulindac and indomethacin. *Biochem Pharmacol* 1983; 32:1995–1998.
77. Kador PF, Goosey JD, Sharpless NE, Kolish J, Miller DD: Stereospecific inhibition of aldose reductase. *Eur J Med Chem* 1981;16:293–298.
78. Kador PF, Sharpless NE: Pharmacophor requirements of the aldose reductase inhibitor site. *Mol Pharmacol* 1983;24:521–531.
79. De Ruiter J, Brubaker AN, Millen J, Riley TN: Design and synthesis of 2-(arylamino)-4-(3H)-quinazolinones as novel inhibitors of rat lens aldose reductase. *J Med Chem* 1986;29:627–629.

Afterword

The Future of Diabetic Complications

The specific long-term small vessel and metabolic complications of diabetes remain a major problem and indeed it is these complications that make diabetes the extremely unpleasant disease that it is. The cynic would suggest that the diabetic physician is a voyeur of the natural history of these complications. This may well be the case with regard to arteriosclerotic degenerative major vessel disease, but this would be an unrealistic and erroneous view to take of the small vessel complications—retinopathy, nephropathy, and neuropathy. At this point it must be emphasised that the major aetiopathological build-up to peripheral nerve damage is indeed a metabolic process, and this is perhaps, at a later stage, complicated by the presence of small vessel disease within nerve.

The best way to describe the enormous task facing diabetes care professionals of preventing complications is to describe the services that should be an integral part of every diabetic clinic—and these are just the minimum of services that should be available.

- Physicians with specific training in the management of diabetes and its complications.
- Nurse specialists with an equally extensive knowledge of diabetes who are trained in patient education.
- Specialists in chiropody and shoe design.
- A diabetes centre available at all times for screening and educational services, and linked to clinical areas for the management of the many organic problems resulting from diabetes.
- Access to and collaboration with ophthalmologists who handle regular retinal screening, recall for review and treatment, and maintain facilities for laser therapy.
- Access to and collaboration with renal physicians and vascular and orthopaedic surgeons.
- A computer register for the diabetic community—whether or not the patient attends a diabetic clinic.

Through educational support and clinical management it is the *aim* of such a service to ensure diabetics the means to maintain their blood glucose levels as near to the normal range as possible, and to minimize the effects leading to morbidity in diabetics who have developed complications.

However, even in societies regarded as affluent, it is all too evident that such comprehensive services are not being provided and moreover, even where reasonable time and facilities are available, normoglycaemia is achieved in a relatively small minority. The difficulty of achieving normoglycaemia is due to the variability of insulin absorption, the unphysiological route of subcutaneous injection of insulin, and the difficulty many diabetics have in coping with the daily "forever" routine. Novel instruments like insulin pumps and pen injectors help to some extent, but they still only form one small part of the complex business of living the diabetic life. Islet cell culture and transplantation, total organ transplantation, and the development of glucose sensors to control external or implanted insulin pumps are still some time away in terms of practical application to the total diabetic population.

For these reasons, at least for the foreseeable future, it would seem that efforts should be directed in three main areas:

- Improved provision of intensive screening and preventative services to be offered to those with already established complications.
- The development of standardised markers to identify those at risk so that they might be offered more intensive services.
- The use of pharmacological agents that would logically prevent or reverse tissue, biochemical, functional and structural abnormalities.

It is to this last area that this publication has addressed itself.

A. Prevention. Screening and early application of laser therapy is now a well established and an effective method of preventing deterioration of the retina. Advanced stages of retinopathy should be a thing of the past.

It seems that the presence of microproteinuria may well be a marker for the development of renal disease and renal failure and soon it may be necessary to offer those with this feature an intensive program for blood glucose and blood pressure control.

Screening, education, shoe design and early therapy can totally prevent neuropathic ulcer, and diabetic neuropathy, the ravages of neuropathic and ischaemic foot ulceration leading to amputation, can certainly be radically reduced.

B. Regrettably at present we do not have adequate markers to identify those likely to develop any of these complications—perhaps with the exception of microproteinuria. Although there is reasonable circumstantial evidence that complications do relate to overall quality of metabolic control, it is all too obvious that there are other important factors involved in the development of complications. A search for these factors, be they biochemical, haematological or rheological or environmental, must continue. A simple marker of those subjects likely to develop complications would certainly allow the concentration of clinical resources to be applied with intensity to a smaller percentage of patients.

C. The aldose reductase inhibitors do seem to be a group of drugs that could logically prevent tissue abnormalities, particularly with regard to peripheral nerve damage. However, it must be reiterated that in human diabetic neuropathy, by the time ARI's are given in current clinical trials to people with established syndromes of diabetic neuropathy, we know that there is considerable damage to the nerve—axonal degeneration and fibre loss, segmental demyelination, small areas of infarction, and considerable occlusion of small vessels. Moreover, it is not apparent that the biochemical pathway is so relevant at this advanced stage in the disease, and in these circumstances such agents may well fail to produce measureable effect.

It seems likely that the major role of aldose reductase inhibitors will be either in administration to earlier clinical features of diabetic neuropathy (although in many of these cases advanced nerve damage may already be quite marked despite the apparent triviality of the clinical syndrome) or, more likely, as a long-term prophylactic agent. Unfortunately, as with all diabetic complications the natural history over years would require clinical studies over time and with great expense. However, because of the unpleasant nature of diabetic neuropathy and its ensuing problems such a therapeutic approach must be strongly considered and pursued in the attempt to achieve any possible benefit. If further evidence is produced regarding the importance of such pathways in eyes and kidneys then even greater pressure will mount for proof of long-term efficacy. While we do not have fully reliable meaningful and reproducible measurements in diabetic neuropathy, objective measurement of the state of the retina and the fairly accurate assessment of early kidney damage and microproteinuria are available. This may well determine that in the future long-term prophylactic studies will focus more on retinopathy and nephropathy.

Lacking additional information as to abnormal pathways that lead to the diabetic complications and which could be beneficially altered, it is most important to continue studies of the aldose reductase inhibitors in all the likely relevant complications.

"Hope is a good breakfast, but a bad supper" (Francis Bacon, 1615). Let us hope that the predictions of the benefits of these agents will be borne out in the next few years.

J.D. Ward, M.D., F.R.C.P., B.Sc.
Royal Hallamshire Hospital
Sheffield, U.K.

Index